Mental Health: Clinical Perspectives

Mental Health: Clinical Perspectives

Editor: John Dalvi

AMERICAN
MEDICAL PUBLISHERS
www.americanmedicalpublishers.com

AMERICAN
MEDICAL PUBLISHERS
www.americanmedicalpublishers.com

Cataloging-in-Publication Data

Mental health : clinical perspectives / edited by John Dalvi.
p. cm.
Includes bibliographical references and index.
ISBN 978-1-63927-440-6
1. Mental health. 2. Mental illness. 3. Psychology. 4. Psychiatry. 5. Psychology, Pathological.
6. Clinical psychology. I. Dalvi, John.
RA790.5 .M46 2022
362.2--dc23

American Medical Publishers,
41 Flatbush Avenue,
1st Floor, New York,
NY 11217, USA

ISBN 978-1-63927-440-6 (Hardback)

Contents

Preface

In my initial years as a student, I used to run to the library at every possible instance to grab a book and learn something new. Books were my primary source of knowledge and I would not have come such a long way without all that I learnt from them. Thus, when I was approached to edit this book; I became understandably nostalgic. It was an absolute honor to be considered worthy of guiding the current generation as well as those to come. I put all my knowledge and hard work into making this book most beneficial for its readers.

Mental health is the state when a person is functioning at a satisfactory level of emotional and behavioral adjustment. It can also be characterized by the absence of any mental illness. As per positive psychology, mental health includes an individual's ability to enjoy life, efforts to achieve psychological resilience and to create a balance between life activities. Mental health also includes subjective well-being, perceived self-efficacy, autonomy, competence, inter-generational dependence, etc. It also provides the ability to adapt, change and cope with hardship. Mental illness is caused by depression, anxiety, loneliness, stress, death of loved ones, etc. Treatments of mental illnesses include pharmacotherapy, psychotherapy, meditation, etc. This book covers in detail some existent theories and innovative concepts revolving around mental health. The topics included herein on mental health are of utmost significance and bound to provide incredible insights to readers. This book will serve as a reference to a broad spectrum of readers.

I wish to thank my publisher for supporting me at every step. I would also like to thank all the authors who have contributed their researches in this book. I hope this book will be a valuable contribution to the progress of the field.

Editor

1

Policy development and challenges of global mental health: a systematic review of published studies of national-level mental health policies

Wei Zhou[1,2], Yu Yu[3], Mei Yang[4], Lizhang Chen[1] and Shuiyuan Xiao[5*]

Abstract

Background: Mental health policy can be an essential and powerful tool to improve a population's mental health. However, around one third of countries do not possess a mental health policy, and there are large disparities in population coverage rates between high- and low-income countries. The goal of this study is to identify the transition and implementation challenges of mental health policies in both high-income countries (HICs) as well as middle- and low-income countries (MLICs).

Methods: PubMed, Cochrane Library and Campbell Library were searched from inception to 31 December 2017, for studies on implemented mental health policies at the national level. Abstracts and the main texts of papers were double screened, and extracted data were analysed through thematic synthesis.

Results: A total of 93 papers were included in this study, covering 24 HICs, 28 MLICs and 5 regions. Studies on mental health policies, especially those of MLICs, kept increasing, but MLICs were still underrepresented in terms of publication quantity and study frequency. Based on the included studies, nine policy domains were summarized: service organizing, service provision, service quality, human resources, legislation and human rights, advocacy, administration, surveillance and research, and financing and budgeting. HICs incrementally enriched their policy content in all domains over centuries of development; following HICs' experience, mental health policies in MLICs have boomed since the 1990s and quickly extended to all domains. Implementation problems in HICs were mainly related to service organizing and service provision; for MLICs, more severe implementation problems converged on financing and budgeting, administration and human resources.

Conclusions: Mental health policy developments in both HICs and MLICs present a process of diversification and enrichment. In terms of implementation, MLICs are faced with more and greater challenges than HICs, especially in funding, human resources and administration. Therefore, future efforts should not only be made on helping MLICs developing mental health policies, but also on promoting policy implementation under MLICs' local context.

Keywords: Global mental health, Policy development, Implementation challenges, Systematic review

* Correspondence: xiaosy@csu.edu.cn
[5]Department of Social Medicine and Health Management, School of Public Health, Central South University, Changsha, China
Full list of author information is available at the end of the article

Background

Mental health policy is a government statement specifying values, principles and objectives for mental health. It can be implemented in the forms of mental health plans, programmes, strategies and legislation at multiple levels [1]. If properly formulated and implemented, mental health policy can be an essential and powerful tool for countries to improve mental health and reduce the burden of mental disorders. Mental health policies have undergone long periods of transition, tracing back to the removal of the chains of lunatics in 1793 by Philippe Pinel, to the second psychiatric revolution in the 1960s thanks to the advent of new psychosocial and biological therapies, to the growth of attention towards mental health policies and finally to a boom of policy statements over the last two decades [2–5]. In 2013, the adoption of the Comprehensive Mental Health Action Plan 2013–2020 by the 66th World Health Assembly would promote further development of mental health policies across the world. Despite the importance of mental health policy, centuries of developments and active promotion by international organizations, by 2011 only 60% of member countries of the World Health Organization (WHO) possessed their own mental health policies, only 71% had mental health plans and just 59% had legislation on mental health. Moreover, large disparities in population coverage rates exist between high- and low-income countries. For example, mental health legislation covers 92% of people living in high-income countries, whereas only 36% are covered in low-income countries [6].

There were international comparative reviews on mental health legislation in the 1950s, 1970s and in 1995 [7–9], as well as reviews of mental health policy in individual countries or certain regions [3, 10–13]. However, these international reviews are mostly outdated and only focused on legislation, and some have a narrow geographic scope. Thus, to update and broaden our understanding on mental health policies, this systematic review aims to present global mental health policy developments and search for the answers to two questions that may be critical to future policy making: (i) What are the focuses of mental health policy content in different countries and at different periods? and (ii) What are the policy implementation problems across the world and throughout the centuries?

To explore these answers, the current review is focused on identifying the differences in mental health policy development trajectories and implementation challenges between high-income countries (HICs) and middle- and low-income countries (MLICs) [14], by using thematic synthesis of published studies of implemented national-level mental health policies. We hope to provide some inspiration to both HICs and MLICs for their future development of mental health policies.

Methods

Search strategy and selection criteria

For inclusion in the review we screened published research on implemented mental health policies at the national level. We searched PubMed, the Cochrane Library, and the Campbell Library from their collections' inception to 31 December 2017. "Policy(ies)", "national plan", "national program(me)", "national strategy(ies)", "legislation", "law", "national reform", and "system", were combined with "mental health" in our search. We set no restriction on the publication date or language. A title search was adopted, as the pilot title/abstract search identified a large amount of irrelevant research whose abstracts only mentioned mental health policy in the studies' background.

Studies were excluded if they: (i) were theoretical studies, describing standards that mental health policies are expected to meet; (ii) focused on only one aspect of policy content (to avoid over-weighted statistics); (iii) studied the process of policy formulation; (iv) were policy interpretation for operation/practice; (v) were news, interviews, editorials, commentaries, letters, personal narratives, speeches, conference abstracts, case reports or research protocols (to guarantee objectivity and research quality).

Screening, abstraction and synthesis

Identified citations were first screened based on their titles and abstracts, and if they met the selection criteria, their full texts were obtained for further screening to determine whether or not they would be included. The screening process was carried out independently by two authors (ZW and YY), and any disagreement was resolved through consensus.

The authors (ZW, YY, YM, CLZ, and XSY) extracted data on publication year, countries/regions being studied, policy time and content, implementation problems, barriers and progress. Extracted data were compiled by country and further grouped into HICs and MLICs.

As all the included papers except for one were qualitative studies, a thematic synthesis was adopted, which is a tested method for qualitative research in systematic reviews [15] and has been used in health policy and systems research and review [16, 17]. Extracted information was first coded line by line into descriptive themes. Like the process of generating analytical themes in classical thematic synthesis [15, 18], the descriptive themes were then summarized into the main domains of mental health policy. This summarizing process was informed by ideas from the 12 areas of action suggested by the WHO [1].

Results

From the initially identified 1751 studies, 1588 references were excluded on the basis of the title or abstract, leaving 163 full-text papers for further scrutiny. Of these, 93 met the selection criteria [3, 4, 8, 10–13, 19–104]. Ten non-English studies were further excluded from analysis (Additional file 1: Appendix A) because their eligibility was difficult for the reviewers to determine (Fig. 1).

Characteristics of included studies

The 93 included papers were published between 1948 and 2017 and covered mental health policies in 24 HICs, 28 MLICs and 5 regions (Additional file 1: Appendix B) on five continents. There was an overall increasing trend in research on mental health policies. Compared to HICs, there was a quick increase of MLICs studies after 2000 (Table 1, Fig. 2).

Despite the rapid increase of studies on MLICs since 2000, there were only 33 publications included in our review. In terms of frequency, HICs were studied 68 times, while MLICs were studied only 44 times. Among HICs, as well as among all 52 countries, the United States was the most frequently studied (18 times); among MLICs, Ghana was studied with the highest frequency (6 times) (Additional file 1: Appendix B).

Policy development

Based on the descriptive themes and action areas suggested by the WHO, nine domains were summarized, and their main features are listed as follows: (i) service organizing, referring to the way in which mental health services are organized; (ii) service provision, including promotion, prevention, treatment, rehabilitation, essential drug provision, service availability and accessibility; (iii) service quality, including accreditation and management of service providers, service standards and guidelines; (iv) human resources, including quantity and quality of workforce, professional training and education; (v) legislation and human rights, including the rights of patients in and outside the health sector, social security and welfare; (vi) advocacy, including awareness raising, anti-stigma, empowering consumers; (vii) administration, including coordination within mental health systems and among all levels of governments, designation of agencies' responsibilities and collaboration across sectors; (viii) surveillance and research, including mental health information systems, monitoring and evaluation of policy implementation and research on service provision; and (ix) financing and budgeting, including government funding arrangements, service payment and health insurance. The detailed list of descriptive themes and their corresponding domains is presented by policy time period and country category in Additional file 1: Appendix C.

Generally, the transition of mental health policy was a process of diversification and enrichment in both HICs and MILCs. The form of mental health policy was diversified from early laws to recent policies, plans, programmes, strategies and legislation, and its content was enriched from the limited focus on institutionalization of patients in asylums to full coverage of all nine policy domains (Fig. 3, Additional file 1: Appendix D). According to the included studies, service organizing, legislation and human rights, service provision and service quality were four domains of traditionally focus across the world.

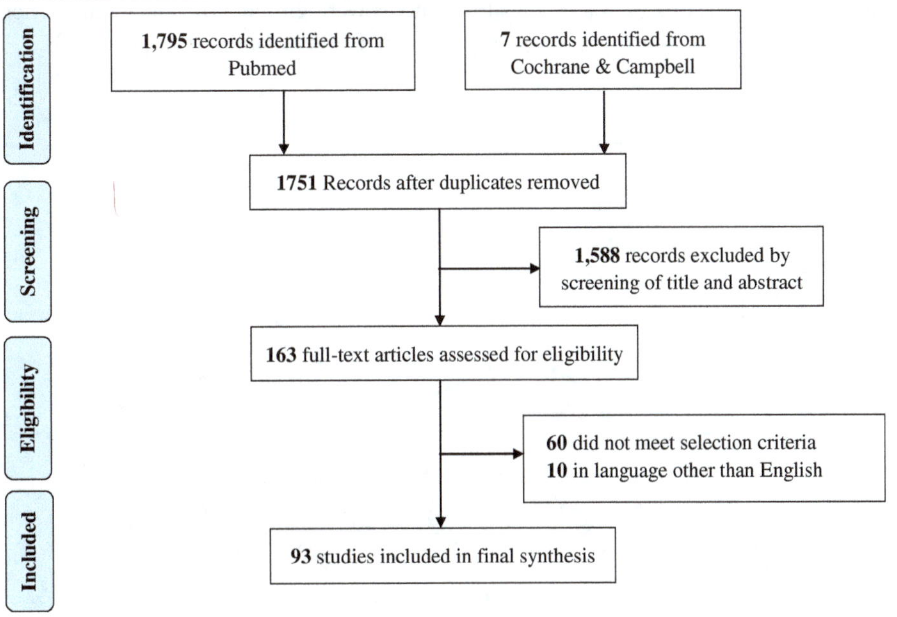

Fig. 1 Process and results of study selection

Table 1 The number of included studies by the country category and publication years

Category	1948-1979	1980-1984	1985-1989	1990-1994	1995-1999	2000-2004	2005-2009[a]	2010-2014[b]	2015-2017	Total
HICs	3	3	6	8	5	6	11	8	6	56
MLICs	0	0	1	0	1	1	4	12	14	33
Regions	1	0	2	1	0	1	0	1	0	6
Total	4	3	9	9	6	8	14	20	20	93

[a]One publication studied both HICs and MLICs
[b]One publication studied both HICs and MLICs

Differences existed in the development trajectories of HICs and MLICs. Many HICs had a much longer history of mental health policy, dating back to the nineteenth century or even earlier, and their policy content transformed incrementally throughout their practical exploration. Before the end of World War II, institutionalization of service organizing and relevant legislation were the most common policy themes. After that, policy debate in service organizing remained heated, as the movement of transferring patients into the community, originating in North America in the 1960s, spread to almost all HICs in the 1990s. At the same time, measures were also proposed for heightened consideration for patients in service provision and service quality; legislation and human rights extended from protecting patients' rights in the health sector to guaranteeing patients' and their families' social welfare. Since the 1990s, community mental health care has been accepted and developed in almost all HICs, and policy debate in service organizing has become less heated. Currently, policy attention is less focused on certain domains. In comparison, HICs' policy expressions place less emphasis on financing and budgeting and human resources (Table 2).

Most MLICs have a shorter history of mental health policy and experienced a boom of development in the 1990s and 2000s. As late arrivers, many followed the experience of HICs. Before 1945, mental health policies in countries like India and Algeria had origin in ones in the United Kingdom and France. Between the late 1940s and the 1980s, some MLICs developed their own mental health policies and sporadically discussed service organizing, provision, quality and legislation. In the 1990s, the policy content of MLICs was further enriched, and every policy domain was mentioned by at least one or two countries, but without obvious focuses. In 2000s, the community-oriented policy was accepted as a trend in MLICs; countries like South Africa and Uganda had comprehensive mental health policies covering all nine domains. In comparison, current MLICs policies contain less expression of financing and budgeting, surveillance and research, and human resources (Table 2).

Implementation challenges

Of the included studies, 64 provided information regarding implementation evaluation [3, 4, 10–13, 19–63, 97–104]. The descriptive themes of implementation problems were categorized into each policy domain, and the unsorted items were grouped by policy time period and country category (Additional file 1: Appendix E).

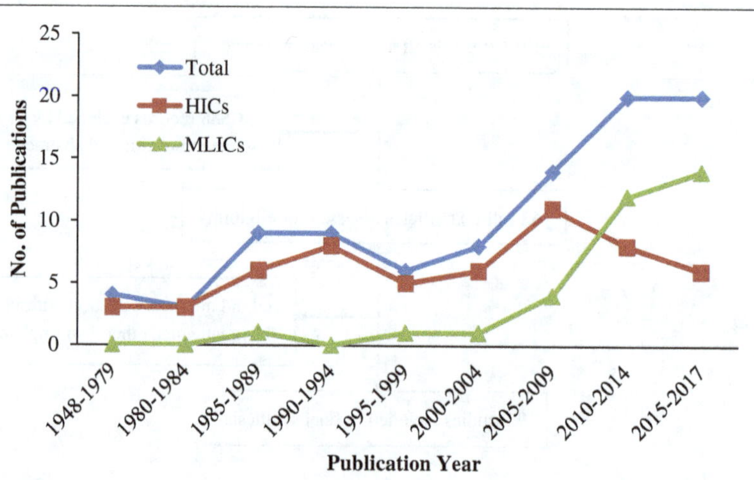

Fig. 2 The number of included studies by country categories & publication years

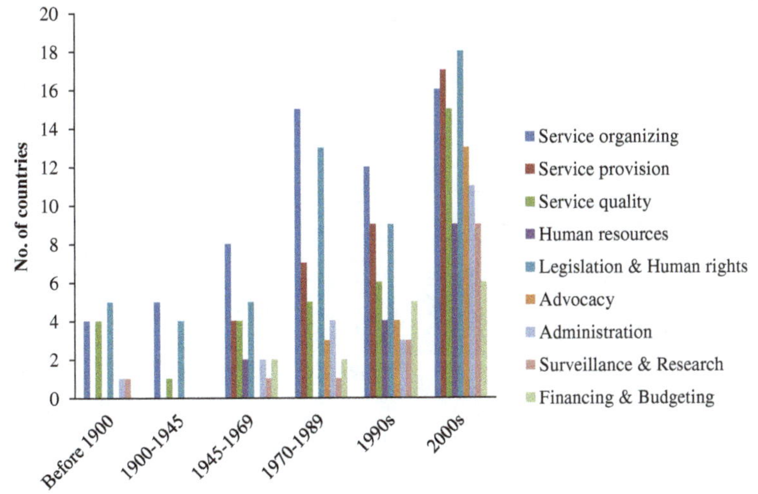

Fig. 3 The number of countries expressing each domain in policies based on included studies

There were some positive evaluation results. For example, many of the HICs effectively closed down mental hospitals and successfully transferred patients to community-based mental health organizations by the 2000s. Some research showed an increase in treatment access as a result of the implementation of community-oriented policies [28]. However, challenges were also present and problems increased as policy content extended. Slow or inconsistent implementation and under-implementation existed in both HICs and MLICs.

The included studies reported implemented problems of HICs between the 1970s and 1990s mostly on domains of service organizing and service provision, which was closely related to their shift towards community mental health care at that time. However, deinstitutionalization, but without sufficient community mental health care to take over discharged patients, once hampered service availability, accessibility and response to certain populations like the severely ill. In the 2000s, few implementation problems were discussed (Table 3).

For MLICs, problems have persistently and commonly existed in financing and budgeting, administration and human resources (Table 3). Though some HICs also listed similar problems in these three domains, the problems' severity was much greater for MLICs. For example, underfunding for many MLICs was so severe that their formulation of mental health policies depended on international funding and the cessation of international funding greatly impacted policy sustainability [44].

Discussion

Reflections on policy development

Mental health policies in many MLICs are developed with financial and technical assistance from HICs and

Table 2 The number of HICs and MLICs expressing each domain in policies based on included studies

Policy domains	HICs						MLICs					
	Before 1900	1900-1944	1945-1969	1970-1989	1990s	2000s	Before 1900	1900-1944	1945-1969	1970-1989	1990s	2000s
Service organizing	3	3	6	11	8	2	1	2	2	4	4	14
Service provision	0	0	3	6	6	3	0	0	1	1	3	14
Service quality	2	0	3	3	4	5	2	1	1	2	2	10
Human resources	0	0	1	0	2	2	0	0	1	0	2	7
Legislation & Human rights	4	3	3	7	6	4	1	1	2	6	3	14
Advocacy	0	0	0	1	1	3	0	0	0	2	3	10
Administration	1	0	2	3	2	3	0	0	0	1	1	8
Surveillance & Research	1	0	1	1	1	2	0	0	0	0	2	7
Financing & Budgeting	0	0	2	1	4	1	0	0	0	1	1	5

Table 3 The number of HICs and MLICs with implementation problems in each domain based on included studies

Policy domains	HICs						MLICs					
	Before 1900	1900-1944	1945-1969	1970-1989	1990s	2000s	Before 1900	1900-1944	1945-1969	1970-1989	1990s	2000s
Service organizing	2	1	3	7	5	1	0	0	0	0	0	2
Service provision	0	0	1	6	4	0	0	0	1	0	1	2
Service quality	0	0	3	2	3	0	0	0	0	0	0	1
Human resources	0	0	2	3	2	0	0	0	1	0	2	9
Legislation & Human rights	2	0	2	2	0	0	0	0	0	0	1	3
Advocacy	0	0	1	0	1	0	0	0	1	0	0	6
Administration	0	0	1	5	3	1	0	0	0	2	2	7
Surveillance & Research	0	0	0	2	3	0	0	0	0	0	1	4
Financing & Budgeting	0	0	0	5	2	2	0	0	0	1	4	11
Unsorted	0	0	0	3	3	2	0	0	0	1	6	7

international organizations. Thus, they follow the experience and policy practices of HICs. This is reflected in their intensive policy attention on community mental health care in the 2000s and in the comprehensiveness of domain coverage as compared to their high-income counterparts. However, the experience of HICs is accumulated through centuries of development and their current practices are based on well-established mental health systems. Seriously under-resourced and under-developed mental health systems are commonly found in many MLICs [105]. Therefore, MLICs should be cautious about potential problems arising from the direct transplantation of HICs' experience [106]. Foreign experience developed in different social and cultural contexts should be carefully selected and MLICs should consider policy feasibility based on their own situations. For example, because funding and resources for mental health are scare in MLICs, excessive policy focus will result in fewer inputs in each domain and a possibly result in underdevelopment.

Reflections on implementation evaluation

Of note is that this review's findings on policy implementation present only a limited understanding of existing problems, as a lack of information and evaluation of policy implementation itself was listed as a problem in both HICs and MLICs.

Moreover, among the limited implementation information provided by the included studies, many were just general comments such as "while significant gains had been made in mental health reform, these had been uneven across and within jurisdictions" [69]. Even for the included assessment studies, different evaluation frameworks and indicators were applied. The WHO-AIMS (WHO's Assessment Instrument for Mental Health Systems) Version 2.2 and the WHO Checklist for Mental Health Policy were the only two internationally recognized evaluation instruments related to mental health policies, but they focus on policy content and formulation [107, 108]. Therefore, exploring evaluative frameworks for policy implementation is an important future research topic in mental health policy.

Limitation

One major limitation is that this review is based on published research rather than first-hand government documents and grey literature. Though advantages of using published research include quick acquisition of policy information from centuries ago, easy determination of a policy's implementation, and the guarantee of basic quality through a peer review mechanism, there may be bias of result representativeness.

Conclusion

Global mental health policy developments present a process of diversification and enrichment. The process in HICs is long and incremental through centuries. Based on HICs' experience, MLICs have quickly developed mental health policies covering domains as comprehensive as HICs, in the recent three decades. In terms of implementation, problems exist in both HICs and MLICs. However, MLICs are faced with more and greater challenges, especially in funding, human resources and administration. Therefore, future efforts should not only be made on helping MLICs developing mental health policies, but also on promoting policy implementation under MLICs' local context.

Abbreviations

HICs: High-income countries; MLICs: Middle- and low-income countries; WHO: World Health Organization; WHO-AIMS: WHO's Assessment Instrument for Mental Health Systems

Funding
This work was supported by the China Medical Board (CMB-14-188) to XSY, the China Postdoctoral Science Foundation (2017 M622618) and the Central South University Postdoctoral Science Foundation (185708) to ZW. Then funding agencies did not take part in the design of the study and collection, analysis, and interpretation of data and in writing the manuscript.

Authors' contributions
ZW and XSY designed this research; ZW and YY screened for inclusion papers; ZW, YY, YM, CLZ and XSY extracted and analysed data; ZW drafted the manuscript and all authors read and approved the final manuscript.

Competing interests
The authors declare that they have no competing interests.

Author details
[1]Department of Epidemiology and Health Statistics, School of Public Health, Central South University, Changsha, China. [2]Hospital Administration Institute, Xinagya Hospital, Central South University, Changsha, China. [3]Evaluation Department, Xiangya Hospital, Central South University, Changsha, China. [4]Department of Addiction Medicine, Shenzhen Kangning Hospital, Shenzhen Mental Health Center, Shenzhen, China. [5]Department of Social Medicine and Health Management, School of Public Health, Central South University, Changsha, China.

References

1. WHO. Mental health policy, plans and programmes. World Health Organization. 2005. Available from: http://www.who.int/mental_health/policy/services/2_policy%20plans%20prog_WEB_07.pdf.
2. Knapp M, McDaid D, Mossialos E, Thornicroft G, editors. Mental health policy and practice across Europe: the future direction of mental health care. Maidenhead: Open University Press; 2007.
3. Grob GN. Mental health policy in the liberal state: the example of the United States. Int J Law Psychiatry. 2008;31:89–100.
4. Lurie S. Comparative mental health policy: are there lessons to be learned? Int Rev Psychiatry. 2005;17:97–101.
5. Haque A. Mental health concepts and program development in Malaysia. J Ment Health. 2005;2:183–95.
6. WHO. Mental Health Atlas 2011. World Health Organization. 2011. Available from: http://apps.who.int/iris/bitstream/10665/44697/1/9799241564359_eng.pdf.
7. Curran WJ. Hospitalization of the mentally Ill. North Carolina L Rev. 1953;31:274.
8. Curran WJ. Comparative analysis of mental health legislation in forty-three countries: a discussion of historical trends. Int J Law Psychiatry. 1978;1:79–92.
9. Bertolote JM. Legislation related to mental health: a review of various international experiences. Rev Saude Publica. 1995;2:152–6. [Article in Portuguese]
10. Alarcon RD, Aguilar-Gaxiola SA. Mental health policy developments in Latin America. Bull World Health Organ. 2000;78:483–90.
11. Mosse P, Maury C, Daumerie N, Roelandt JL. Mental health in France, policies and actors: developing administrative knowledge in a segmented world. Int J Health Plann Manag. 2013;28:e242–55.
12. Hamid H, Abanilla K, Bauta B, Huang KY. Evaluating the WHO assessment instrument for mental health systems by comparing mental health policies in four countries. Bull World Health Organ. 2008;86:467–73.
13. Draper CE, Lund C, Kleintjes S, Funk M, Omar M, Flisher AJ, et al. Mental health policy in South Africa: development process and content. Health Policy Plan. 2009;24:342–56.
14. World Bank. Country and lending groups. 2018. Available from: https://datahelpdesk.worldbank.org/knowledgebase/articles/906519.
15. Thomas J, Harden A. Methods for the thematic synthesis of qualitative research in systematic reviews. BMC Med Res Methodol. 2008;8:45.
16. Baker P, Friel S, Kay A, Baum F, Strazdins L, Mackean T. What enables and constrains the inclusion of the social determinants of health inequities in government policy agendas? A narrative review. Int J Health Policy Manage. 2017;2:101 11.
17. Reeve E, Thow AM, Bell C, Engelhardt K, Gamolo-Naliponguit EC, Go JJ, et al. Implementation lessons for school food policies and marketing restrictions in the Philippines: a qualitative policy analysis. Glob Health. 2018;1:8.
18. Barnett-Page E, Thomas J. Methods for the synthesis of qualitative research: a critical review. BMC Med Res Methodol. 2009;9:59.
19. Surles R, Mazade N. Federal policies which influence the planning of local community mental health programs. J Community Psychol. 1978;6:45–7.
20. Brown P. The transfer of care: U.S. mental health policy since world war II. Int J Health Serv. 1979;9:645–62.
21. Andrulis DP, Mazade NA. American mental health policy: changing directions in the 80s. Hosp Community Psychiatry. 1983;34:601–6.
22. Merwin MR, Ochberg FM. The long voyage: policies for progress in mental health. Health Aff. 1983;2:96–127.
23. Goldman HH, Morrissey JP. The alchemy of mental health policy: homelessness and the fourth cycle of reform. Am J Public Health. 1985;75:727–31.
24. Jansen MA. Mental health policy: observations from Europe. Am Psychol. 1986;41:1273–8.
25. Bloche MG, Cournos F. Mental health policy for the 1990s: tinkering in the interstices. J Health Polit Policy Law. 1990;15:387–411.
26. Goldie N, Freden L. A 'crisis' of closure and openness: the present state of the Swedish mental health system in the light of a policy of sectorisation. Soc Sci Med. 1991;32:499–506.
27. Grob GN. Mental health policy in America: myths and realities. Health Aff. 1992;11:7–22.
28. Kiesler CA. U.S. mental health policy: doomed to fail. Am Psychol. 1992;47:1077–82.
29. VandenBos GR. U.S. mental health policy: proactive evolution in the midst of health care reform. Am Psychol. 1993;48:283–90.
30. Levav I, Restrepo H, Guerra de Macedo C. The restructuring of psychiatric care in Latin America: a new policy for mental health services. J Public Health Policy. 1994;15:71–85.
31. Yfantopoulos J. Economic and legal aspects of mental health policies in Greece. Int J Soc Psychiatry. 1994;40:296–305.
32. Mandiberg JM. The Japanese mental health system and law: social and structural impediments to reform. Int J Law Psychiatry. 1996;19:413–35.
33. Pearson V. The Chinese equation in mental health policy and practice: order plus control equal stability. Int J Law Psychiatry. 1996;19:437–58.
34. Barbato A. Psychiatry in transition: outcomes of mental health policy shift in Italy. Aust N Z J Psychiatry. 1998;32:673–9.
35. Bindman J, Beck A, Glover G, Thornicroft G, Knapp M, Leese M, et al. Evaluating mental health policy in England: care programme approach and supervision registers. Br J Psychiatry. 1999;175:327–30.
36. McCulloch A, Muijen M, Harper H. New developments in mental health policy in the United Kingdom. Int J Law Psychiatry. 2000;23:261–76.
37. Silfverhielm H, Kamis-Gould E. The Swedish mental health system: past, present, and future. Int J Law Psychiatry. 2000;23:293–307.
38. Whiteford H, Thompson I, Casey D. The Australian mental health system. Int J Law Psychiatry. 2000;23:403–17.
39. Shera W, Aviram U, Healy B, Ramon S. Mental health system reform: a multi country comparison. Soc Work Health Care. 2002;35:547–75.
40. Simmons LA, Wright DW. National practice guidelines for mental health care: a comparative policy analysis of the United Kingdom and the United States. J Health Soc Policy. 2004;19:59–80.
41. Grob GN. Public policy and mental illnesses: Jimmy Carter's presidential commission on mental health. Milbank Q. 2005;83:425–56.
42. Goldman HH. Making progress in mental health policy in conservative times: one step at a time. Schizophr Bull. 2006;32:424–7.
43. Keste D, Lazeri L, Demi N, Severoni S, Lora A, Saxena S. Mental health system and services in Albania. Epidemiol Psichiatr Soc. 2006;15:194–201.
44. Jenkins R, Heshmat A, Loza N, Siekkonen I, Sorour E. Mental health policy and development in Egypt: integrating mental health into health sector reforms 2001-9. Int J Ment Heal Syst. 2010;4:17.

45. Kahng SK, Kim H. A developmental overview of mental health system in Korea. Soc Work Public Health. 2010;25:158–75.
46. Omar MA, Green AT, Bird PK, Mirzoev T, Flisher AJ, Kigozi F, et al. Mental health policy process: a comparative study of Ghana, South Africa, Uganda and Zambia. Int J Ment Heal Syst. 2010;4:24.
47. Salvador-Carulla L, Costa-Font J, Cabases J, McDaid D, Alonso J. Evaluating mental health care and policy in Spain. J Ment Health Policy Econ. 2010;13:73–86.
48. Faydi E, Funk M, Kleintjes S, Ofori-Atta A, Ssbunnya J, Mwanza J, et al. An assessment of mental health policy in Ghana, South Africa, Uganda and Zambia. Health Res Policy Syst. 2011;9:17.
49. Jenkins R, Mussa M, Haji SA, Haji MS, Salim A, Suleiman S, et al. Developing and implementing mental health policy in Zanzibar, a low income country off the coast of East Africa. Int J Ment Heal Syst. 2011;5:6.
50. Liu J, Ma H, He YL, Xie B, Xu YF, Tang HY, et al. Mental health system in China: history, recent service reform and future challenges. World Psychiatry. 2011;10:210–6.
51. Munizza C, Gonella R, Pinciaroli L, Rucci P, Picci RL, Tibaldi G. CMHC adherence to National Mental Health Plan standards in Italy: a survey 30 years after national reform law. Psychiatr Serv. 2011;62:1090–3.
52. Abel WD, Kestel D, Eldemire-Shearer D, Sewell C, Whitehorne-Smith P. Mental health policy and service system development in the English-speaking Caribbean. West Indian Med J. 2012;61:475–82.
53. Banfield MA, Gardner KL, Yen LE, McRae IS, Gillespie JA, Wells RW. Coordination of care in Australian mental health policy. Aust Health Rev. 2012;36:153–7.
54. Dlouhy M. Mental health policy in Eastern Europe: a comparative analysis of seven mental health systems. BMC Health Serv Res. 2014;14:42.
55. Lora A. An overview of the mental health system in Italy. Annali dell'Istituto superiore di sanita. 2009;45:5–16.
56. Puzynski S, Moskalewicz J. Evolution of the mental health care system in Poland. Acta Psychiatr Scand. 2001;104:69–73.
57. Roberts M, Mogan C, Asare JB. An overview of Ghana's mental health system: results from an assessment using the World Health Organization's assessment instrument for mental health systems (WHO-AIMS). Int J Ment Heal Syst. 2014;8:16.
58. Lovell AM. The paradoxes of reform: reevaluating Italy's mental health law of 1978. Hosp Community Psychiatry. 1986;37:802–8.
59. Ofori-Atta A, Read UM, Lund C, MHaPP research Programme consortium. A situation analysis of mental health services and legislation in Ghana: challenges for transformation. Afr J Psychiatry. 2010;13:99–108.
60. Kelly BD. Mental health law in Ireland, 1945 to 2001: reformation and renewal. Medico-legal J. 2008;76:65–72.
61. Kelly BD. Mental health law in Ireland, 1821 to 1902: building the asylums. Medico-legal J. 2008;76:19–25.
62. Mosher LR. Italy's revolutionary mental health law: an assessment. Am J Psychiatry. 1982;139:199–203.
63. Felix RH. The national mental health program: a progress report. Public Health Rep. 1948;63:837–47.
64. Grob GN. The forging of mental health policy in America: world war II to new frontier. J Hist Med Allied Sci. 1987;42:410–46.
65. Grob GN. Mental health policy in post-world war II America. New Dir Ment Health Serv. 1987;1987(36):15–32.
66. Mangen SP. Mental health policies in Europe: an analysis of priorities and problems. Int J Soc Psychiatry. 1987;33:76–82.
67. Walsh D. Mental health policy developments in Ireland. Int J Soc Psychiatry. 1987;33:111–4.
68. Grob GN. From hospital to community: mental health policy in modern America. Psychiatr Q. 1991;62:187–212.
69. Whiteford HA. Australia's national mental health policy. Hosp Community Psychiatry. 1993;44:963–6.
70. Ramsay J. The National Mental Health strategy. Aust J Rural Health. 1996;4:53–6.
71. Ganju V. The mental health system in India: history, current system, and prospects. Int J Law Psychiatry. 2000;23:393–402.
72. Attah Johnson FY. Mental health care and the law in developing countries: the independent state of Papua New Guinea. Med Law. 1988; 7:359–63.
73. Whiteford H, Buckingham B, Manderscheid R. Australia's national mental health strategy. Br J Psychiatry. 2002;180:210–5.
74. Joseph R, Birchwood M. The national policy reforms for mental health services and the story of early intervention services in the United Kingdom. J Psychiatry Neurosci. 2005;30:362–5.
75. Asai K. From mental health law to mental health and welfare law. Psychiatry Clin Neurosci. 1998;52(Suppl):S247–9.
76. Crosbie DW. Mental health policy–stumbling in the dark? Med J Aust. 2009; 190:S43–5.
77. Awenva AD, Read UM, Ofori-Attah AL, Doku VC, Akpalu B, Osei AO, et al. From mental health policy development in Ghana to implementation: what are the barriers? Afr J Psychiatry. 2010;13:184–91.
78. Kiima D, Jenkins R. Mental health policy in Kenya: an integrated approach to scaling up equitable care for poor populations. Int J Ment Heal Syst. 2010;4:19.
79. Muga FA, Jenkins R. Health care models guiding mental health policy in Kenya 1965-1997. Int J Ment Heal Syst. 2010;4:9.
80. Ssebunnya J, Kigozi F, Ndyanabangi S. Developing a national mental health policy: a case study from Uganda. PLoS Med. 2012;9:e1001319.
81. Narayan CL, Shikha D. Indian legal system and mental health. Indian J Psychiatry. 2013;55:S177–81.
82. Qureshi NA, Al-Habeeb AA, Koenig HG. Mental health system in Saudi Arabia: an overview. Neuropsychiatr Dis Treat. 2013;9:1121–35.
83. Nicaise P, Dubois V, Lorant V. Mental health care delivery system reform in Belgium: the challenge of achieving deinstitutionalisation whilst addressing fragmentation of care at the same time. Health Policy. 2014;115:120–7.
84. Liverpool N. A survey of mental health legislation in the eastern Caribbean. Int J Law Psychiatry. 1986;8:119–31.
85. Abdulmalik J, Kola L, Gureje O. Mental health system governance in Nigeria: challenges, opportunities and strategies for improvement. Global Mental Health. 2016;3:e9.
86. Aboaja A, Arroyo GR, Grant L. Mental health law in Bolivia. BJPsych Int. 2015;4:89–92.
87. Alhassani G, Osman OT. Mental health law profile: the United Arab Emirates. BJPsych Int. 2015;3:70–2.
88. Benmebarek Z. Mental health legislation in Algeria. BJPsych Int. 2017;14:12–5.
89. Chaskel R, Shultz JM, Gaviria SL, Taborda E, Vanegas R, Garcia NM, et al. Mental health law in Colombia. BJPsych Int. 2015;4:92–4.
90. Dos Santos PF, Wainberg ML, Caldas-de-Almeida JM, Saraceno B, Mari JJ. Overview of the mental health system in Mozambique: addressing the treatment gap with a task-shifting strategy in primary care. Int J Ment Heal Syst. 2016;10:1.
91. Grace FC, Meurk CS, Head BW, Hall WD, Carstensen G, Harris MG, et al. An analysis of policy levers used to implement mental health reform in Australia 1992-2012. BMC Health Serv Res. 2015;15:479.
92. Grace FC, Meurk CS, Head BW, Hall WD, Harris MG, Whiteford HA. An analysis of policy success and failure in formal evaluations of Australia's National Mental Health Strategy (1992-2012). BMC Health Serv Res. 2017;1:374.
93. Karam E, El Chammay R, Richa S, Naja W, Fayyad J, Ammar W. Lebanon: mental health system reform and the Syrian crisis. BJPsych Int. 2016;4:87–9.
94. Ndetei DM, Muthike J, Nandoya ES. Kenya's mental health law. BJPsych Int. 2017;4:96–7.
95. Tareen A, Tareen KI. Mental health law in Pakistan. BJPsych Int. 2016;3:67–9.
96. Walker GH, Osei A. Mental health law in Ghana. BJPsych Int. 2017;2:38–9.
97. Datta A, Frewen J. Mental health law profile on the Republic of Ireland. BJPsych Int. 2016;1:15–7.
98. Firdosi MM, Ahmad ZZ. Mental health law in India: origins and proposed reforms. BJPsych Int. 2016;3:65–7.
99. Ho RC, Ho CS, Khan N, Kua EH. An overview of mental health legislation in Singapore. BJPsych Int. 2015;2:42–4.
100. Khan NN, Yahya B, Abu Bakar AK, Ho RC. Malaysian mental health law. BJPsych Int. 2015;2:40–2.
101. Shao Y, Wang J, Xie B. The first mental health law of China. Asian J Psychiatr. 2015;13:72–4.
102. Soosay I, Kydd R. Mental health law in New Zealand. BJPsych Int. 2016;2:43–5.
103. Stevovic LI, Jovanovic TP, Raznatovic A. Mental health law in Montenegro. BJPsych Int. 2016;4:94–5.
104. Upadhaya N, Jordans MJD, Pokhrel R, Gurung D, Adhikari RP, Petersen I, et al. Current situations and future directions for mental health system governance in Nepal: findings from a qualitative study. Int J Ment Heal Syst. 2017;11:37.

105. Knapp M, Funk M, Curran C, Prince M, Grigg M, McDaid D. Economic barriers to better mental health practice and policy. Health Policy Plan. 2006;3:157–70.
106. Kopinak JK. Mental health in developing countries: challenges and opportunities in introducing western mental health system in Uganda. Int J MCH AIDS. 2015;1:22–30.
107. WHO. Monitoring and evaluation of mental health policies and plans. World Health Organization. 2007. Available from: http://www.who.int/mental_health/policy/services/14-monitoring%20evaluation_HKprinter.pdf.
108. World Health Organization. World Health Organization Assessment Instrument for Mental Health Systems (AIMS) Version 2.2. 2005. World Health Organization. Available from: http://www.who.int/mental_health/evidence/AIMS_WHO_2_2.pdf?ua=1.

2

Mental health supported accommodation services: a systematic review of mental health and psychosocial outcomes

Peter McPherson*, Joanna Krotofil and Helen Killaspy

Abstract

Background: Post-deinstitutionalisation, mental health supported accommodation services have been implemented widely. The available research evidence is heterogeneous in nature and resistant to synthesis attempts, leaving researchers and policy makers with no clear summary what works and for whom. In this context, we undertook a comprehensive systematic review of quantitative studies in order to synthesise the current evidence on mental health and psychosocial outcomes for individuals residing in mental health supported accommodation services.

Methods: Using a combination of electronic database searches, hand searches, forward-backward snowballing and article recommendations from an expert panel, 115 papers were identified for review. Data extraction and quality assessments were conducted, and 33 articles were excluded due to low quality, leaving 82 papers in the final review. Variation in terminology and service characteristics made the comparison of service models unfeasible. As such, findings were presented according to the following sub-groups: 'Homeless', 'Deinstitutionalisation' and 'General Severe Mental Illness (SMI)'.

Results: Results were mixed, reflecting the heterogeneity of the supported accommodation literature, in terms of research quality, experimental design, population, service types and outcomes assessed. There is some evidence that supported accommodation is effective across a range of psychosocial outcomes. The most robust evidence supports the effectiveness of the permanent supported accommodation model for homeless SMI in generating improvements in housing retention and stability, and appropriate use of clinical services over time, and for other forms of supported accommodation for deinstitutionalised populations in reducing hospitalisation rates and improving appropriate service use. The evidence base for general SMI populations is less developed, and requires further research.

Conclusions: A lack of high-quality experimental studies, definitional inconsistency and poor reporting continue to stymie our ability to identify effective supported accommodation models and practices. The authors recommend improved reporting standards and the prioritisation of experimental studies that compare outcomes across different service models.

Keywords: Supported accommodation, Supported housing, Rehabilitation, Recovery, Effectiveness

* Correspondence: p.mcpherson@ucl.ac.uk
Division of Psychiatry, Faculty of Brain Sciences, UCL, 6th Floor, Maple House, 149 Tottenham Court Road, London W1T 7NF, UK

Background

In Western Europe and North America, the process of de-institutionalisation, defined as "*...the practice of caring for individuals in the community rather than in an institutional environment*" (p.47), has led to a significant increase in community based care for people with severe mental illness (SMI) [1]. Housing-based support, or supported accommodation, operates as a component of the broader mental health 'care pathway' and attempts to meet the needs of service users by providing focussed, flexible support. In this context, support aims to address functional impairment, develop practical living skills, improve social functioning and promote recovery and independence [2]. Mental health supported accommodation services have been implemented widely; recent estimates indicate that, in the UK alone, over 60,000 individuals are currently receiving support in these settings [3]. Due to high rates of service use, and expenditure related to staffing, support and infrastructure, this form of intervention is also extremely costly. However, despite the broad implementation of these services and the associated financial burden, little is known about their effectiveness.

Definitional issues are well documented in the literature, and present a significant obstacle to the assessment of the effectiveness of supported accommodation. Both within and between countries, supported accommodation services vary widely in terms of physical structure, staffing arrangements, levels of support, recovery focus, and discharge and move-on policies, contributing to confusion as to what exactly a supported accommodation service 'looks' like. Despite these issues being discussed in the literature for over 20 years, there have been few meaningful attempts to address them. As a result, the available literature is heterogeneous in nature and resistant to synthesis attempts, leaving researchers and policy makers with no clear summary of the bigger picture; that is, what works and for whom.

For these reasons, previous attempts to summarise the evidence base have been largely unsatisfactory. O'Malley and Croucher [4] conducted a scoping study of supported accommodation services for people with mental health problems in the UK, aiming to explore evidence for models of good practice. After reviewing 131 studies from an original pool of 2506, the authors concluded that most services are based on the assumption that service users will progress from higher to lower levels of supported accommodation over time, however they could not identify any "*concrete evidence to support any particular model of housing support*" (p.841). Due to the methodology used, the authors did not undertake an assessment of the quality of the publications, thus significantly limiting the validity of the findings. In addition, the study focussed solely on UK papers and is also now more than 10 years old. More recently, a Cochrane Review (initially conducted in 2002, and updated in 2006) [5, 6] compared the efficacy of supported housing schemes, outreach support and standard care. The systematic review considered only randomised controlled trials (RCT) and quasi-randomised trials. A thorough search identified 139 potential studies for inclusion, but after review, none fulfilled the inclusion criteria. While the superiority of RCTs as a 'gold standard' for providing evidence for effectiveness is widely acknowledged, there is also a growing argument for considering other quantitative evidence beyond RCT studies. This is particularly salient in cases where RCTs are not possible due to ethical or pragmatic concerns, as is typically the case in in supported accommodation research. The Cochrane review provides a stark comment on the state of the literature in the field, however it does little to describe the existing evidence base.

In light of these observations, it is clear that there is an urgent need to summarise the current evidence as it relates to mental health supported accommodation services. We therefore undertook a comprehensive systematic review of data from quantitative studies in the field, incorporating evidence beyond that derived from RCTs alone. Our aim was to synthesise the current evidence on mental health and psychosocial outcomes for individuals residing in mental health supported accommodation, making comparisons between different models, where the quality of evidence allowed. Our objective was to report findings likely to be of interest to those providing and commissioning mental health supported accommodation, as well as policy makers, and to highlight areas for future research.

This review follows the PRISMA guidelines [7]. The PRISMA checklist and review protocol are available and can be requested directly from the authors.

Methods

Inclusion criteria

The review included quantitative studies, and quantitative components of mixed-method studies, that evaluated the effectiveness of supported accommodation on the mental health and psychosocial outcomes of people with mental health problems, published after 1990. No country-based limitations were imposed. The review considered all relevant papers published in Latin alphabet text. Non-English papers were translated prior to data extraction. A separate review was carried out by our research team that focussed on studies that used qualitative methods.

Definition of supported accommodation

There is large variation in the terminology used in the supported accommodation sector internationally. For the purpose of this review, we defined mental health supported accommodation as any service that provided support, delivered predominately by non-professionally qualified staff, to people with mental health problems living in community-based accommodation, either alone or in shared settings. The components of this definition are common in the literature, and aim to distinguish supported accommodation from specialist, inpatient rehabilitation services, such as community-based rehabilitation units (e.g. 'ward in the community') and statutory mental health teams, where staff are required to possess appropriate professional qualifications. All studies that investigated mental health and psychosocial outcomes in these settings were included. Cost-effectiveness papers, and studies examining specific interventions within these settings (e.g. token economies), were excluded.

Study design

The review examined studies with a broad range of designs, including experimental, quasi-experimental, cohort, case control and observational studies with and without comparison groups. Systematic reviews, clinical guidance, book chapters, conference proceedings and general commentaries or discussion papers were excluded.

Population

We included studies that reported outcomes on individuals with a primary mental health diagnosis, aged 18 to 65. Studies reporting outcomes for service users with a primary diagnosis of dementia, learning disability, personality disorder, substance misuse, eating disorder or physical disability were excluded. Studies with an explicit focus on mental health-substance misuse dual diagnosis populations, or those that included a sample with fewer than 50% of participants with a mental health problem were also excluded.

Outcomes

Due to the heterogeneity of studies, it was necessary to consider a wide range of mental health and psychosocial outcomes. These were grouped into four categories:

- Service use: Housing stability, including maintaining tenancy/being evicted from tenancy; hospitalisation; imprisonment; psychiatric service contact; move-on to more independent accommodation.
- Mental health and wellbeing: Symptoms of mental illness; death/suicide; self-esteem; mental well-being
- Function: Social functioning (including employment); autonomy; quality of life (QoL); recovery
- Service user satisfaction with care

Search strategy

An electronic database search was conducted in January 2015 using MEDLINE, EMBASE, PsycINFO, CINAHL Plus, International Bibliography of the Social Sciences (IBSS), Applied Social Sciences Index and Abstracts (ASSIA), Sociological Abstracts, Web of Science and The Cochrane Library. Terms and concepts relating to 'mental illness', 'supported accommodation' and key outcomes, such as quality of life, housing retention and social functioning, were combined with MeSH terms, subject headings or thesaurus terms (depending on database). Searches were conducted again in June 2017 to ensure comprehensiveness. Limits relating to age (18–65 years) and publication date (> 1990) were applied. The original search strategy, organised according to database, is provided in Additional file 1.

Four journals returning the highest number of retained articles in the electronic search were selected for hand-searching: Community Mental Health Journal, Psychiatric Services, Psychiatric Rehabilitation Journal and International Journal of Social Psychiatry. Two authors (PM, JK) reviewed all issues of these journals to identify any articles not retrieved through the formal search. An expert panel, comprised of the Programme Management Group of the Quality and Effectiveness of Supported Tenancies (QuEST) research project (a national programme of research into mental health supported accommodation funded by the National Institute of Health Research [NIHR], Ref. RP-PG-0610-10,097), were also asked to provide key publications. Reference lists from six key papers [8–13] were also reviewed in order to identify any articles missed through the other search strategies.

After the initial database search results were collated, and duplicates omitted, a relevance review of 10% of articles ($n = 1066$) was conducted by the reviewers (PM, JK) to ensure fidelity to the inclusion criteria. There was 2.5% discrepancy between the two raters ($n = 27$ articles). These 27 publications were reviewed and discussed until consensus regarding inclusion was reached.

Data extraction

A data extraction form was created to facilitate recording of key study information. Data extraction was carried out by two researchers (PM, JK), with the following information recorded from each included article:

- Article characteristics: Country of origin; language; population; subject and context.
- Study characteristics: Aims of the study; study design; theoretical framework; outcomes; methods; participant numbers by group (N); participant eligibility; sampling method; recruitment procedures; data collection procedures; data analysis.

- Findings: Reported results; interpretation of results; summary of findings; recommendations; policy and practice implications.

For non-English language articles, researchers at UCL that were native-speakers were employed to extract the data. JK and PM instructed these individuals on the process of data extraction.

Quality assessment

Quality appraisal of articles was carried out to assess bias and inform the relative weighting of results. The Quality Assessment Tool for Quantitative Studies (QATQS) [14] was used to assess article quality; the tool is recommended for use in systematic reviews by Deeks and colleagues [15] and displays acceptable psychometric properties [14]. The QATQS assesses the methodological strength of a study across eight domains (selection bias; study design; confounders; blinding; data collection methods; withdrawals and dropouts; intervention integrity; and analysis) and provides a global quality rating of 'strong' (high quality), 'moderate' (moderate quality) and 'weak' (low quality). Due to the scoring system, it is possible for well-designed and executed non-experimental studies to be rated as high quality (e.g. cohort analytic, case control, and interrupted time series rated as 'moderate' in the design domain). Any papers assessed as 'weak' were excluded from the synthesis (see below).

Data synthesis

Due to the heterogeneity of the literature, a narrative synthesis method was employed. The synthesis was structured using guidelines published by Popay and colleagues [16], and included developing a preliminary synthesis, exploring the relationships in the data, and assessing the robustness of the final synthesis product.

Results

Descriptives

The initial return comprised of 16,080 articles from electronic databases, and 601 articles from hand-searches and snowballing. After the removal of duplicates, and the application of inclusion-exclusion criteria, the final sample consisted of 115 articles. A PRISMA diagram, illustrating the retrieval procedure and returns, is presented in Fig. 1. The majority of the retrieved papers focussed on American populations, with smaller numbers considering Canadian, United Kingdom, Italian, Australian and German contexts (see Table 1). In terms of experimental design, the review considered cohort (n = 85), quasi-experimental (n = 15), randomised control (n = 11) and case-control (n = 4) studies. Quality assessment,

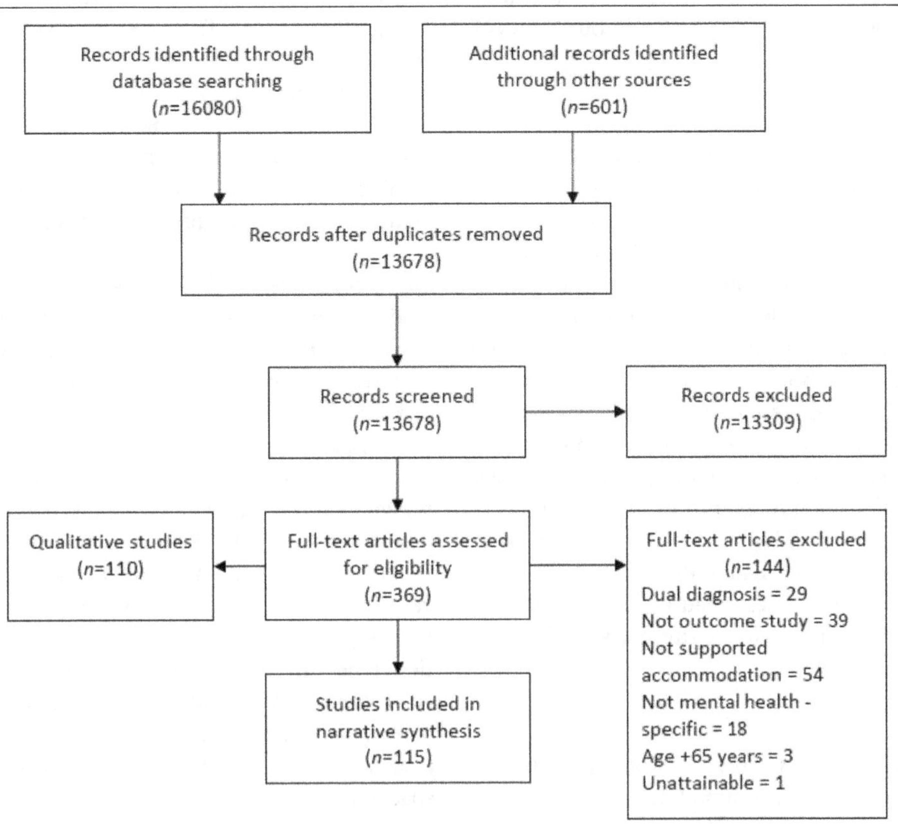

Fig. 1 PRISMA diagram: Retrieval process

Table 1 Retrieved papers by country of origin

Country	Number of papers
USA	50
Canada	14
UK	11
Italy	8
Australia	6
Germany	6
Denmark	3
Hong Kong	3
Israel	3
Japan	3
Holland	2
Albania	1
Finland	1
Greece	1
India	1
New Zealand	1
Taiwan	1
Total	115

using the QATQS, indicated that the majority of studies were rated as moderate quality ($n = 62$), with a smaller number rated as high quality ($n = 20$). In total, 33 studies were assessed as low quality and, in line with our protocol, excluded from the synthesis.

Initially, the review was intended to assess and contrast outcomes according to supported accommodation service types. However, the significant variation in terminology and service characteristics in the reviewed papers made this approach unfeasible. Consequently, we examined the characteristics of individual studies, in line with guidance by Popay and colleagues [16], and identified specific study populations. Two clear sub-groups emerged; homeless individuals with mental illness, and former patients of large hospitals that had been resettled in the community. The remaining papers considered supported accommodation for non-specified mentally ill populations. Based on these characteristics, it was decided to present the findings according to the following population sub-groups: 'Homeless', 'Deinstitutionalisation' and 'General Severe Mental Illness (SMI)'. These three groups of studies are described in the sub-sections below. See Additional file 2 for a summary table of all reviewed studies.

Homeless

This group of papers comprised of studies examining outcomes of supported accommodation focussed on homeless individuals with SMI. These studies were typically from the USA or Canada, and included permanent supported housing projects (such as Housing First [HF]) and the 'HUD-VASH' program (Department of Housing and Urban Development - Veterans Affairs Supportive Housing Program), which caters to military veterans in the USA. These studies are unique, not only for their population-focus but also for the type of supported accommodation examined; the bulk of the 'homeless' papers examined the permanent supported housing approach which aims to support homeless individuals to achieve housing stability or permanent accommodation, as well providing support with mental health issues. Specifically, this approach *"provides individuals with immediate housing, client choice is emphasized in every aspect of treatment, housing is separated from treatment, and a harm reduction approach is followed"* [13] (p.2). It contrasts with traditional continuum models whereby service users progress through 'levels' of support (of lessening intensity), with the intention of achieving stable, permanent housing as an end-point.

Study design, quality and outcomes

The 'homeless' group comprised of the largest number of examined studies; 40 papers in total were reviewed. Of this, 11 were rated as high quality [8, 13, 17–24, 44] and 20 moderate quality [9, 25–43]. Nine papers were omitted from the synthesis due to low quality. Of the retained papers, the majority were cohort studies ($n = 16$), followed by RCTs ($n = 8$), quasi-experimental studies ($n = 6$), and a single case control study ($n = 1$) (see Additional file 2 for detail). The outcomes assessed varied, but reflect the high number of HF studies and their primary foci; the most common outcomes were housing stability, service use, symptoms of mental illness, substance misuse, social functioning, and QoL.

Supported accommodation types

The structure of the examined supported accommodation services varied considerably, as did the detail in which they were reported. The majority of the papers on homeless supported accommodation services were based on the permanent supported housing model [9, 13, 17, 18, 21–23, 25–27, 30, 31, 33, 36–44]. Projects adhering to this model included, among others, HF [13, 17, 18, 26, 27, 31–33, 36, 37, 40, 41], Pathways to Housing [34, 44], At Home/Chez Soi [42], and projects using Section 8 housing certificates [39]. The principles of permanent supported housing are implemented in various forms; accommodation types include group homes [24, 35, 43], individual apartments [24, 35, 38, 43], community residences (residences in buildings with single or shared rooms, or studio apartments, and common dining, meeting, and services space) [21]. The permanent supported housing projects also varied according to intensity and nature of support (including intensive case management, assertive community treatment and different levels of on-site staff support), level of integration between housing and mental health service providers, fidelity to the principle of separation between housing and treatment, and restrictions around sobriety [9]. Traditional housing available to homeless populations with SMI, such as homeless shelters [29], nursing homes [20], board and care homes [28] and residential care facilities [35] were used as comparison conditions in some studies.

Housing stability In total, 19 studies of supported accommodation for homeless populations assessed housing stability as an outcome, comprising 7 high quality [8, 18, 19, 21–23, 44] and 12 moderate quality studies [9, 25, 26, 30–35, 37, 39, 42]. Supported accommodation appears to be effective in promoting housing retention for homeless adults with mental illness; high quality studies consistently reported high rates of housing retention, with 37 to 84% of participants still housed at follow-up (6 months to 5 years) [19, 21, 23, 44, 45]. Moderate quality studies generally supported these findings, reporting high rates of housing stability [9, 34, 35], reductions in nights spent homeless [26, 33, 37], and increases in nights spent in own apartment [26, 42].

A number of factors appear to be related to housing stability including gender, with women more likely to be housed and less likely to be evicted [18, 30], age (being older associated with longer tenure) [19, 34] and income [9], with higher income increasing the probability of a 'positive' move-on. Other related factors include access to housing subsidies [39], neighbourhood quality [9], supportive relationships with support staff [9], case manager support to access appropriate benefits [18], self-harm behaviours [30], chronic pain/illness [30], improvements in housing problems [8] and past [9, 19] and current substance misuse [30]. Intensity of case management [39] and service users' preference for housing type and satisfaction with support were not found to be predictive of housing stability [31, 32].

Service use Eight studies of supported accommodation for homeless populations examined the association between the supported accommodation service and appropriate service use (two high quality studies [8, 21] and six moderate quality studies [28, 29, 35–37, 42]). There was generally consistent evidence that supported accommodation for homeless individuals lead to an increased use of appropriate support services, such as outpatient clinics and medication visits [36, 37], a reduction in hospitalisations [28], homeless shelter use [29] and the use of crisis services [21] for adult homeless populations. In contrast, a single moderate quality study [42] found no difference in hospital days or emergency service use between HF participants and those receiving treatment as usual (TAU). One high quality study found a positive association between neighbourhood quality and length of hospital admissions, and between housing problems and service needs [8]. One moderate quality study [35] demonstrated a significant relationship between housing stability and appropriate service use.

Symptoms of mental illness Eight studies of homeless supported accommodation services investigated mental health symptoms (five high quality [13, 21, 23, 44, 45] and three moderate quality studies [32, 33, 42]). Symptom assessment methods varied (across all studies in this review), and included clinical assessments, staff-rated and self-report instruments. All high quality studies suggested that supported accommodation was associated with significant improvements in, or stability of, mental health symptoms [13, 21, 23, 44, 45]. No deterioration in symptoms was reported. Results of moderate quality studies were inconsistent; one study found no differences in symptoms over time between HF and TAU groups [42], while another reported that improvements in symptoms were not consistently observed and, where they did occur they were slight [33].

One high quality study [13] reported all findings, including symptoms, in terms of "expected trajectory", referring to an improvement or no change in key variables. This presented a challenge in interpreting the results, as improvements, and lack of change in outcomes, were not presented separately. Although this study suggested that 71% of participants followed the expected trajectory for improvements in symptomology, no data were provided to distinguish what proportion of this group improved, or did not change. This observation pertains to all subsequent reporting of findings from this study.

One study reported a greater improvement in psychiatric symptoms in supported housing settings where mental health services are integrated (see descriptions above) [23]. Paradoxically, one high quality study found that a diagnosis of alcohol or substance abuse or dependence was associated with a reduction in psychiatric symptoms [13].

Substance use In total, six homeless supported accommodation service studies examined the association between the supported accommodation and substance use (four high quality [13, 23, 44, 45] and two moderate quality studies [33, 42]). There was no clear evidence that supported accommodation was associated with reduction in drug and alcohol use for homeless populations. The majority of high quality studies reported no change in this outcome over time [23, 44, 45]. A single high quality study reported improvement or no change in this outcome, with 72% of the sample meeting the expected trajectory for change [13]. A single moderate quality paper reported a small but significant reduction in ratings of alcohol abuse, and in the proportion of participants who reported illicit substance misuse [33]. Similarly, a moderate study reported a significant reduction number of days experiencing alcohol-related problems at 12 and 24 months, and in the amount of money spent on alcohol at 24 months, in the HF group compared to TAU [42]. Although we did not find evidence that supported accommodation was associated with reduction in substance misuse, it is important to note that it was not associated with any increase amongst homeless individuals either.

Social functioning, family support and community integration Across the seven studies (two high quality [13, 45], five moderate quality [31, 33, 38, 41, 42]) that examined this outcome, there was inconsistent evidence to suggest that supported accommodation was associated with improvements in social functioning, family support or community integration. A single high quality study reported significant improvement in satisfaction with family relationships, perceived availability of family and frequency of family interactions over time [45]. Study 13 provides perhaps the strongest evidence in support of improvements in these outcomes: 60, 62 and 67% of participants followed the 'expected trajectory' of improvement for physical community integration (actual participation in community activity and use of community resources), psychological community integration (how an individual perceives themselves as a member of their community) and community functioning respectively [13]. However, as described previously, the method of reporting in this study limits our ability to confidently interpret the findings. One study [41] demonstrated significant improvements in psychological community integration at 12-month follow-up for HF participants, when compared to TAU, however they found no change between groups or over time in physical community integration. Similar results were reported in another moderate quality paper [42]. A moderate quality study found a small but statistically significant increase in overall community participation over time [33], however, for nine of the 18 activities assessed, there was no significant change; the authors reported that *"Participants ...remained socially isolated and showed limited improvement in other domains of social integration"* (p.427).

Quality of life The data were inconsistent in demonstrating any association between supported accommodation for homeless individuals and QoL. In total, nine papers reported on this outcome (four high quality studies [13, 21, 23, 44] and five moderate quality studies [27, 31, 37, 40, 42]). Amongst the high quality papers, one study reported improvement in QoL at 18-months [23], one reported 66% of participants meeting the "expected trajectory" for change in QoL [13], and one reported no change over time [21]. Another high quality study reported no significant difference in QoL between participants receiving HF and controls at six months follow-up, however, baseline data were not reported so change over time could not be assessed [44]. One moderate quality study demonstrated initial improvement in QoL in a HF group, compared to TAU, however the effect was not sustained, with no group differences in QoL observed at 24 month follow-up [42]. Data from other moderate quality studies suggested that supported accommodation is associated with improvements in QoL for homeless adults [27, 40], but the experimental design of another moderate quality study did not allow examination of change over time [37]. Time in independent housing was significantly associated with QoL [27]. The same study showed QoL was negatively associated with severity of symptoms but it was not associated with participation in community activities [27]. Another study found service users having choice over living environment predicted QoL at six and 12-month follow up, albeit weakly [31].

Deinstitutionalisation

The 'deinstitutionalisation' subgroup of papers is comprised of studies examining outcomes of people previously residing longer term in large mental hospitals who were resettled in the community following the closure of these institutions and the development of community based mental health services. These individuals were typically older, with a long illness history and had been in hospital for an extended period of time.

Study design, quality and outcomes

In total, 35 deinstitutionalisation papers were reviewed; five were rated as high quality [46–50] and 23 as moderate quality [51–73]. Seven were omitted from the synthesis due to a low quality rating. The included articles were typically cohort studies ($n = 24$), with a smaller number of quasi-experimental ($n = 2$) and a single case-control ($n = 1$) and randomised controlled trial ($n = 1$) (see Additional file 2 for detail). Common outcomes assessed for this group were rates of hospitalisation, symptoms, social functioning, employment and QoL.

Supported accommodation types

Due to the naturalistic nature of the deinstitutionalisation process and the associated research, the majority of the studies were uncontrolled, and often considered a range of community-based accommodation settings within a single study; this contributed, at times, to descriptions of services that lacked detail. Identifiable service types included nursing homes [47, 56, 65], residential care units or high-support hostels with 24 h staffing [46–48, 51, 52, 54, 55, 57, 59, 60, 62, 63, 66], supported group homes [48, 49, 55, 56, 61, 64, 67], apartments with flexible support [46, 48, 56, 60], halfway houses [50, 53, 58, 68, 71, 73], and boarding/rooming houses [56, 59, 61]. Some studies refer to 'supported housing' or 'supported accommodation' services without providing further detail [70, 72].

Rates of hospitalisation Twelve studies, including one high quality [48] and 12 moderate quality studies [51–53, 56, 58, 60, 63, 67–69, 71, 72], examined rates of hospitalisation as an outcome. Unfortunately, the single high quality study did not report data assessing change over time [48]. Amongst the moderate quality studies, however, supported accommodation appeared to be related to reduce rates of hospitalisation [51, 53, 60] and duration of hospital admissions [53, 69, 71] over time. There was, across almost all studies, clear evidence of high rates of rehospitalisation; a number of moderate quality studies [52, 53, 56, 58, 63, 67, 68, 72] indicated between 35 and 87% of participants required inpatient treatment at least once during the follow-up period (range 4–10 years). The single high quality study reported a rehospitalisation rate of 22% during the follow-up period [48]. There is some evidence to suggest that participants from more highly supported settings were more likely to hospitalised, than those in more independent settings [56].

Symptoms There was strong evidence for improvement or a lack of deterioration in the severity of symptoms of mental illness for patients who were discharged to community-based supported accommodation settings from large institutions. In total, 15 studies examined this outcome, including four high quality [46–49] and 11 moderate quality studies [52, 54, 56, 57, 62, 63, 65, 66, 70, 72, 73]. The majority of high quality studies reported improvements in symptoms over time [46, 47, 49]. Improvement in positive symptoms was most common [47, 50]. Findings from the moderate quality papers were less consistent; most reported no change [52, 62, 63, 65, 66, 70, 72, 73], or mixed results [54, 56, 57].

A number of high and moderate quality studies seemed to indicate that more restrictive settings, such as nursing homes were associated with poorer outcomes, with some demonstrating a worsening of symptoms in patients discharged to these environments [47, 73].

Social functioning Fifteen studies examined social functioning as an outcome, including four high quality [47–50] and 11 moderate quality studies [52, 54–58, 62, 63, 65, 66, 70]. Evidence for an association between supported accommodation and improvement in social functioning amongst the 'deinstitutionalisation' sub-group was mixed, although findings suggested a trend toward improvement. Two high quality studies reported significant improvements in performance of socially expected activities [50], social competence and social interest [49], and a significant reduction in behavioural problems, such as hostility, over/under activity and inappropriate sexual behaviour [50]. Two high quality studies, however, found no improvements in social functioning over time [47, 48]. Data from the moderate quality studies contributed to the mixed picture; while some studies reported significant improvements over time [54, 63, 65], the evidence was complicated by poor methodologies and, occasionally, a lack of inferential data [55, 62]. In addition, several moderate quality studies reported no change in this domain [52, 65, 66]. Several studies showed no change in the size of social networks over time [57, 70], while others demonstrated a reduction in the frequency of contacts with family and friends, with a parallel increase in contacts with fellow residents [58]. Similar to the findings reported previously for symptoms, one study reported a deterioration in global social adjustment in individuals discharged to more restrictive settings, such as psychiatric nursing homes [47].

Employment There was some evidence supporting an association between supported accommodation and employment in the deinstitutionalised population, however the number and quality of studies was limited. Employment rates ranged from 0 to 17% in the three moderate quality studies that assessed this outcome [56, 68, 72]. One moderate study reported an unspecified reduction in rates of unemployment at the time of discharge [53]. No high quality papers examined this outcome.

Quality of life A relatively small proportion of the reviewed studies examined QoL as an outcome in the deinstitutionalised subgroup; in total, eight studies, including two high quality [47, 50] and six moderate quality studies [54, 61, 63, 66, 72, 73], examined this variable. There was a lack of clear evidence for any improvement in QoL over time for this population but most studies reported that it remained stable. The high quality papers suggested an inverse relationship between QoL and restrictiveness of setting, with studies reporting significant reduction in QoL for patients discharged to psychiatric nursing homes [47, 50]. Similarly, one moderate quality paper found that moving into 'inappropriate' residential settings resulted in a deterioration in QoL [61]. The lack of association between supported accommodation and subjective QoL over time reported in the high quality papers was consistent with the evidence from the moderate quality papers [54, 72, 73].

General SMI

Although this group is largely defined by non-inclusion in the Homeless and Deinstitutionalisation groups, a number of characteristics make it distinct. The General SMI group represents service users of the post-deinstitutionalisation rehabilitation pathway; generally, they present with complex needs associated with psychotic illness and will have entered the supported accommodation system through various pathways (e.g. referred from acute inpatient units, deteriorated after independent community living, or moved-on from community-based rehabilitation units / forensic services etc). Importantly, as opposed to the deinstitutionalisation group, they will generally not present with the clinical, social and behavioural impairments associated with long-term hospitalisation.

Study design, quality and outcomes

In total, 40 general SMI papers were reviewed. The majority were of moderate quality ($n = 19$) [74–91, 96], with a smaller number rated as high quality ($n = 4$) [92–95]. However, 17 papers were not included in this synthesis due to low quality. As with the previous subgroups, the majority of the studies were cohort designs ($n = 18$), with one quasi-experimental ($n = 1$) and one matched case control study ($n = 1$) (see Additional file 2 for detail). There was a wide variety of outcomes assessed in these papers, however the most common were rates of hospitalisation, symptoms, social functioning, and QoL.

Supported accommodation types

For this group of papers, service types ranged from intensive congregate residential care settings, with 24 h staffing [76, 78–80, 87, 89, 93, 95], to less intensively supported accommodation, including group homes and supervised individual apartments (e.g. staffed 9 am-5 pm daily) [74, 78, 81, 82, 90, 92–94], to individual tenancies with outreach support (staff based off-site) [75, 81, 83, 87, 88, 90, 96]. Other service descriptions lacked detail and were unable to be confidently categorised, including "sheltered housing" [77], "sheltered-care facilities" [86], "community-based housing" [91], "transitional, high-expectation, sheltered care environment" [85] and "support house" [84].

Rates of hospitalisation Twelve papers, including two high quality [92, 94] and ten moderate quality studies [74, 77, 78, 81, 82, 84, 88–90, 96], reported data relating to changes in rates of hospitalisation. The findings were mixed. Generally, it appeared that supported accommodation was associated with a reduction in days spent in hospital [78, 81, 82, 89, 90], and duration of hospital stays [96], over time. One study demonstrated a significant reduction in mean number of hospital and crisis centre admissions from pre-entry into a residential program to one-year post-discharge [89]. Similarly, another moderate quality study demonstrated a significant reduction in mean number of days in hospital from baseline year (pre-entry) to the first year in community living arrangement facilities [78]. In spite of these positive findings, other studies, including a single high quality article [94], reported no change in this outcome over time [74, 88]. One high quality study found that specialist case management, which was reserved for SUs with a history of repeated hospitalisations, was the only predictor of future hospitalisations [92], while another moderate quality study found that severity of symptoms predicted both hospitalisations and duration of stay [77].

Symptoms Nine papers assessed changes in symptoms over time (two high quality [94, 95] and seven moderate quality studies [74, 76, 80, 82, 84, 86, 88]. There was mixed evidence for an association between supported accommodation and symptoms in general SMI populations. Although some moderate quality papers demonstrated significant improvements in symptoms over time [82, 84, 95], a number, including a single high quality study, reported no change [86, 94], or a worsening of symptoms [74, 80] amongst this group. In examining change over time, one moderate quality study showed a significant improvement in symptoms for a small sub-group of participants who had been discharged from a residential facility, but no change for those participants who had remained in place [76]. One study demonstrated improvement in depression and anxiety over time, however this was assessed using a scale assessing social behaviours as opposed to a symptom inventory [88].

Social functioning In total, 12 general SMI studies examined the association between supported accommodation and social functioning, including one high quality [94] and eleven moderate quality papers [74–76, 79, 82, 83, 85–88, 96]. Again, the findings related to this outcome are best described as mixed. Some moderate quality studies demonstrated significant improvements in social integration [82] and community participation [96], increases in friendships and supportive relationships [82, 83] and reductions in social disability over time [79]. However, the majority of studies found no change in key social variables over time, such as social functioning [74, 76, 82], social networks [74, 75, 82] and satisfaction with social support [94]. One study, examining the effectiveness of outreach support, found a significant reduction in the size of social networks over time [88]. Another study reported a reduction in independent social functioning and an increase in assisted social functioning over time [86]. In contrast, a single moderate quality study found that SUs receiving home care reported significantly higher levels of social activity compared to SUs residing in half-way house [87]. Severity of symptoms and number of hospitalisations was found, in one study, to negatively influence the quality of social networks [85].

Quality of life Six moderate quality papers [74, 79, 80, 82, 87, 88] examined changes in QoL with the general SMI group. The findings were mixed; half reported a significant improvement in QoL over time [79, 82] or a non-significant trend towards improvement [88], and half indicated no change [74, 80, 87], suggesting a limited, or inconsistent, relationship between supported accommodation and this outcome. In one study, QoL was positively associated with specific life skills, including budgeting, self-care, ability to go out, and work performance [82].

Discussion

This systematic review attempted to synthesise the literature on mental health and psychosocial outcomes associated with mental health supported accommodation services. Despite the initial aim of comparing and contrasting outcomes across supported accommodation models, the wide variation in accommodation services, in terms of structure, staffing and related variables, required us to group our findings by population sub-groups.

Homeless

The strongest evidence for supported accommodation comes from research with homeless mentally ill populations and the permanent supported housing model. Studies in this area demonstrate consistent evidence for improvements in housing retention and stability, and appropriate use of clinical services over time. There is also some indication that this form of support for this group is associated with improvements in symptoms, QoL and social functioning, but this evidence is inconsistent. The majority of studies reviewed found no change in substance use over time. As stated by Tsermberis [97], "*Housing First and other supportive housing interventions may end homelessness but do not cure psychiatric disability, addiction, or poverty*" (p.52). These findings are in line with the conclusions of a recent review of HF [98].

Although the permanent supported housing approach has been shown to be effective in some domains, the intervention specifically targets mentally ill homeless populations, and the characteristics of the studied cohorts make generalising to other mental health populations troublesome. First, many of the samples used in these studies have relatively low rates of serious psychiatric illness. In the current review, we utilised a > 50% with psychiatric diagnosis cut-off point to ensure we included appropriate studies. However, even with this approach, it remains difficult to confidently apply the synthesised findings to other groups of people with mental health problems. Second, the presence of long term homelessness amongst the target population conflates the findings when considering the applicability to general SMI populations. It remains difficult to establish whether positive changes in psychosocial outcomes are attributable to intervention components that impact on homelessness (such as housing), or mental health (such as medication management) or both. Third, participants in the permanent supported housing studies typically present with higher rates of drug and alcohol use than comparable, non-homeless samples. There is danger that, due to the large and growing evidence base for these services, policy makers will attempt a wholesale import of the permanent supported housing model for use with psychiatric populations, without a reliable evidence base.

Deinstitutionalisation

Research on outcomes in supported accommodation for deinstitutionalised populations provided good evidence for improvement or non-deterioration in psychiatric symptoms, social functioning and rates of rehospitalisation. There was limited evidence for improvement in QoL and employment. Notably, a number of studies highlighted a consistent association between more restrictive settings and poorer outcomes, across psychiatric, social and QoL outcomes, for this group. Although, these findings are somewhat inconsistent, the threshold of 'success' for this population is radically different than for other groups. Due to the severity of clinical presentations and duration of institutionalised care, most researchers and clinicians consider the absence of deterioration as indicative of successful transition to community care. Indeed, one of the greatest challenges of the deinstitutionalisation process was to address the chronic psychiatric, social and behavioural difficulties of patients, while simultaneously maintaining their tenure in the community [1]. Supported accommodation services appear to have contributed to the achievement of these goals; the reported findings, while not consistently demonstrating improvements across domains do, for the most part, highlight stability.

In reality, the deinstitutionalisation 'story' has already been told; in most European and north American countries, the deinstitutionalisation process commenced the late 1980s and early 1990s and, as such, the majority of the studies cited in this review are old, or report on longer-term follow-ups. It is generally accepted that community based settings are more humane and offer a better QoL than long term hospitalisation [99]. The transition of people from long-stay wards to community-based care has been successful, and the evidence suggests that this group, for the most part, can be maintained in community settings without any significant deterioration [100]. This is an important and well established finding but does little to guide us in the development and implementation of contemporary supported accommodation services.

General SMI

The reviewed papers in this group presented less clear evidence between supported accommodation and psychosocial outcomes for general SMI populations. While there was a trend toward reductions in rates of hospitalisation over time, the evidence was mixed with regards to symptoms, social functioning and QoL, with studies variously demonstrating improvement, no-change, or deterioration in these outcomes over time. These findings may reflect the heterogeneous nature of the literature.

This sub-group had the fewest number of studies overall, the fewest number of high-quality papers and the largest number of omitted low-quality studies, yet this population is growing rapidly, reflecting the broad adoption of the supported accommodation model, current approaches to community-based rehabilitation and the rejection of long-term hospitalisation as a form of treatment.. This observation highlights an urgent need for increased research in this area. As mentioned above, there is a genuine danger that due to the growing evidence base, the HF model is applied to this group despite the problems in generalising the research findings.

Strengths and limitations

The current review had a number of strengths. We applied a thorough search strategy, utilising a broad date range, and included a range of psychosocial outcomes and a variety of quantitative designs beyond RCTs. These methodological decisions enabled us to be comprehensive in our review and confident in capturing all key outcome studies.

As the reviewed studies relate to supported accommodation only, it must be acknowledged that, by examining the outcomes in relation to subgroups, broader findings related to these groups may have been overlooked. For example, many of the Team for the Assessment of Psychiatric Services (TAPS) studies, and other programmes of research investigating outcomes for deinstitutionalised groups, were not included in this review as they did not explicitly consider supported housing, however data from these studies would have expanded and contextualised the reported findings as they relate to the deinstitutionalisation sub-group. The population-based conclusions, therefore, must be considered strictly in relation to supported accommodation.

As we were unable to examine differences in outcomes across models, the current review cannot comment on their relative merits in relation to outcomes. As described, there is a large variation in housing models; within each of the population sub-groups considered above, service models ranged from independent tenancies with outreach support to high-staffed, congregate residential settings. Inevitably, the characteristics of a service, such as the physical structure, staffing arrangements, levels of support, recovery focus, and discharge and move-on policies, will impact on service user outcomes, possibly beyond the influence of population characteristics. As a result, this review is limited in its ability to fully consider the effectiveness of mental health supported accommodation services.

By comparing services from different national contexts, we aimed to enhance our understanding of the critical components of these interventions and how contextual factors impact outcomes. However, due to the aforementioned variation in service models (evident even within countries), it was difficult to discern the impact of national level factors, such as legislation, funding barriers or statutory responsibilities. The international focus of this review makes it challenging to provide any specific recommendations for local policy makers and commissioners. A more targeted study, focusing on one country or region, would be better suited for this purpose. In line with the recovery approach, however, it is likely that any high-quality supported accommodation provision will comprise of a range of accommodation options, with the delivery of flexible, personalised support.

Finally, as we have considered evidence from non-RCT designs, the data presented herein, even from studies rated as 'high quality', should be interpreted with caution.

Conclusion

The mixed results of this study highlight the heterogeneity of the supported accommodation literature, in terms of research quality, experimental design, population, service types and outcomes assessed. There is some evidence that supported accommodation is effective across a range of psychosocial outcomes, with the most robust evidence showing the effectiveness of the HF model for homeless SMI and for other forms of supported accommodation for deinstitutionalised populations in reducing hospitalisation rates and improving appropriate service use. The evidence base for general SMI populations is less developed, and requires further research. Unfortunately, these broad observations reinforce the conclusions of Chilvers and colleagues [5] in their recent

Cochrane review: "*In the absence of evidence of their relative efficacy, decisions on the provision of alternative forms of accommodation and continued support for people with mental illness can only be based on a combination of professional judgement, patient preference and availability*" (p.6).

The intention of the current review was to compare and contrast the effectiveness of various models of supported accommodation, across a range of psychosocial outcomes. However, as noted, this attempt was stymied by the large variation in service models, the lack of definitional consistency and, at times, poor reporting practices in the literature. In order to make assertions regarding the effectiveness of various models of supported accommodation, it is clear that a simple method of service categorisation, based on current reporting practices, is required. A taxonomy that can be applied retrospectively to existing research, and utilised in future studies, would allow effective synthesis of outcome data, facilitate an examination of efficacy and effectiveness, and strengthen follow-up/replication studies [101]. While some attempts have been made to develop a supported accommodation taxonomy [102, 103], these models are complex and have not been widely utilised. Recently, a new, simple classification system for supported accommodation services has been developed (The Simple Taxonomy for Supported Accommodation [STAX- SA] [104]). Future research should consider utilising this tool to synthesise the available effectiveness evidence, comparing service user outcomes across service models.

Mental health supported accommodation services are widely implemented, however, currently we have no clear research base articulating what works and for whom. There is a clear need for high quality effectiveness research, improved reporting standards and consistent and meaningful descriptions of supported accommodation services in the literature. Researchers must prioritise experimental studies that compare outcomes across different service models. These developments should inform and improve mental health commissioning and service development decisions in the future.

Abbreviations

HF: Housing First; HUD-VASH: Department of Housing and Urban Development - Veterans Affairs Supportive Housing Program; NIHR: National Institute of Health Research; QATQS: Quality Assessment Tool for Quantitative Studies; QoL: Quality of life; QuEST: Quality and effectiveness of supported tenancies for people with mental health problems; RCT: Randomised controlled trial; SMI: Severe mental illness; TAU: Treatment as usual

Acknowledgements

We would like to acknowledge current and past members of the Quality and Effectiveness of Supported Tenancies (QuEST) research group at UCL/QMUL (Christian Dalton-Locke, Sarah Dowling, Isobel Harrison, Rose McGranahan, Sima Sandhu,) and the QuEST programme management group (Maurice Arbuthnott, Sarah Curtis, Sandra Eldridge, Michael King, Gerry Leavey, Gavin McCabe, Paul McCrone, Stefan Priebe and Geoff Shepherd) for their support with this project.

Funding

This paper presents independent research funded by the National Institute for Health Research (NIHR) under its Programme Grants for Applied Research scheme (RP-PG-0610-10,097). The views expressed in this publication are those of the authors and not necessarily those of the National Health Service, the NIHR or the Department of Health.

Authors' contributions

PM designed the study, undertook searches, extracted data and drafted the manuscript. JK designed the study, undertook searches, extracted data and critically commented on drafts of the manuscript. HK conceived and supervised the study, contributed to interpretation of the data, and critically commented on drafts of the manuscript. All authors read and approved the final manuscript.

Competing interests

The authors declare that they have no competing interests.

References

1. Shen GC, Snowden LR. Institutionalization of deinstitutionalization: a cross-national analysis of mental health system reform. Int J Ment Health Syst. 2014;8:47. https://doi.org/10.1186/1752-4458-8-47.
2. Pleace N, Wallace A. Demonstrating the effectiveness of housing support services for people with mental health problems: a review: The University of York - Centre for Housing Policy; 2011. https://www.york.ac.uk/media/chp/documents/2011/NHF%20final.pdf. Accessed 01 Mar 2014
3. Sandhu S, Killaspy H, Krotofil J, McPherson P, Harrison I, Dowling S, et al. Development and psychometric properties of the client's assessment of treatment scale for supported accommodation (CAT-SA). BMC Psychiatry. 2016;16:43.
4. O'Malley L, Croucher K. Supported housing services for people with mental health problems: a scoping study. Hous Stud. 2005;20:831–45.
5. Chilvers R, Macdonald G, Hayes A. Supported housing for people with severe mental disorders. Cochrane Database Syst Rev. 2002. Issue 4. Art. No.: CD000453. https://doi.org/10.1002/14651858.CD000453.
6. Chilvers R, Macdonald G, Hayes A. Supported housing for people with severe mental disorders. Cochrane Database Syst Rev. 2006 (update). Issue 4. Art. No.: CD000453. https://doi.org/10.1002/14651858.CD000453.pub2.
7. Liberati A, Altman DG, Tetzlaff J, Mulrow C, Gøtzsche PC, Ioannidis JPA, et al. The PRISMA statement for reporting systematic reviews and meta-analyses of studies that evaluate health care interventions: explanation and elaboration. PLoS Med. 2009;6:e1000100. https://doi.org/10.1371/journal.pmed.1000100.
8. Newman SJ, Reschovsky JD, Kaneda K, Hendrick AM. The effects of independent living on persons with chronic mental illness: an assessment of the section 8 certificate program. Milbank Q. 1994;72:171–98.
9. Lee S, Wong Y-LI, Rothbard AB. Factors associated with departure from supported independent living programs for persons with serious mental illness. Psychiatr Serv. 2009;60:367–73.

10. Hurlburt MS, Hough RL, Wood PA. Effects of substance abuse on housing stability of homeless mentally ill persons in supported housing. Psychiatr Serv. 1996;47:731–6.
11. Gulcur L, Stefancic A, Shinn M, Tsemberis S, Fischer SN. Housing, hospitalization, and cost outcomes for homeless individuals with psychiatric disabilities participating in continuum of care and housing first programmes. J Community Appl Soc Psychol. 2003;13:171–86. https://doi.org/10.1002/casp.723.
12. Dunn M, O'Driscoll C, Dayson D, Wills W, Leff J. The TAPS project. 4: an observational study of the social life of long-stay patients. Br J Psychiatry. 1990;157:842–8. 852
13. Stergiopoulos V, Gozdzik A, O'Campo P, Holtby AR, Jeyaratnam J, Tsemberis S. Housing first: exploring participants' early support needs. BMC Health Serv Res. 2014;14:167.
14. Thomas BH, Ciliska D, Dobbins M, Micucci S. A process for systematically reviewing the literature: providing the research evidence for public health nursing interventions. Worldviews Evidence-Based Nurs. 2004;1:176–84. https://doi.org/10.1111/j.1524-475X.2004.04006.x.
15. Deeks JJ, Dinnes J, D'Amico R, Sowden AJ, Sakarovitch C, Song F, et al. Evaluating non-randomised intervention studies. Health Technol Assess. 2003;7(iii–x):1–173.
16. Popay J, Roberts H, Sowden A, Petticrew M, Arai L, Rodgers M, et al. Guidance on the Conduct of Narrative Synthesis in Systematic Reviews A Product from the ESRC Methods Programme. 2006. https://www.researchgate.net/profile/Mark_Rodgers4/publication/233866356_Guidance_on_the_conduct_of_narrative_synthesis_in_systematic_reviews_A_product_from_the_ESRC_Methods_Programme/links/02e7e5231e8f3a6183000000/Guidance-on-the-conduct-of-narrative-synthesis-in-systematic-reviews-A-product-from-the-ESRC-Methods-Programme.pdf. Accessed 15 Aug 2017.
17. Henwood BF, Derejko K-S, Couture J, Padgett DK. Maslow and mental health recovery: a comparative study of homeless programs for adults with serious mental illness. Adm Policy Ment Heal Ment Heal Serv Res. 2015;42: 220–8. https://doi.org/10.1007/s10488-014-0542-8.
18. Kasprow WJ, Rosenheck RA, Frisman L, DiLella D. Referral and housing processes in a long-term supported housing program for homeless veterans. Psychiatr Serv. 2000;51:1017–23.
19. Lipton FR, Siegel C, Hannigan A, Samuels J, Baker S. Tenure in supportive housing for homeless persons with severe mental illness. Psychiatr Serv. 2000;51:479–86.
20. McCarthy JF, Szymanski BR, Karlin BE, Katz IR. Suicide mortality following nursing home discharge in the Department of Veterans Affairs health system. Am J Public Health. 2013;103:2261–6.
21. Siegel CE, Samuels J, Tang DI, Berg I, Jones K, Hopper K. Tenant outcomes in supported housing and community residences in new York City. Psychiatr Serv. 2006;57:982–91.
22. Wood PA, Hurlburt MS, Hough RL, Hofstetter CR. Longitudinal assessment of family support among homeless mentally ill participants in a supported housing program. J Community Psychol. 1998;26:327–344. doi:10.1002/(sici)1520-6629(199807)26:4<327::aid-jcop3>3.0.co;2-q.
23. McHugo GJ, Bebout RR, Harris M, Cleghorn S, Herring G, Xie HY, et al. A randomized controlled trial of integrated versus parallel housing services for homeless adults with severe mental illness. Schizophr Bull. 2004;30:969–82.
24. Seidman LJ, Schutt RK, Caplan B, Tolomiczenko GS, Turner WM, Goldfinger SM. The effect of housing interventions on neuropsychological functioning among homeless persons with mental illness. Psychiatr Serv. 2003;54:905–8.
25. Gabrielian S, Burns AV, Nanda N, Hellemann G, Kane V, Young AS. Factors associated with premature exits from supported housing. Psychiatr Serv. 2016;67:86–93. https://doi.org/10.1176/appi.ps.201400311.
26. Gilmer TP, Stefancic A, Katz ML, Sklar M, Tsemberis S, Palinkas LA. Fidelity to the housing first model and effectiveness of permanent supported housing programs in California. Psychiatr Serv. 2014;65:1311–7.
27. Henwood BF, Matejkowski J, Stefancic A, Lukens JM. Quality of life after housing first for adults with serious mental illness who have experienced chronic homelessness. Psychiatry Res. 2014;220:549–55.
28. Mares A, McGuire J. Reducing psychiatric hospitalization among mentally ill veterans living in board-and-care homes. Psychiatr Serv. 2000;51:914–21.
29. Metraux S, Marcus SC, Culhane DP. The New York-New York housing initiative and use of public shelters by persons with severe mental illness. Psychiatr Serv. 2003;54:67–71. https://doi.org/10.1176/appi.ps.54.1.67.
30. Montgomery AE, Cusack M, Szymkowiak D, Fargo J, O'Toole T. Factors contributing to eviction from permanent supportive housing: Lessons from HUD-VASH. Eval Program Plann. 2017;61:55–63. https://doi.org/10.1016/j.evalprogplan.2016.11.014.
31. Tsai J, Rosenheck RA. Consumer choice over living environment, case management, and mental health treatment in supported housing and its relation to outcomes. J Heal Care Poor Underserved. 2012;23:1671–7.
32. Tsai J, Mares AS, Rosenheck RA. Housing satisfaction among chronically homeless adults: identification of its major domains, changes over time, and relation to subjective well-being and functional outcomes. Community Ment Health J. 2012;48:255–63. https://doi.org/10.1007/s10597-011-9385-x.
33. Tsai J, Mares AS, Rosenheck RA. Does housing chronically homeless adults lead to social integration? Psychiatr Serv. 2012;63:427–34.
34. Tsemberis S, Eisenberg RF. Pathways to housing: supported housing for street-dwelling homeless individuals with psychiatric disabilities. Psychiatr Serv. 2000;51:487–93.
35. Dickey B, Gonzalez O, Latimer E, Powers K, Schutt R, Goldfinger S. Use of mental health services by formerly homeless adults residing in group and independent housing. Psychiatr Serv. 1996;47:152–8.
36. Gilmer TP, Stefancic A, Tsemberis S, Ettner SL. Full-service partnerships among adults with serious mental illness in California: impact on utilization and costs. Psychiatr Serv. 2014;65:1120–5. https://doi.org/10.1176/appi.ps.201300380.
37. Gilmer TP, Stefancic A, Ettner SL, Manning WG, Tsemberis S. Effect of full-service partnerships on homelessness, use and costs of mental health services, and quality of life among adults with serious mental illness. Arch Gen Psychiatry. 2010;67:645. https://doi.org/10.1001/archgenpsychiatry.2010.56.
38. Schutt RK, Seidman LJ, Caplan B, Martsinkiv A, Goldfinger SM. The role of neurocognition and social context in predicting community functioning among formerly homeless seriously mentally ill persons. Schizophr Bull. 2007;33:1388–96. https://doi.org/10.1093/schbul/sbm037.
39. Hurlburt MS, Wood PA, Hough RL. Providing independent housing for the homeless mentally ill: a novel approach to evaluating long-term longitudinal housing patterns. J Community Psychol. 1996;24:291–310.
40. Patterson M, Moniruzzaman A, Palepu A, Zabkiewicz D, Frankish CJ, Krausz M, et al. Housing first improves subjective quality of life among homeless adults with mental illness: 12-month findings from a randomized controlled trial in Vancouver, British Columbia. Soc Psychiatry Psychiatr Epidemiol. 2013:1245–59. https://doi.org/10.1007/s00127-013-0719-6.
41. Patterson ML, Moniruzzaman A, Somers JM. Community participation and belonging among formerly homeless adults with mental illness after 12 months of housing first in Vancouver, British Columbia: a randomized controlled trial. Community Ment Health J. 2014;50:604–11. https://doi.org/10.1007/s10597-013-9672-9.
42. Stergiopoulos V, Gozdzik A, Misir V, Skosireva A, Connelly J, Sarang A, et al. Effectiveness of ousing first with intensive case management in an ethnically diverse sample of homeless adults with mental illness: a randomized controlled trial. PLoS One. 2015;10:e0130281. https://doi.org/10.1371/journal.pone.0130281.
43. Caplan B, Schutt RK, Turner WM, Goldfinger SM, Seidman LJ. Change in neurocognition by housing type and substance abuse among formerly homeless seriously mentally ill persons. Schizophr Res. 2006;83:77–86. https://doi.org/10.1016/j.schres.2005.11.013.
44. Tsemberis SJ, Asmussen SM, Moran L, Shern DL, Shinn M. Consumer preference programs for individuals who are homeless and have psychiatric disabilities: a drop-in center and a supported housing program. Am J Community Psychol. 2003;32(3/4):305–17.
45. Tsai J, Lapidos A, Rosenheck RA, Harpaz-Rotem I. Longitudinal association of therapeutic alliance and clinical outcomes in supported housing for chronically homeless adults. Community Ment Health J 2013;49:438–443. doi:10.1016/j.eurpsy.2008.12.015http://dx.doi.org/10.1007/s10597-012-9518-x.
46. Furlan PM, Zuffranieri M, Stanga F, Ostacoli L, Patta J, Picci RL. Four-year follow-up of long-stay patients settled in the community after closure of italy's psychiatric hospitals. Psychiatr Serv. 2009;60:1198–202.
47. Kallert TW, Leisse M, Winiecki P. Comparing the effectiveness of different types of supported housing for patients with chronic schizophrenia. J Public Health (Bangkok). 2007;15:29–42.
48. Barbato A, D'Avanzo B, Rocca G, Amatulli A, Lampugnani D. A study of long-stay patients resettled in the community after closure of a psychiatric hospital in Italy. Psychiatr Serv. 2004;55:67–70.

49. Grinshpoon A, Naisberg Y, Weizman A. A six-month outcome of long-stay inpatients resettled in a hostel. Psychiatr Rehabil J. 2006;30:89–95.
50. Chan H, Inoue S, Shimodera S, Fujita H, Fukuzawa K, Kii M, et al. Residential program for long-term hospitalized persons with mental illness in Japan: randomized controlled trial. Psychiatry Clin Neurosci. 2007;61:515–21. https://doi.org/10.1111/j.1440-1819.2007.01701.x.
51. Cohen BZ, Hatib A. The effect of placement in a hostel on the post-hospitalization rehabilitation of psychiatrically disabled persons in Israel. Int J Rehabil Res. 1999;22:61–3.
52. Hornblow A, Baird K. From hospital to community: a follow up of community placement of the long term mentally ill. N Z Med J. 1992;105:348–50.
53. Meissner A. Rehabilitation by a halfway house for mentally ill - A catamnestic study. [German]Wiedereingliederung durch eine ubergangseinrichtung fur psychisch kranke - Eine katamnestische untersuchung. Rehabilitation. 1998;37: 199–204.
54. Crosby C, Barry M, Carter MF, Lowe CF. Psychiatric rehabilitation and community care: resettlement from a North Wales hospital. Health Soc Care Community. 1993;1:355–63.
55. Dayson D, Lee-Jones R, Chahal KK, Leff J. The TAPS project 32: social networks of two group homes ... 5 years on. Soc Psychiatry Psychiatr Epidemiol. 1998;33:438–44.
56. Dewees M, Pulice RT, McCormick LL. Community integration of former state hospital patients: outcomes of a policy shift in Vermont. Psychiatr Serv. 1996;47:1088–92.
57. Duurkoop P, van Dyck R. From a "state mental hospital" to new homes in the city: longitudinal research into the use of intramural facilities by long-stay care-dependent psychiatric clients in Amsterdam. Community Ment Health J 2003;39:77–92.
58. Eikelmann B, Reker T. Rehabilitation of the chronically mentally ill in the community: five-year follow-up. [German]Ergebnisse Der Extramuralen rehabilitation Chronisch Psychisch Kranker: 5-Jahres-follow-up. Rehabilitation. 1993;32:171–6.
59. Hadley TR, McGurrin MC, Fye DM. Community residential services and community tenure. Psychosoc Rehabil J. 1993;16:41–53. https://doi.org/10.1037/h0095676.
60. Lerner Y, Hornik-Lurie T, Zilber N. The effect of the implementation of the rehabilitation of the mentally disabled in the community law in Israel on the pattern of psychiatric hospitalizations: a National Case Register Study. Int J Ment Health. 2012;41:45–59. https://doi.org/10.2753/IMH0020-7411410303.
61. Baker F, Douglas C. Housing environments and community adjustment of severely mentally ill persons. Community Ment Health J. 1990;26:497–505. https://doi.org/10.1007/BF00752454.
62. Higgins A, Webb M, O'Neill G, Brosnan R, Keane J. The needs for care of the chronic mentally ill relocating from psychiatric hospital to the community: a pilot study. Irish J Psychol. 1997;18:307–20.
63. Okin RL, Borus JF, Baer L, Jones AL. Long-term outcome of state hospital patients discharged into structured community residential settings. Psychiatr Serv. 1995;46:73–8.
64. Salokangas RKR, Honkonen T, Stengard E, Koivisto AM. Subjective life satisfaction and living situations of persons in Finland with long-term schizophrenia. Psychiatr Serv. 2006;57:373–81. https://doi.org/10.1176/appi.ps.57.3.373.
65. Shields D, McGuinness J, MacFlynn G. Moving long-stay patients from hospital to community: effects on mental state and social functioning. J Ment Health. 1995;4:281–7.
66. Trauer T, Farhall J, Newton R, Cheung P. From long-stay psychiatric hospital to community care unit: evaluation at 1 year. Soc Psychiatry Psychiatr Epidemiol. 2001;36:416–9.
67. Trieman N, Smith HE, Kendal R, Leff J. The TAPS project 41: homes for life? Residential stability five years after hospital discharge. Team for the assessment of psychiatric services. Community Ment Health J. 1998;34:407–17.
68. Vaslamatzis G, Katsouyanni K, Markidis M. The efficacy of a psychiatric halfway house: a study of hospital recidivism and global outcome measure. Eur Psychiatry. 1997;12:94–7.
69. Kaiser W, Hoffmann K, Isermann M, Priebe S. Long-term patients in supported housing after deinstitutionalisation - part V of the berlin deinstitutionalisation study. Psychiatr Prax. 2001;28:235–43. https://doi.org/10.1055/s-2001-15577.
70. Anderson J, Dayson D, Wills W, Gooch C, Margolius O, O'Driscoll C, et al. The TAPS project. 13: clinical and social outcomes of long-stay psychiatric patients after one year in the community. Br J Psychiatry Suppl. 1993;19:45–56.
71. Volfing BE, Vogel A. Evaluation of group homes for the mentally ill in the county of Copenhagen–1980-1995. A study of a time-limited stay in the group home assessed by the development of the social situation and duration of hospitalization before and after. Ugeskr Laeger. 2002;164:1357–60.
72. Meehan T, Stedman T, Robertson S, Drake S, King R. Does supported accommodation improve the clinical and social outcomes for people with severe psychiatric disability? The project 300 experience. Aust New Zeal J Psychiatry. 2011;45:586–92. https://doi.org/10.3109/00048674.2011.559634.
73. Chan GWL, Ungvari GS, Shek DTL, Leung JP. Impact of deinstitutionalisation on the quality of life of Chinese patients with schizophrenia: A longitudinal pilot study. Hong Kong J Psychiatry. 2003;13:2–5+32.
74. Hodgins S, Cyr M, Gaston L. Impact of supervised apartments on the functioning of mentally disordered adults. Community Ment Health J. 1990;26:507–16.
75. Boydell KM, Everett B. What makes a house a home? An evaluation of a supported housing project for individuals with long-term psychiatric backgrounds. Can J Commun Ment Health. 1992;11(1):109–23.
76. Candini V, Buizza C, Ferrari C, Boero ME, Giobbio GM, Goldschmidt N, et al. Is psychiatric residential facility discharge possible and predictable? A multivariate analytical approach applied to a prospective study in Italy. Soc Psychiatry Psychiatr Epidemiol. 2014;49:157–67.
77. de Mooij LD, Kikkert M, Lommerse NM, Theunissen J, de Koning MB, de Haan L, et al. Homesick: residential and care patterns in patients with severe mental illness. BMC Psychiatry. 2016;16:431. https://doi.org/10.1186/s12888-016-1137-6.
78. Hanrahan P, Luchins DJ, Savage C, Goldman HH. Housing satisfaction and service use by mentally ill persons in community integrated living arrangements. Psychiatr Serv. 2001;52(9):1206.
79. Law KKP, Yau SB, Wan DLY, Chan CCH. Relationship between perceived quality of life, social functioning, and life skills performance of patients with chronic psychiatric conditions in a long stay care home. Hong Kong. J Psychiatry. 2002;12:2–7.
80. Lora A, Contartese A, Franco M, Lo Maglio MC, Molteni E, Pallavicin A, et al. An observational study of effectiveness in community residential facilities. Epidemiol Psichiatr Soc. 2004;13:198–208.
81. McDermott S, Bruce J, Muir K, Ramia I, Fisher KR, Bullen J. Reducing hospitalisation among people living with severe mental illness. Aust Health Rev. 2016;40:124. https://doi.org/10.1071/AH15073.
82. Middelboe T. Prospective study of clinical and social outcome of stay in small group homes for people with mental illness. Br J Psychiatry. 1997;171:251–5.
83. Muir K, Fisher KR, Abello D, Dadich A. "I didn"t like just sittin' around all day': facilitating social and community participation among people with mental illness and high levels of psychiatric disability. J Soc Policy. 2010;39:375–91.
84. Sakiyama S, Iida J, Minami Y, Kishimoto T. Factors of good outcome after discharge from support house (engoryou) for schizophrenia. Psychiatry Clin Neurosci. 2002;56:609–15.
85. Segal SP, Holschuh J. Effects of sheltered care environments and resident characteristics on the development of social networks. Hosp Community Psychiatry. 1991;42:1125–31.
86. Segal SP, Kotler PL. Sheltered care residence: ten-year personal outcomes. Am J Orthop. 1993;63:80–91.
87. Shu BC, Lung FW, Lu YC, Chase GA, Pan P. Care of patients with chronic mental illness: comparison of home and half-way house care. Int J Soc Psychiatry. 2001;47:52–62.
88. Clarkson P, McCrone P, Sutherby K, Johnson C, Johnson S, Thornicroft G. Outcomes and costs of a community support worker service for the severely mentally ill. Acta Psychiatr Scand. 1999;99:196–206.
89. Hawthorne WB, Fals-Stewart W, Lohr JB. A treatment outcome study of community-based residential care. Hosp Community Psychiatry. 1994;45:152–5.
90. Malinovsky I, Lehrer P, Silverstein SM, Shankman SA, O'Brien W, Samuelson T, et al. An empirical evaluation of recovery transformation at a large community psychiatric rehabilitation organization. Psychol Serv. 2013;10: 428–41. https://doi.org/10.1037/a0032747.
91. Nelson G, Hall GB, Walsh-Bowers R. The relationship between housing characteristics, emotional well-being and the personal empowerment of psychiatric consumer/survivors. Community Ment Health J. 1998;34:57–69. https://doi.org/10.1023/A:1018764229147.
92. Casper ES, Clark D. Service utilization, incidents, and hospitalizations among people with mental illnesses and incarceration histories in a supportive housing program. Psychiatr Rehabil J. 2004;28:181–4.

93. D'Avanzo B, Battino RN, Gallus S, Barbato A. Factors predicting discharge of patients from community residential facilities: a longitudinal study from Italy. Aust New Zeal J Psychiatry. 2004;38:619–28.
94. Grant JG, Westhues A. Choice and outcome in mental health supported housing. Psychiatr Rehabil J. 2010;33:232–5.
95. Guazzelli M, Palagini L, Giuntoli L, Pietrini P. Rehab rounds: outcomes of patients with schizophrenia in a family-style, residential, community-based program in Italy. Psychiatr Serv. 2000;51:1113–5.
96. Muir K, Fisher KR, Dadich A, Abello D. Challenging the exclusion of people with mental illness: the mental health housing and accommodation support initiative (HASI). Aust J Soc Issues. 2008;43:271–90.
97. Tsemberis S. Housing first: ending homelessness, promoting recovery and reducing cost. In: How to house the homeless; 2010. p. 37–56.
98. Woodhall-Melnik JR, Dunn JR. A systematic review of outcomes associated with participation in housing first programs. Hous Stud. 2016;31:287–304. https://doi.org/10.1080/02673037.2015.1080816.
99. Lamb HR, Bachrach LL. Some perspectives on deinstitutionalization. Psychiatr Serv. 2001;52:1039–45. https://doi.org/10.1176/appi.ps.52.8.1039.
100. Leff J, Trieman N, Gooch C. Team for the assessment of psychiatric services (TAPS) project 33: prospective follow-up study of long-stay patients discharged from two psychiatric hospitals. Am J Psychiatry. 1996;153:1318–24. https://doi.org/10.1176/ajp.153.10.1318.
101. Schulz R, Czaja SJ, McKay JR, Ory MG, Belle SH. Intervention taxonomy (ITAX): describing essential features of interventions. Am J Health Behav. 2010;34:811–21.
102. Leff HS, Chow CM, Pepin R, Conley J, Allen IE, Seaman CA. Does one size fit all? What we can and can't learn from a meta-analysis of housing models for persons with mental illness. Psychiatr Serv. 2009;60:473–82.
103. Siskind D, Harris M, Pirkis J, Whiteford H. A domains-based taxonomy of supported accommodation for people with severe and persistent mental illness. Soc Psychiatry Psychiatr Epidemiol. 2013;48:875–94. https://doi.org/10.1007/s00127-012-0590-x.
104. McPherson P, Krotofil J, Killaspy H. What Works? Toward a New Classification System for Mental Health Supported Accommodation Services: The Simple Taxonomy for Supported Accommodation (STAX-SA). Int J Environ Res Public Health. 2018;15(2). https://doi.org/10.3390/ijerph15020190.

3

Associations between loneliness and perceived social support and outcomes of mental health problems

Jingyi Wang[1], Farhana Mann[1], Brynmor Lloyd-Evans[1], Ruimin Ma[1] and Sonia Johnson[1,2*]

Abstract

Background: The adverse effects of loneliness and of poor perceived social support on physical health and mortality are established, but no systematic synthesis is available of their relationship with the outcomes of mental health problems over time. In this systematic review, we aim to examine the evidence on whether loneliness and closely related concepts predict poor outcomes among adults with mental health problems.

Methods: We searched six databases and reference lists for longitudinal quantitative studies that examined the relationship between baseline measures of loneliness and poor perceived social support and outcomes at follow up. Thirty-four eligible papers were retrieved. Due to heterogeneity among included studies in clinical populations, predictor measures and outcomes, a narrative synthesis was conducted.

Results: We found substantial evidence from prospective studies that people with depression who perceive their social support as poorer have worse outcomes in terms of symptoms, recovery and social functioning. Loneliness has been investigated much less than perceived social support, but there is some evidence that greater loneliness predicts poorer depression outcome. There is also some preliminary evidence of associations between perceived social support and outcomes in schizophrenia, bipolar disorder and anxiety disorders.

Conclusions: Loneliness and quality of social support in depression are potential targets for development and testing of interventions, while for other conditions further evidence is needed regarding relationships with outcomes.

Keywords: Loneliness, Perceived social support, Outcomes, Mental health problems, Systematic review

Background

There is increasing interest in the effects of social relations on health, and in the service delivery and policy implications of such effects [1]. Loneliness has been a particularly prominent focus in recent research on physical health [2–4]. For instance, two meta-analytic reviews have reported that loneliness and poor social support are associated with higher mortality rates, and that the effect is comparable with some well-established risk factors such as obesity, physical inactivity, and smoking [5, 6]. They are also predictive of development of coronary heart disease and stroke [7], increases in systolic blood pressure [8, 9], and chronic pain [10, 11] in longitudinal studies. The effect of loneliness on physical health may be via biological, psychological and/or behavioural mechanisms, including physiological functioning, neuroendocrine effects, gene effects, immune functioning, perception of stressful events, health behaviours and sleep quality [2, 12, 13]. In contrast, while loneliness and lack of social support are well-documented problems among mental health service users [14], they have not been prominent in research, mental health service delivery and policy. Until recently, there has tended to be less focus on the social determinants of mental health than on genetics and neurobiology, but recent integrated aetiological models,

* Correspondence: s.johnson@ucl.ac.uk
[1]Division of Psychiatry – University College London, 6th Floor, Maple House, 149 Tottenham Court Road, London W1T 7NF, England
[2]Camden and Islington NHS Foundation Trust, St Pancras Hospital, 4 St Pancras Way, London NW1 0PE, England

such as the integrated sociodevelopmental-cognitive model, bring social factors into the neuroscientific mainstream, with increasing evidence that such factors need to be included to achieve models of good explanatory value [15–17]. An increasing focus on loneliness has also been driven by recognition of its high prevalence, and of its wide ranging impacts on physical health and mental well-being [17]. Despite this increasing recognition of its importance, to date no systematic synthesis of the evidence on the relationship between loneliness and the outcomes of mental health problems has been published.

Loneliness has been defined as a negative emotional state that occurs when there is "a discrepancy between... the desired and achieved patterns of social interaction" [18]. Loneliness is sometimes seen as an essentially unidimensional concept, sometimes as comprising two dimensions. Weiss [19] proposed a multidimensional concept of loneliness, categorising loneliness into social and emotional dimensions. Social loneliness derived from "the absence of socially integrative relationships", while emotional loneliness stemmed from the absence of "a close emotional attachment" [19]. Social loneliness occurs when a person does not have a wider social network as desired, which can lead to the feelings of boredom, exclusion and marginality [19, 20]. In contrast, emotional loneliness occurs when someone is missing an intimate relationship, which can result in distress and apprehension [19, 20]. Psychometrically robust self-report measures of loneliness have been developed and used extensively in research on physical health and on older people, including the University of California at Los Angeles (UCLA) Loneliness Scale [21] and the de Jong-Gierveld Loneliness Scale [22]. Feelings of loneliness are more prevalent among people with mental illness than in the general population [23, 24]. In a study of older adults with major depression, dysthymia, or minor depression, 83% of the respondents reported loneliness and 38% reported severe loneliness [25]. By comparison, only 32% of non-depressed elderly people were lonely and 4% severely lonely using the same loneliness scale [26]. In a comparison of people with psychosis and a general population sample with similar demographic characteristics, the prevalence of loneliness among people with psychosis was 79.9% compared with 35% in the general population [27]. For people with depression, cross-sectional studies have found up to 40% of respondents feeling lonely most of the time [28], with a tenfold increase in the odds of being lonely compared to the general population [29].

Given the high prevalence of loneliness among people with mental health problems and the evidence for its harmful effects in other populations, good quality evidence is needed on its impact on recovery from mental health problems and on the health and social functioning of mental health service users. This has potential to inform the development of preventive and therapeutic interventions for which there is not as yet an evidence base. An important question in evaluating the available evidence is how far loneliness is conceptually and empirically distinct from other concepts and measures related to social relationships. Loneliness has been shown to be only moderately correlated with more objectively measured concepts such as social isolation, social network size and objective social support received from others [30, 31]. However, subjectively rated concepts related to social relationships are less easy to distinguish clearly from loneliness [32]. For example, perceived social support refers to people's beliefs about how much support is potentially available from their relationships and social contacts and about the quality of this support [33, 34]. This is distinct from received social support, a rating of how often someone reports receiving particular supportive behaviours [33, 34]. Measures of perceived social support assess the quality or adequacy of social support from a subjective perspective. For instance, the two widely used measures, the Multi-dimensional Scale of Perceived Social Support (MSPSS) [35] and the Subjective Support Subscale of Duke Social Support Index (DSSI) [36], consist of items such as "How often do you feel lonely?", "Can you talk about your deepest problems?", "I have friends with whom I can share joys and sorrows", which have a high degree of overlap with loneliness measures. Likewise, measures of confiding relationships assess the extent to which people feel close to and able to talk intimately with other people [37, 38]. Studies have found large negative correlations between loneliness and perceived social support [39–42]. Thus these concepts resemble loneliness as subjective evaluations of the quality and impact of social relationships: given this conceptual overlap, this paper includes them along with loneliness.

Three previous systematic reviews have explored the relationship between social relations and depression in general population [43, 44], or older adults [45], but included both cross-sectional and prospective studies. One further review looked at the relationship between social networks and support and early psychosis in people with first episode psychosis and in general population samples, but included no prospective studies [46]. To our knowledge, there is no systematic review which summarises and synthesises the evidence regarding the relationship between loneliness and perceived social support and the course of existing mental health problems, and which includes only prospective studies, from which inferences about the direction of causation may be drawn. Our review will fill this gap, and will provide useful evidence about how far and in what context loneliness and perceived social support may influence mental health recovery. Thus the aim of the current paper is to synthesise the available evidence as to whether higher levels of loneliness and poorer perceived social support have an adverse effect on outcomes in adults of all ages with existing mental health problems.

Methods

A systematic review was conducted of the scientific literature addressing the question of whether loneliness and low perceived social support are associated longitudinally with poorer outcomes among adults of all ages with a range of mental health problems. The review's protocol was registered on PROSPERO, which is an international database of prospective systematic reviews with health related outcomes (registration number: CRD42015014784) [47].

Inclusion criteria

Types of study: The review included longitudinal studies in which the relationship between baseline measures of loneliness and poor perceived social support and outcomes at follow up was examined using quantitative measures.

Participants: Participants in the included studies were adults with mental illnesses, specifically schizophrenia and schizoaffective disorder, psychosis in general, depression, bipolar disorder, and anxiety disorders. Clinical populations were included however diagnosis was made, for example clinical diagnoses, ratings according to the criteria of the Diagnostic and Statistical Manual of Mental Disorders (DSM) or the International Classification of Diseases (ICD), or use of reliable and valid instruments such as the Mini-International Neuropsychiatric Interview (M.I.N.I.). We excluded studies with samples of children under 16 years old, people with intellectual disabilities or organic mental disorders including dementia, or cohorts assembled on the basis of a primary physical illness diagnosis.

Exposure variables: Included studies used quantitative measures of loneliness or of related concepts that involve a subjective rather than objective appraisal of social relationships, such as perceived social support or confiding relationships. Concepts based on objective ratings of the size and functioning of social networks, such as social isolation and social network size, were excluded. Social capital was also excluded as it relates to characteristics of society or communities as a whole as well as individuals' appraisal of their relationships, and is conceptually distinct from loneliness [32]. We included studies only if exposure variables assessed subjective appraisal of overall social connectedness, rather than the quality of specific relationships: therefore, measures of support from partner and quality of a specific significant relationship were excluded.

Outcomes: The review included a wide variety of outcomes, ranging from clinical outcomes to functioning outcomes. Studies in which any of the following outcomes were measured at follow-up were eligible for inclusion:

1) Relapse: recurrent episodes following recovery at baseline of mental illness meeting the criteria of DSM or ICD, or of other reliable and valid instruments such as the Center for Epidemiologic Studies Depression Scale (CES-D), and proxy measures of acute relapse such as admission to psychiatric hospital/crisis services/acute mental health services.
2) Measures of functioning or of recovery: recovery of function, social functioning, self-rated recovery, quality of life, and disability.
3) Symptom severity: level of symptoms, symptom improvement or deterioration.
4) Global outcome: overall outcome rating combining different aspects of mental health and functioning, such as the Health of the Nation Outcome Scales (HoNOS).

Search strategy

A systematic search of the following six electronic databases was undertaken: Medline, PsycINFO, Embase, Web of Science, CINAHL and Cochrane Library (1891 to April 2016). No language and publication period restrictions were applied. Search terms for loneliness and related concepts were combined with terms for mental disorders and outcomes. Searches were conducted using both subject headings (MeSH terms) and text words within title and abstract. Search terms were adapted as required for different databases (for full details, see Additional file 1). The search terms used in Medline are as follows:

1) Loneliness: loneliness [MeSH] OR loneliness OR lonely OR social support adj5 (subjective or personal or perceived or quality) OR confiding relationship*
2) Mental disorders: mental disorders [MeSH]. exp. OR mental OR psychiatr* OR schizo* OR psychosis OR psychotic OR depress* OR mania* OR manic OR bipolar adj5 (disorder or disease or illness) OR anxiety disorders [MeSH]. exp.
3) Outcomes: prognosis [MeSH] OR outcome* OR recurren* OR relapse OR admission OR hospitali?ation OR crisis OR admitted OR detained OR detention OR recovery of function [MeSH] OR "social functioning" OR "self-rated recovery" OR "quality of life" OR "symptom severity" OR disability

Apart from outcome terms, we searched "onset" and related terms as searches were conducted simultaneously for this and a companion systematic review on loneliness as a risk factor for the onset of psychiatric disorders in the general population. Reference lists of studies identified through the electronic search for inclusion in the review and of review articles were manually searched for further relevant studies. Relevant studies reported in dissertations, conference reports or other sources other than published journals were searched using the free text and keyword searches from the following two sources: Zetoc (indexing and abstracting database of conference proceedings) and OpenGrey (system for information on grey literature in Europe). When necessary and possible, we sent emails to authors to request full text or clarify some uncertainties.

Selection of studies for inclusion in the review was made independently by two reviewers (J.W. & F.M.). Titles of all identified studies were screened. The abstracts of potentially relevant studies were read; the full text of studies still considered potentially relevant was then retrieved and read. All studies included by one assessor were confirmed by the other reviewer to check adherence to inclusion criteria in study selection. 800 studies excluded by one assessor were checked by the other reviewer to establish reliability of our study selection. The agreement between reviewers was higher than 99%. Queries about inclusion/exclusion were resolved through discussion with a third reviewer (S.J.).

Data extraction, quality assessment and synthesis

A structured template was developed to extract relevant data from eligible papers. Two review authors (J.W. & F.M.) independently extracted data and assessed their methodological quality. Extracted data and quality assessment scores were checked by a second reviewer for 20% of papers. Disagreements between the two assessors were resolved through discussion with a third review author (S.J.). The methodological quality of each study included in the review was assessed using a standard form adapted from the Mixed Methods Appraisal Tool (MMAT) – Version 2011 [48]. The MMAT has been designed for appraisal of the methodological quality for qualitative, quantitative and mixed methods studies. For quantitative studies it includes criteria relevant to randomised controlled, non-randomised, and descriptive studies. For the purposes of our review, we used the criteria for the quantitative non-randomised domain (Cohort study version). As there are four criteria for this domain following two screening questions, the overall quality score was presented using descriptors *, **, ***, and ****, ranging from * (one criterion met) to **** (all criteria met). The four criteria related to selection bias, measurement quality, adjustment for confounders, and percentage of complete outcome data/response rate/follow-up rate (see Additional file 2). We conducted a narrative synthesis of results as the anticipated heterogeneity of included studies, for example in samples, predictor measures and outcomes, made a meta-analysis inappropriate. The main results have been stratified by type of mental health problem investigated and tables and text were used to summarise the data.

Results

Literature search

Our initial database search retrieved 13,076 records (see Fig. 1). After excluding duplicates and screening titles and abstracts to exclude obviously irrelevant papers, 797 full-text articles were assessed for eligibility. 734 studies were excluded because: i) they were not longitudinal quantitative studies; ii) they assessed a form of social relationships conceptually distinct from loneliness or perceived social support; iii) they analysed the relationship between change scores in loneliness and outcome variables, rather than baseline loneliness as a predictor of outcome; or iv) they investigated a sample consisting of children under 16 years old or of people with primary diagnoses of drug and alcohol disorders, personality disorders, post-traumatic stress disorder (PTSD), learning disabilities or organic mental disorders, or of people recruited as having specific physical illnesses. Twenty-two further papers were retrieved by hand-searching the reference lists of the papers already identified. Of the resulting 85 studies, 34 articles about outcomes of mental disorders among people with existing mental health problems were included in this review. The other 51 papers will be reported in a companion systematic review regarding the relationship between loneliness and onset of mental health problems in the general population. The search results are reported as a Prisma diagram in the Fig. 1.

Eligible papers

The 34 eligible papers were from seven countries, including 23 from North America, 10 from Europe and one from Israel. These papers consisted of 23 studies with samples of people with depression, two focusing on schizophrenia or schizoaffective disorders, four on bipolar disorder, and three on anxiety disorders. Two further studies included people with a mixture of mental health problems (Table 1). Only two studies directly assessed loneliness, and most of the studies used various scales to measure perceived social support. Nearly half of included papers studied symptom severity as an outcome, a third of the papers assessed recovery/remission, and a third of the papers included other outcomes such as quality of life, disability pension qualification, functional impairment or life satisfaction. The sample sizes of six studies in our review exceeded 400, 22 were between 100 and 400, and six were less than 100. Six studies had

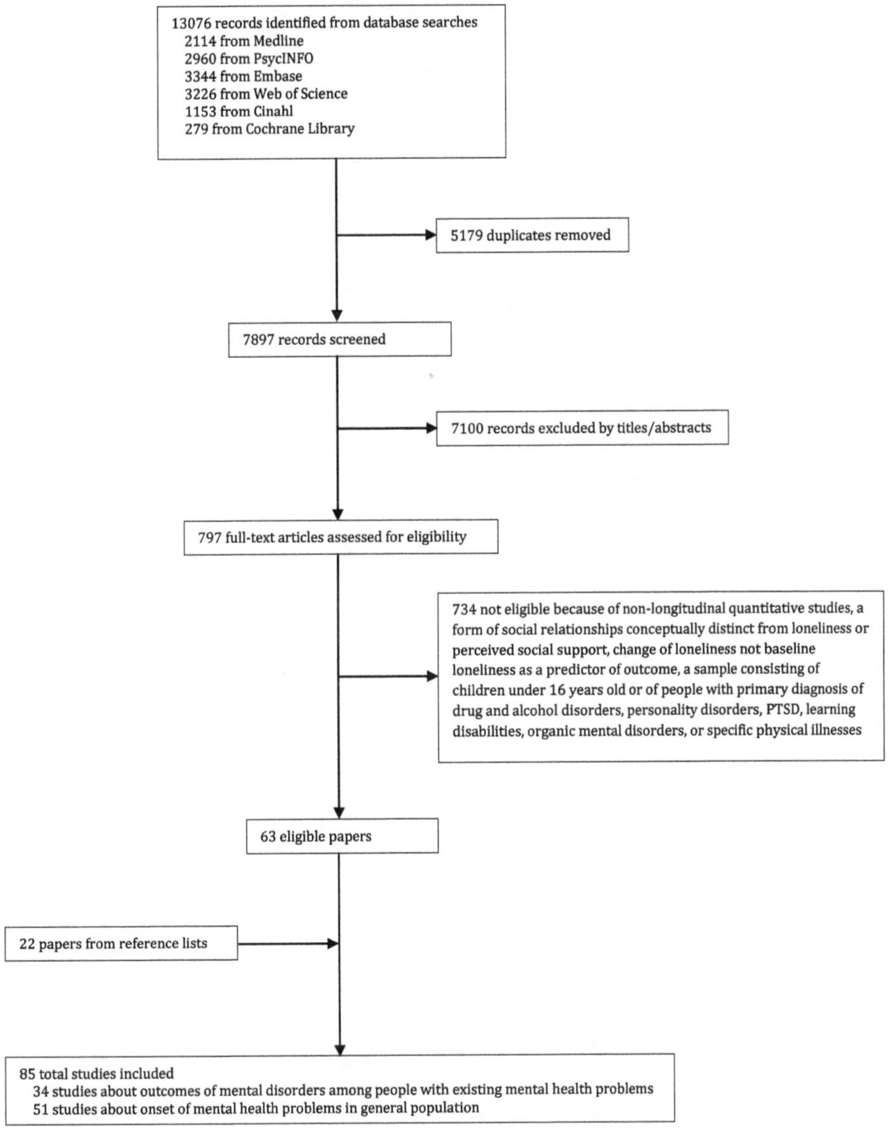

Fig. 1 Studies selection flowchart

short length of follow-up (less than one year), 23 following up the cohorts for one to two years, and five for over two years. With regard to quality assessment, five studies were assigned a maximum score of four (****) as their overall quality scores, 16 studies had a score of three (***) and 13 papers had two (**) according to the appraisal criteria of MMAT. Most studies had lower quality assessment ratings because they did not report the percentage of complete outcome data, response rate or follow-up rate (for full details, see Additional file 2).

Depression

Among the 23 papers with samples of people with depression, 13 studies assessed depression severity as an outcome. Eleven of these found that poorer perceived social support or greater loneliness at baseline was a significant predictor of higher depressive symptom severity at follow-ups (Table 2). Nine of these eleven papers conducted multivariable analyses including adjusting for baseline depression severity. In eight of these nine papers, the relationship between baseline loneliness and depressive symptom outcome remained significant. For example, among the three studies with high quality scores (****), Blazer and colleagues [49] and Brugha and colleagues [50] followed cohorts of adults with depression in America and the UK respectively. They reported that poorer subjective social support at baseline was predictive of poorer outcomes at follow-up, outcomes including poorer life satisfaction (beta = 0.10, B = 0.37), worse depressive symptoms (beta = 0.10, B = 0.30) [49], and more severe psychiatric status (regression coefficient = – 1.46) [50]. In the third study rated as high

Table 1 Summary of characteristics of included studies

Condition studied	Predictor variable	Outcomes	Sample size range (median)	Length of follow-up[a]	Follow-up rate range (median)	Quality score
Depression ($n = 23$)	Perceived social support ($n = 22$) Loneliness ($n = 1$)	Symptom severity ($n = 13$) Recovery/remission ($n = 7$) Functional outcomes ($n = 5$)	66–604 (239)	Short ($n = 4$) Medium ($n = 14$) Long ($n = 5$)	60.6–100% (81.9%)	**** ($n = 4$) *** ($n = 11$) ** ($n = 8$)
Schizophrenia/schizoaffective disorders ($n = 2$)	Perceived social support ($n = 2$)	Functional outcomes ($n = 2$)	139–148 (143.5)	Medium ($n = 2$)	71.9–100% (86.0%)	*** ($n = 1$) ** ($n = 1$)
Bipolar disorder ($n = 4$)	Perceived social support ($n = 4$)	Symptom severity ($n = 3$) Recovery/remission ($n = 2$) Functional outcomes ($n = 2$)	42–173 (55.5)	Short ($n = 1$) Medium (n = 3)	71.1–100% (86.4%)	*** ($n = 2$) ** ($n = 2$)
Anxiety disorders ($n = 3$)	Perceived social support ($n = 3$)	Symptom severity ($n = 1$) Recovery/remission ($n = 1$) Functional outcomes ($n = 1$)	134–1004 (1004)	Short ($n = 1$) Medium ($n = 2$)	80–87% (81.0%)	**** ($n = 1$) *** ($n = 1$) ** ($n = 1$)
Mixed samples with various mental health problems (n = 2)	Perceived social support ($n = 1$) Loneliness ($n = 1$)	Symptom severity ($n = 1$) Functional outcomes ($n = 1$)	352–743 (547.5)	Medium ($n = 2$)	79.9–84.4% (82.2%)	*** ($n = 1$) ** ($n = 1$)

[a]Length of follow-up: Short = < 1 year; Medium = 1–2 years; Long = > 2 years. ** = two criteria of MMAT met. *** = three criteria of MMAT met. **** = all criteria of MMAT met

Table 2 Summary of findings on depression

Reference	Predictor variable	Outcome variable	Results (++ < 0·05 adjusted; + < 0·05 unadjusted; – non-significant)	
Hybels et al. (2016) [79]	Perceived social support	Trajectory class (quick recovery, slow recovery, persistent moderate, and persistent high)	++	Patients in the persistent moderate depression class had lower levels of baseline subjective social support compared with patients in the quick recovery class (OR (95%CI) = 0.91 (0.83, 0.98)). Patients in the persistent high depression class had lower levels of baseline subjective social support compared with those in the quick recovery class (OR (95%CI) = 0.83 (0.75, 0.92))
Holvast et al. (2015) [25]	Loneliness	Symptom severity; Remission	++ ++	In the fully adjusted model, a 1-point higher baseline loneliness score predicted a 0·61-point higher depressive symptom severity score at follow-up (Beta = 0.61, 95% CI 0.12–1.11, $p = 0.02$). Logistic regression analysis showed that while adjusting for social network size and potential confounders, the very severely lonely respondents were less likely to achieve remission from their depressive disorder compared with the non-lonely respondents (OR = 0.25, 95% CI 0.08–0.80, $p = 0.02$).
Holma et al. (2012) [54]	Perceived social support	Disability pensions	+	Lower perceived social support at baseline predicted greater likelihood of being granted a disability pension over 5 year follow-up on univariate analysis ($p = 0.031$), but not significant in multivariate analyses where the outcome was the interval time to the date the pension was granted
Backs-Dermott et al. (2010) [80]	Perceived social support	Relapse versus stable remitted	++	Lower perceived social support from a significant other (standardized discriminant function coefficient 0.48) and lower perceived social support from friends (standardized coefficient 0.35) at baseline predicted greater likelihood of depressive relapse at one-year follow-up. The Discriminant Function Analysis was significant, Wilk's Lambda = 0.69, x^2 (5) = 16.35, $p = 0.006$
Bosworth et al. (2008) [81]	Perceived social support	Depression severity	++	Poorer subjective social support was a significant predictor of more severe depression at 12 months. Standardized beta = – 0.13, $p = 0.05$
Rytsala et al. (2007) [55]	Perceived social support	Work disability allowances	+	Lower perceived social support at 6 month was a significant predictor of greater likelihood of being granted disability allowances at 18 months (F = 6.3, $p = 0.013$), but not significant in multivariate analysis
Rytsala et al. (2006) [56]	Perceived social support	Functional disability; Social and work adjustment; Days spent ill in bed or not	++ ++ –	Lower perceived social support at baseline was a significant predictor of more severe functional disability at 6 months (B = 0.232, $\beta = 0.210$, $p = 0.002$, 95% CI 0.084 to 0.379), and poorer social and work adjustment at 6 months (B = – 0.008, $\beta = -0.222$, $p = 0.001$, 95% CI -0.013 to – 0.003). Lower perceived social support at 6 months was one of the most significant factors predicting more severe functional disability at 18 months (B = 0.240, $\beta = 0.215$, $p = 0.002$, 95% CI 0.088 to 0.393), and poorer social and work adjustment at 18 months (B = – 0.011, $\beta = -0.303$, $p<0.001$, 95% CI -0.015 to – 0.006). But perceived social support did not predict any days spent ill in bed or not
Leskela et al. (2006) [51]	Perceived social support	Severity of depression	+	Lower perceived social support at 6 months predicted more severe depression at 18 months in original zero-order correlation ($r = -0.392$, $p < 0.001$) and within-group standardised correlation ($r = -0.230$, $p = 0.001$) among all patients, but not significant in multivariate analysis. In full remission group at 6 months ($n = 67$), lower perceived social support at 6 months predicted higher level of depressive symptoms at 18 months in multivariate analysis ($r = -0.321$, $p = 0.012$)
Steffens et al. (2005) [82]	Perceived social support	Severity of depression	++	Lower subjective social support at baseline predicted more severe depression over time (estimate – 0.5641, $p = 0.0002$)
Ezquiaga et al. (2004) [83]	Perceived social support	Episode remission	–	Higher perceived social support at baseline did not predict remission at 12 months in univariate analysis ($p = 0.33$), and it was not included in multivariate analysis

Table 2 Summary of findings on depression *(Continued)*

Reference	Predictor variable	Outcome variable	Results (++ < 0·05 adjusted; + < 0·05 unadjusted; – non-significant)
Reference	Predictor variable	Outcome variable	Results (++ < 0·05 adjusted; + < 0·05 unadjusted; – non-significant)
Gasto et al. (2003) [84]	Perceived social support	Severity of residual symptoms	++ Lower subjective social support at baseline predicted higher intensity of residual symptoms at 9 months in remitters (standardized $\beta = 0.41$, $p < 0.001$)
Bosworth et al. (2002) [53]	Perceived social support	Time-to-remission	++ Lower subjective social support at baseline (Hazard Ratio = 0.47, 95% CI: 0.31–0.71, $p = 0.003$) was a significant predictor of longer time to remission
Bosworth et al. (2002) [52]	Perceived social support	Remission	++ Lower baseline levels of subjective social support (OR = 1.21, 95% CI: 1.09–1.35, $p < 0.001$) predicted poorer recovery one year later
Triesch (2002) [85]	Perceived social support	Severity of depressive symptoms; Quality of life	– – Lower perceived social support at baseline did not predict more severe depression ($\beta = -0.17$) or poorer quality of life ($\beta = -0.12$) at 3 months
Hays et al. (2001) [57]	Perceived social support	Activities of daily living	++ There was modest support for hypothesis that baseline subjective social support predicted functional declines at 1 year. There was partial support for hypothesis that the buffering effects of social support against functional decline would be strongest among the most severely depressed patients
Oxman and Hull (2001) [86]	Perceived social support	Depression severity	++ Greater perceived social support predicted subsequent decreases in depression among participants randomly assigned to placebo group (6-week depression – 0.18, $p < 0.05$; 11-week depression – 0.22, $p < 0.05$), but not significant among paroxetine group or Problem-Solving Treatment for Primary Care group
Brummett et al. (2000) [87]	Perceived social support	Depressive symptoms	– Higher levels of received support at baseline significantly predicted decreases in depressive symptoms at both 6 months and 1 year, whereas subjective support did not significantly predict changes in depressive symptoms at either point in time
Sherbourne et al. (1995) [88]	Perceived social support	Number of depressive symptoms	++ Decreased number of depressive symptoms between baseline and 2-year follow-up was predicted by social support at baseline (standardised regression coefficients = 0.12, zero-order Pearson product-moment correlations = 0.16, $p < 0.05$). Among the subset of patients who had current depressive disorder at baseline, perceived social support was not significantly related to remission. Among patients without current depressive disorder at baseline (subthreshold depression), patients with higher level of perceived social support were less likely to experience a new depressive episode during 2-year period: odds ratio = 0.96 (CI:0.95, 0.98)
Blazer et al. (1992) [49]	Perceived social support	Decreased life satisfaction symptoms; Endogenous symptoms	++ Impaired subjective support at baseline was predictive of poorer outcome at 12-month follow-up in both models: decreased life satisfaction symptoms (b = 0.10, B = 0.37, $p \leq 0.001$), endogenous symptoms (b = 0.10, B = 0.30, $p \leq 0.01$)
Blazer et al. (1991) [89]	Perceived social support	Depressive symptoms	+ Intercorrelation between social support at baseline and depression score at 6 months: – 0.41, $p < 0.001$. Intercorrelation between social support at baseline and depression score at 12 months: – 0.34, $p < 0.001$
Brugha et al. (1990) [50]	Perceived social support	Symptom severity	++ After controlling for the two significant clinical predictors, a significant main effect was found in total sample for lower satisfaction with support at baseline on more severe psychiatric status at 4 months (regression coefficient = – 1.46, $p < 0.05$)

Table 2 Summary of findings on depression *(Continued)*

Reference	Predictor variable	Outcome variable	Results (++ < 0·05 adjusted; + < 0·05 unadjusted; – non-significant)	
George et al. (1989) [90]	Perceived social support	Depressive symptoms	++	Impaired subjective social support at baseline is a significant predictor of higher numbers of CES-D symptoms at follow-up (b = 8.88, B = 0.20, $p \leq 0.05$)
Krantz and Moos (1988) [91]	Perceived social support	Remitted, partially remitted, and nonremitted	+	Lower quality of relationships at baseline predicted poorer remission status after 1 year ($\chi^2 = 10.21$, $p < 0.01$)

quality, Leskela and colleagues [51] assessed adults with major depressive disorder and found that lower perceived social support six months after initial assessment predicted more severe depression at 18 months among all participants, although this relationship only remained significant in multivariable analysis for the group who had remitted following initial assessment ($r = -0.321$). The only study using loneliness as a predictor of depression outcomes was conducted by Holvast and colleagues [25] among Dutch older adults. They found that a 1-point higher loneliness score was predictive of a 0.61-point higher depressive symptom severity score at follow-up (Beta = 0.61, 95% CI 0.12–1.11). For studies which reported beta as the effect size, beta ranged from 0.10 to 0.61. Among the 13 studies, three articles had high quality (****), four had medium quality (***), and the other six received low quality ratings (**). However, no obvious relationship was found between study quality and whether results were significant.

Six out of seven articles which used recovery/remission of depression as their outcomes reported lower perceived social support or higher loneliness at baseline as a significant predictor of lower rates of recovery/remission at follow-up. Three of the seven studies adjusted for baseline depression severity, and all of them reported significant results. For example, in the study of Holvast et al. [25], the lonely respondents at baseline were reported to be less likely to achieve remission from their depressive disorder at follow-up compared with the non-lonely respondents (OR = 0.25, 95% CI 0.08–0.80). Similarly, poorer perceived social support at baseline was a significant predictor of poorer recovery one year later (OR = 1.21, 95% CI 1.09–1.35) [52], and of longer time-to-remission in a study of initially depressed elderly individuals (Hazard Ratio = 0.47, 95% CI 0.31–0.71) [53]. However, none of the seven studies had high quality scores (****), with five receiving medium (***), and two low scores (**).

With regard to functional outcomes (five articles), three studies have found that lower perceived social support at baseline was a significant predictor of greater likelihood of being granted disability pensions during the follow-up period (no effect size reported) [54, 55] and of more severe functional disability (beta 0.210 to 0.215, 95% CI 0.084–0.393) [56]. There is also evidence that greater perceived social support predicted better social and work adjustment (beta – 0.222 to – 0.303, 95% CI -0.013 to – 0.006) [56], and buffered functional declines in performance on activities of daily living (no effect size reported) [57]. However, after adjustment for potential confounders only two [56, 57] of the five studies had significant results.

Schizophrenia/schizoaffective disorders

Two studies assessed patients with schizophrenia or schizoaffective disorders to identify psychosocial predictors of health-related quality of life and functional outcomes (Table 3). Ritsner and colleagues [58] followed a sample of inpatients with schizophrenia or schizoaffective disorders for 16 months and found that greater support from friends at baseline predicted better satisfaction with life quality after 16 months (accounted for 2.9% of quality of life index scores at follow up examination). In an American study, greater perceived social support was

Table 3 Summary of findings on schizophrenia and schizoaffective disorders

Reference	Predictor variable	Outcome variable	Results (++ < 0·05 adjusted; + < 0·05 unadjusted; – non-significant)	
Ritsner et al. (2006) [58]	Perceived social support	Quality of life	++	Higher friend support at baseline predicted better satisfaction with life quality after 16 months (accounted for 2.9% of quality of life index scores at follow up examination)
Brekke et al. (2005) [59]	Perceived social support	Global functional outcome (work, social functioning, and independent living); Social functioning domain	– ++	Higher social support did not significantly predict better global functional outcome at 12 months ($p < 0.10$). But social support became a much stronger and statistically significant predictor of social functioning domain

a strong predictor of better scores on a social functioning domain (no effect size reported), although it did not predict the global functioning score (a composite of vocational and social functioning, and independent living) [59].However, neither of these studies adjusted for the outcome variable baseline scores.

Bipolar disorder

We found four papers that studied adults with a diagnosis of bipolar disorder (Table 4). The evidence regarding depressive symptoms was consistent and showed that lower perceived social support predicted greater depression over time (beta − 0.14 to − 0.25, regression coefficient − 1.33) [60–62]. Lower perceived support was also found to be a significant predictor of greater impairment in functioning (beta − 0.14 to − 0.67) [60, 61], and longer time to recovery (no effect size reported) [62]. Among remitted patients with prior diagnosis of bipolar I disorder, greater perceived social support reduced risk of recurrence of any type (depressive or manic) at one year (OR = 0.92, 95% CI 0.85–0.99) [63]. With regard to severity of manic symptoms, however, the results were not so consistent. In one study lower perceived support significantly predicted more severe manic symptoms on follow-up assessment (beta = − 0.32) [61], but in other two studies it was not linked with subsequent manic symptomatology [60, 62]. Apart from the study of recurrence, the other three had adjustment for baseline score on the outcome measure.

Anxiety disorders

The three studies of patients with anxiety disorders all reported significant associations between perceived social support at baseline and outcomes at follow-up (Table 5). Two studies included people with diagnoses of generalised anxiety disorder, panic disorder, social anxiety disorder or post-traumatic stress disorder. One study found that lower perceived social support was predictive of more severe anxiety (beta = − 0.15, CI [− 0.30, − 0.06], Ratios 8.85%) and depressive symptoms (beta = − 0.16, CI [− 0.28, − 0.08], Ratios 10.51%) at subsequent time points [33], and the other one found that greater perceived social support predicted a higher rate of remission at 6-month follow-up (OR = 1.38, 95% CI Wald 1.09–1.75) [64]. In a study of older adults with generalised anxiety disorder, Shrestha et al. [65] found that individuals with greater perceived social support at baseline reported greater average quality of life over time (beta = 0.41), albeit without adjustment for the outcome variable baseline score.

Mixed samples with various mental health problems

Two studies examined mixed samples of people with a variety of diagnoses (Table 6). Beljouw et al. [66] analysed data from primary care patients with current anxiety

Table 4 Summary of findings on bipolar disorder

Reference	Predictor variable	Outcome variable	Results (++ < 0·05 adjusted; + < 0·05 unadjusted; – non-significant)	
Koenders et al. (2015) [60]	Perceived social support	Depressive symptomatology; Depression related functional impairment; Manic symptomatology; Manic related functional impairment	++ ++ – –	Lower perceived support predicted more depression related functional impairment during the subsequent 3 months (*β* (SE) = − 0.14 (0.03), $p < 0.001$), and with more depressive symptomatology at the subsequent time point (*β* (SE) = − 0.14 (0.04), $p = 0.002$). No significant associations between perceived social support and manic symptoms and impairment were observed
Cohen et al. (2004) [63]	Perceived social support	Recurrence	++	After controlling for clinical variables, lower social support of any kind significantly predicted recurrence of any type at one year (β (SE) = − 0.09 (0.04), $p = 0.03$, OR = 0.92, 95% CI 0.85–0.99)
Daniels (2000) [61]	Perceived social support	Depressive symptomatology; Manic symptomatology; Functional impairment	++ ++ ++	Lower perceived support was a significant predictor of more severe depressive symptomatology after controlling for initial levels of depression ($R^2 = 0.67$, F = 34.15, $\Delta R^2 = 0.05$, ΔF = 5.24, beta = − 0.25). Lower perceived support significantly predicted more severe manic symptomatology over three months ($R^2 = 0.18$, F = 3.74, $\Delta R^2 = 0.10$, ΔF = 4.18, beta = − 0.32). Lower perceived social support significantly predicted impairment in functioning in the participants who completed their life charts for 90 consecutive days, after controlling for initial levels of functional impairment ($R^2 = 0.44$, F = 5.48, $\Delta R^2 = 0.41$, ΔF = 10.22, beta = − 0.67).
Johnson et al. (1999) [62]	Perceived social support	Time to recovery; Severity of depressive symptoms; Severity of manic symptoms	++ ++ –	Lower social support was a significant predictor of longer time to recovery in Cox regression survival analyses ($\chi 2$ (1, *N* = 52) change = 5.89, one-tailed $p < 0.01$). In hierarchical multiple regression analyses, low social support predicted higher depression over time (regression coefficient = − 1.33, $p < 0.01$, R^2 change = 0.07, F change = 11.70). Social support did not have significant impact on mania score at 6-month follow-up

Table 5 Summary of findings on anxiety disorders

Reference	Predictor variable	Outcome variable	Results (++ < 0·05 adjusted; + < 0·05 unadjusted; – non-significant)
Jakubovski and Bloch (2016) [64]	Perceived social support	Remission; Response (a reduction of at least 40% symptoms at 6 months)	++ ++ Generalised anxiety disorder: Greater amount of social support predicted a higher rate of remission (OR = 1.38, 95% CI Wald 1.09–1.75, $p = 0.0067$) and a greater rate of response (OR = 1.33, 95% CI Wald 1.10–1.62, $p = 0.0040$) at 6-month follow-up. Social anxiety disorder: Greater amount of social support predicted a higher rate of remission (OR = 1.716, 95% CI Wald 1.028–2.867, $p = 0.0391$) at 6-month follow-up, but social support did not predict response. Social support did not predict remission or response for panic disorder or post-traumatic stress disorder
Shrestha et al. (2015) [65]	Perceived social support	Quality of life	++ Main effect of social support was significant such that those with higher baseline social support reported higher average quality of life over time (b (SE) = 0.41 (0.08), $p < 0.001$)
Dour et al. (2014) [33]	Perceived social support	Anxiety symptoms; Depressive symptoms	++ ++ Direct effects: Relations between perceived social support and depression were bidirectional at all follow-ups, whereas they were unidirectional between perceived social support and anxiety at 6- and 12-month follow-ups. Indirect effects: Intervention led to changes in 6- and/or 12-month perceived social support, that in turn led to subsequent changes in 18-month depression ($b = -0.16$, CI [−0.28, −0.08], Ratios 10.51%) and anxiety ($b = -0.15$, CI [−0.30, −0.06], Ratios 8.85%)

or depressive disorders, and found that greater loneliness at baseline was predictive of more severe depressive (beta = 0.89) or anxiety symptoms (beta = 0.40) at 1-year follow-up. However, after adjustment for baseline severity of depression or anxiety, only the relationship with depression severity remained significant (beta = 0.39). Fleury and colleagues [67] conducted a study among individuals with severe mental health problems including schizophrenia and other psychotic disorders and severe mood disorders. They reported that greater perceived social support was significantly predictive of higher subjective quality of life at 18 months (beta 0.136 to 0.196, 95% CI 0.255 to 3.410). However, adjustments for baseline measures included functional ability in the community and diagnosis, but not baseline quality of life.

Discussion

Main findings

We found 34 studies that reported quantitatively on the longitudinal relationship between perceived social support/loneliness at baseline and various outcomes of mental illness at follow-up. Although substantial heterogeneity exists in the identified articles, some generalisations can be made. There is substantial evidence that less perceived social support at baseline tends to predict greater symptom severity, poorer recovery/remission and worse functional outcomes at follow-up among people with depression, and preliminary evidence of a similar relationship for people with bipolar disorder, or anxiety disorders. There is also some evidence that greater loneliness is associated with more severe

Table 6 Summary of findings on mixed samples with various mental health problems

Reference	Predictor variable	Outcome variable	Results (++ < 0·05 adjusted; + < 0·05 unadjusted; – non-significant)
Fleury et al. (2013) [67]	Perceived social support	Subjective quality of life	++ Social support variables at baseline accounted for 7.9% of quality of life at 18-month follow-up. Among social support dimensions, higher perception of availability of social integration ($\beta = 0.196$, $t = 3.472$, $p = 0.001$, 95% CI [0.942, 3.410]) and reassurance of worth supports ($\beta = 0.136$, $t = 2.397$, $p = 0.017$, 95% CI [0.255, 2.597]) at baseline predicted better quality of life at 18-month follow-up
Van Beljouw et al. (2010) [66]	Loneliness	Severity of depression; Severity of anxiety	++ + A higher symptom severity in depression at 1-year follow-up was predicted by more loneliness at baseline in both multilevel univariate linear regression analyses ($\beta = 0.89$, SE = 0.17, $p < 0.001$) and multilevel multivariate linear regression analyses ($\beta = 0.39$, SE = 0.16, $p < 0.05$). Positive associations were found between more symptom severity in anxiety at 1-year follow-up and loneliness at baseline by multilevel univariate linear regression analyses ($\beta = 0.40$, SE = 0.12, $p < 0.01$) (but not significant in multivariate analyses)

depression and anxiety symptoms and poorer remission from depression. An important consideration in interpreting findings is that depression is very likely to make people more likely to appraise their social support as inadequate and to feel emotionally lonely. However, a persistent effect on outcomes is found in many studies with adjustment for baseline depression severity. With regard to schizophrenia/schizoaffective disorders, only functional outcomes have been studied and the small amount of available evidence suggests that greater perceived social support is predictive of better subjective quality of life and social functioning. This review, to our knowledge, is the first to systematically examine longitudinal studies regarding the relationship between loneliness and closely related concepts and outcomes for adults of all ages and all types of mental illness.

Strengths and limitations of the included studies and of this review

Generally, the quality of included studies is acceptable and most studies were assigned at least *** as their overall quality scores in accordance with the methodological quality criteria of MMAT. However, some methodological issues in the published literature may limit what can be inferred from the studies. Many studies did not have comprehensive information about percentage of complete outcome data, baseline response rate, or follow-up rate, resulting in lower quality assessment ratings. We did assess whether studies adjusted for baseline measurements on the outcomes. Some did not, increasing uncertainty about the direction of causation (although if the baseline outcome measure which included random errors was introduced as a covariate, regression to the mean might lead to biased results according to Lord's paradox [68]). A large majority of the 23 studies that did adjust for baseline outcome measures still found loneliness/perceived social support to be predictive of outcomes. This suggests that there is a real effect of loneliness/lack of social support on outcomes. However, it is likely that the relationship can be a circular one, with loneliness/lack of social support resulting in more severe symptoms, and more severe symptoms exacerbating loneliness/lack of social support.

The consistency of findings across a variety of settings, measures of the exposure, and population groups increases confidence in the generalisability of the review's findings. The retrieved articles encompassed varying populations including older and younger groups, and people recruited in primary care, inpatient and outpatient settings, and were carried out around the world. Most studies of perceived social support used well-developed scales where psychometric properties have been established. The measures used varied regarding the dimensions and types of social support assessed, although they all measure individuals' subjective appraisal of adequacy or impact of their relationships rather than objective or structural social support. Both loneliness studies used a published measure of loneliness with well-established psychometric properties, but this review shows that knowledge about the relationship between loneliness and outcomes of mental health problems is still very limited. Finally, the studies in our review had sample sizes ranging from 42 to 1004, and diverse follow-up periods from a few months to ten years. The sample size of most studies is under 400 with less than 100 participants in six articles. However, the consistency of positive findings from included studies, irrespective of their sample size, provides some confidence that studies were not underpowered.

Other limitations of this review relate to the search strategy. Although our literature search was conducted in six databases and a variety of search terms were applied, the search might not be exhaustive. Some relevant studies may have been missed if they did not use "subjective or personal or perceived or quality" five or fewer words apart from "social support". Some very old papers might not be indexed in electronic databases, and thus cannot be searched. Eligible studies are only from seven countries and most of them were conducted in North America. Very few papers in other languages were retrieved and none of them could be included in our review, although we did search for them and read their abstracts. It is also worth noting that the extent of any reporting bias is uncertain as studies which did not find a positive result might not be published. Another limitation refers to the scope of our review. We restricted the search to the most common mental disorders, including schizophrenia and schizoaffective disorder, psychosis in general, depression, bipolar disorder, and anxiety disorders. The associations between loneliness and perceived social support and other mental health problems need further investigation. Additionally, we focused on one direction of causation only: the effect of baseline loneliness and poor perceived social support on mental health outcomes at follow up. Psychiatric symptoms probably also influence loneliness and perceived social support, but this was not the research question on which we focused in this review.

Research implications

Most studies included in our review focused on depression, with other types of mental health problems represented by fewer than five studies each. Nevertheless, some significant relationships have been found between loneliness and/or perceived social support and outcomes of those mental disorders. Gayer-Anderson and Morgan [46] systematically examined evidence on social networks and social support in early psychosis. They found some tentative evidence that deficits in social networks and support preceded the onset of psychosis, but it was difficult to disentangle direction of causation as almost all the studies included were cross-sectional and they did not report whether social relationships influence outcomes of psychosis. Given that the prevalence of loneliness in people with psychosis was comparable to that in people with depression, it is surprising that research about impact of loneliness/perceived social support on psychosis is scarce. Similarly, social relationships were shown to be related to bipolar disorder and anxiety disorders, but there is a lack of evidence to discern cause and effect [69, 70]. Therefore more systematic exploration is needed about how loneliness and perceived social support affect conditions such as psychosis, bipolar disorder and anxiety disorders.

Additionally, more longitudinal research with long-term follow-up (and repeated measures) is essential to untangle the direction of effect in the relationship between loneliness/perceived social support and poor outcomes. Among the 34 eligible studies only five articles involve a long-term follow-up period (over 2 years). Thus there is a need to establish the longer term associations of loneliness and perceived social support. As well its effects on longer term mental health outcomes, loneliness may contribute to the adverse physical health outcomes and increased mortality of people with severe mental health problems.

We also found that the relationship between perceived social support and depression was studied far more often and is thus far more clearly established than the relationship between loneliness and depression. Only two studies retrieved for our review included loneliness as an independent variable for outcomes of mental disorders. They found that loneliness at baseline predicted depression and anxiety severity and remission from depression [25, 66]. However, the few longitudinal studies of loneliness do not allow definitive conclusions. Therefore more longitudinal research is needed in clinical samples to try to achieve a clear understanding of the impact of loneliness on the course of mental health problems.

Clinical and policy implications

There are a number of clinical and policy implications from the finding that poor perceived social support has a significant impact on outcomes in depression. Firstly, it highlights the need to pay sufficient attention to the social relationships and social support needs of people with mental health problems. Social activities, or thinking about relationships, can be overlooked in clinical consultations – in favour of medications or psychological therapies, and there have been recent calls to raise the profile of social factors in mental health care and mental health research [16]. Raising practitioners' awareness of the beneficial effects of good perceived social support on symptoms, recovery, and functioning is an important first step, but also promoting awareness amongst service users and the wider public – so that people may feel more motivated to seek relevant help or to try to change their own situation, particularly in depression but probably in other mental health problems studied too.

The development of effective interventions to promote social support and reduce loneliness is required to address the current evidence gap, manifested by the absence of recommendations in this important social domain in current policy guidance. In the UK for example, the National Health Service (NHS) Five Year Forward View [71] refers to a series of plans to improve the quality of mental health services and reduce 'burden' on the NHS. Access to psychological therapies, waiting standards and better physical healthcare are highlighted but there is no specific mention of managing the significant problems of loneliness or limited social relationships. International evidence that poor perceived support from social relationships leads to increased service use and poorer outcomes across a range of diagnostic groups should inform future policy in this area. Also in the UK, the latest National Institute for Clinical Excellence (NICE) guidance on illnesses such as depression and schizophrenia, does not recommend social interventions apart from employment support [72, 73].

Clinicians may doubt whether loneliness and limited support from interpersonal relationships are appropriate or feasible as targets for intervention. However, potential interventions are becoming available in a variety of sectors. Around the world, approaches are being developed to try to reduce loneliness among older people in the general population, with potential to be adapted to other groups in the population at risk of adverse effects from poor social support. In the UK, a variety of approaches to social relationships and social participation are being developed primarily in the charitable sector and in primary care [74]. Social prescribing projects have proliferated in the UK in recent years [75]. Social prescribing is not precisely defined, but typically refers to: navigation - the process of linking support for people to access community activities helpful to wellbeing and participation; and/or funding and providing these activities in a community or group setting [76]. As yet however, social prescribing models are numerous and poorly defined [75], and there is a lack of robust evidence regarding their effectiveness [76]. Psychological approaches, such as Cognitive Behavioural Therapy and Mindfulness, have also been used to help people change their thinking about social relationships: some promising results have been reported, especially with older adult populations [77]. Thus there are approaches available with potential to be adapted and tested for people with mental health problems, to try to alleviate the adverse effects identified in this paper. There is also a need to consider public understanding of the importance of nurturing social relationships, as the high prevalence of loneliness is not only an individual but necessarily also a community and societal level problem. Thus people with mental health problems, like other groups in the population who are vulnerable to the effects of loneliness, are likely to benefit from an approach to loneliness that also takes account of community resources and how they might be enhanced [78].

Conclusions

This systematic review has identified prospective studies in the area of loneliness/perceived social support and outcomes of mental health problems. We found substantial evidence that in depression, poorer perceived social support is associated with poorer outcomes in terms of symptoms, recovery and functioning. There is some preliminary evidence of a similar relationship in bipolar and anxiety disorders, and of a relationship between greater perceived social support and better quality of life and functioning in schizophrenia. Loneliness and its impact on mental health outcomes are still insufficiently addressed compared to perceived social support, but there is some evidence that greater loneliness is related to more severe depression and anxiety symptoms and poorer remission from depression. Further research, including long-term follow-up and repeated measures, is required to longitudinally investigate the direction of effect between loneliness/perceived social support and poor mental health outcomes among service users from different diagnostic groups. There is also a case, especially in depression, for raising public awareness of the importance of reducing public health, and for developing, testing and implementing strategies to improve perceived social support and reduce loneliness in people with mental health problems.

Abbreviations

CES-D: Center for Epidemiologic Studies Depression Scale; DSM: Diagnostic and Statistical Manual of Mental Disorder; HoNOS: Health of the Nation Outcome Scales; ICD: International Classification of Diseases; M.I.N.I. : Mini-International Neuropsychiatric Interview; MMAT: Mixed Methods Appraisal Tool; NHS: National Health Service; NICE: National Institute for Clinical Excellence; PTSD: post-traumatic stress disorder; UCLA: University of California at Los Angeles Loneliness Scale

Acknowledgments

We are grateful for the help of UCL Library staff for consultation and guidance in the search strategy. We would like to thank the authors of screened papers who responded to our emails for their support.

Authors' contributions

SJ, JW and BLE conceived the review. SJ and BLE commented on search strategy and review protocol. JW developed the search strategy and review protocol, did the systematic search, and wrote the first draft and co-ordinated further drafts. JW and FM independently screened and selected papers for inclusion, extracted data, and assessed the methodological quality of each study. RM helped screen reference lists of included studies and extract data from relevant studies. SJ resolved queries about inclusion/exclusion and disagreements between JW and FM during the review process. SJ, BLE, FM, and RM contributed comments and suggestions to the drafts. All authors read and approved the final manuscript.

Competing interests

The authors declare that they have no competing interests.

References

1. Umberson D, Montez JK. Social relationships and health: a flashpoint for health policy. J Health Soc Behav. 2010;51:S54–66.
2. Hawkley LC, Cacioppo JT. Loneliness matters: a theoretical and empirical review of consequences and mechanisms. Ann Behav Med. 2010;40(2):218–27.
3. Petitte T, Mallow J, Barnes E, Petrone A, Barr T, Theeke L. A systematic review of loneliness and common chronic physical conditions in adults. Open Psychol J. 2015;8(Suppl 2):113–32.
4. Uchino BN. Understanding the links between social support and physical health: a life-span perspective with emphasis on the Separability of perceived and received support. Perspect Psychol Sci. 2009;4(3):236–55.
5. Holt-Lunstad J, Smith TB, Baker M, Harris T, Stephenson D. Loneliness and social isolation as risk factors for mortality: a meta-analytic review. Perspect Psychol Sci. 2015;10(2):227–37.
6. Holt-Lunstad J, Smith TB, Layton JB. Social Relationships and mortality risk: a meta-analytic review. PLoS Med. 2010;7(7)
7. Valtorta NK, Kanaan M, Gilbody S, Ronzi S, Hanratty B. Loneliness and social isolation as risk factors for coronary heart disease and stroke: systematic review and meta-analysis of longitudinal observational studies. Heart. 2016; 102(13):1009–16.
8. Hawkley LC, Thisted RA, Masi CM, Cacioppo JT. Loneliness predicts increased blood pressure: 5-year cross-lagged analyses in middle-aged and older adults. Psychol Aging. 2010;25(1):132–41.
9. Yang YC, Boen C, Harris KM. Social relationships and hypertension in late life: evidence from a nationally representative longitudinal study of older adults. J Aging Health. 2015;27(3):403–31.
10. Jaremka LM, Andridge RR, Fagundes CP, Alfano CM, Povoski SP, Lipari AM, Agnese DM, Arnold MW, Farrar WB, Yee LD, et al. Pain, depression, and fatigue: loneliness as a longitudinal risk factor. Health Psychol. 2014;33(9):948–57.
11. Hughes S, Jaremka LM, Alfano CM, Glaser R, Povoski SP, Lipari AM, Agnese DM, Farrar WB, Yee LD, Carson WE, et al. Social support predicts inflammation, pain, and depressive symptoms: longitudinal relationships among breast cancer survivors. Psychoneuroendocrinology. 2014;42:38–44.
12. House JS, Landis KR, Umberson D. Social relationships and health. Science. 1988;241(4865):540–5.
13. Cacioppo JT, Cacioppo S, Boomsma DI. Evolutionary mechanisms for loneliness. Cogn Emot. 2014;28(1):3–21.
14. Perese EF, Wolf M. Combating loneliness among persons with severe mental illness: social network interventions' characteristics, effectiveness, and applicability. Issues Ment Health Nurs. 2005;26(6):591–609.
15. Howes OD, Murray RM. Schizophrenia: an integrated sociodevelopmental-cognitive model. Lancet. 2014;383(9929):1677–87.
16. Johnson S. Social interventions in mental health: a call to action. Soc Psychiatry Psychiatr Epidemiol. 2017;52(3):245–7.
17. Reininghaus U, Morgan C. Integrated models in psychiatry: the state of the art. Soc Psychiatry Psychiatr Epidemiol. 2014;49(1):1–2.
18. Peplau LA, Perlman D. Loneliness: A Sourcebook of current theory, Research, and Therapy. New York: Wiley Interscience; 1982.
19. Weiss RS. Loneliness: the experience of emotional and social isolation. Cambridge, MA. In: US: the MIT press; 1973.
20. Gierveld JD, Van Tilburg T. A 6-item scale for overall, emotional, and social loneliness - confirmatory tests on survey data. Res Aging. 2006;28(5):582–98.
21. Russell DW. UCLA loneliness scale (version 3): reliability, validity, and factor structure. J Pers Assess. 1996;66(1):20–40.
22. Dejonggierveld J, Kamphuis F. The development of a rasch-type loneliness scale. Appl Psychol Meas. 1985;9(3):289–99.
23. Borge L, Martinsen EW, Ruud T, Watne O, Friis S. Quality of life, loneliness, and social contact among long-term psychiatric patients. Psychiatr Serv. 1999;50(1):81–4.
24. Lauder W, Sharkey S, Mummery K. A community survey of loneliness. J Adv Nurs. 2004;46(1):88–94.

25. Holvast F, Burger H, de Waal MMW, van Marwijk HWJ, Comijs HC, Verhaak PFM. Loneliness is associated with poor prognosis in late-life depression: longitudinal analysis of the Netherlands study of depression in older persons. J Affect Disord. 2015;185:1–7.
26. van Tilburg TG, de Jong Gierveld J. Reference standards for the loneliness scale. Tijdschr Gerontol Geriatr. 1999;30(4):158–63.
27. Badcock JC, Shah S, Mackinnon A, Stain HJ, Galletly C, Jablensky A, Morgan VA. Loneliness in psychotic disorders and its association with cognitive function and symptom profile. Schizophr Res. 2015;169(1–3):268–73.
28. Victor CR, Yang KM. The prevalence of loneliness among adults: a case study of the United Kingdom. Aust J Psychol. 2012;146(1–2):85–104.
29. Meltzer H, Bebbington P, Dennis MS, Jenkins R, McManus S, Brugha TS. Feelings of loneliness among adults with mental disorder. Soc Psychiatry Psychiatr Epidemiol. 2013;48(1):5–13.
30. Routasalo PE, Savikko N, Tilvis RS, Strandberg TE, Pitkala KH. Social contacts and their relationship to loneliness among aged people - a population-based study. Gerontology. 2006;52(3):181–7.
31. Coyle CE, Dugan E. Social isolation, loneliness and health among older adults. J Aging Health. 2012;24(8):1346–63.
32. Wang JY, Lloyd-Evans B, Giacco D, Forsyth R, Nebo C, Mann F, Johnson S. Social isolation in mental health: a conceptual and methodological review. Soc Psychiatry Psychiatr Epidemiol. 2017;52(12):1451–61.
33. Dour HJ, Wiley JF, Roy-Byrne P, Stein MB, Sullivan G, Sherbourne CD, Bystritsky A, Rose RD, Craske MG. Perceived social support mediates anxiety and depressive symptom changes following primary care intervention. Depress Anxiety. 2014;31(5):436–42.
34. Hupcey JE. Clarifying the social support theory-research linkage. J Adv Nurs. 1998;27(6):1231–41.
35. Zimet GD, Dahlem NW, Zimet SG, Farley GK. The multidimensional scale of perceived social support. J Pers Assess. 1988;52(1):30–41.
36. Koenig HG, Westlund RE, George LK, Hughes DC, Blazer DG, Hybels C. Abbreviating the Duke social support index for use in chronically ill elderly individuals. Psychosomatics. 1993;34(1):61–9.
37. Brown GW, Harris T. Social origins of depression. London: Tavistock; 1978.
38. Murphy E. Social origins of depression in old-age. Br J Psychiatry. 1982;141:135–42.
39. Salimi A, Bozorgpour F. Percieved Social Support and Social-Emotional Loneliness. In: International Conference on Education & Educational Psychology. Volume 69 ed. Amsterdam: Elsevier Science Bv; 2012. p. 2009–13.
40. Pamukcu B, Meydana B. The role of empathic tendency and perceived social support in predicting loneliness levels of college students. In: Wcpcg 2010. Volume 5 ed. Amsterdam: Elsevier Science Bv; 2010. p. 905–9.
41. Lasgaard M, Nielsen A, Eriksen ME, Goossens L. Loneliness and social support in adolescent boys with autism Spectrum disorders. J Autism Dev Disord. 2010;40(2):218–26.
42. Chrostek A, Grygiel P, Anczewska M, Wciorka J, Switaj P. The intensity and correlates of the feelings of loneliness in people with psychosis. Compr Psychiatry. 2016;70:190–9.
43. Gariepy G, Honkaniemi H, Quesnel-Vallee A. Social support and protection from depression: systematic review of current findings in western countries. Br J Psychiatry. 2016;209(4):286–95.
44. Santini ZI, Koyanagi A, Tyrovolas S, Mason C, Haro JM. The association between social relationships and depression: a systematic review. J Affect Disord. 2015;175:53–65.
45. Schwarzbach M, Luppa M, Forstmeier S, Konig HH, Riedel-Heller SG. Social relations and depression in late life - a systematic review. Int J Geriatr Psychiatry. 2014;29(1):1–21.
46. Gayer-Anderson C, Morgan C. Social networks, support and early psychosis: a systematic review. Epidemiol Psychiatr Sci. 2013;22(2):131–46.
47. Wang J, Mann F, Lloyd-Evans B, Ma R, Johnson S. Loneliness as a predictor of outcomes in mental disorders: a systematic review. PROSPERO International prospective register of systematic reviews. 2014; http://www.crd.york.ac.uk/PROSPERO/display_record.asp?ID=CRD42015014784. Accessed 19 Oct 2016
48. Pluye P, Robert E, Cargo M, Bartlett G, O'Cathain A, Griffiths F, Boardman F, Gagnon MP, Rousseau MC. Proposal: A Mixed Methods Appraisal Tool for Systematic Mixed Studies Reviews. Canada: Department of Family Medicine, McGill University, Montreal; 2011. http://mixedmethodsappraisaltoolpublic.pbworks.com. Accessed 19 Oct 2016
49. Blazer D, Hughes DC, George LK. Age and impaired subjective support. Predictors of depressive symptoms at one-year follow-up J Nerv Ment Dis. 1992;180(3):172–8.
50. Brugha TS, Bebbington PE, Maccarthy B, Sturt E, Wykes T, Potter J. Gender, social support and recovery from depressive disorders: a prospective clinical study. Psychol Med. 1990;20(1):147–56.
51. Leskela U, Rytsala H, Komulainen E, Melartin T, Sokero P, Lestela-Mielonen P, Isometsa E. The influence of adversity and perceived social support on the outcome of major depressive disorder in subjects with different levels of depressive symptoms. Psychol Med. 2006;36(6):779–88.
52. Bosworth HB, Hays JC, George LK, Steffens DC. Psychosocial and clinical predictors of unipolar depression outcome in older adults. Int J Geriatr Psychiatry. 2002;17(3):238–46.
53. Bosworth HB, McQuoid DR, George LK, Steffens DC. Time-to-remission from geriatric depression: psychosocial and clinical factors. Am J Geriatr Psychiatry. 2002;10(5):551–9.
54. Holma I, Holma K, Melartin T, Rytsala H, Isometsa E. A 5-year prospective study of predictors for disability pension among patients with major depressive disorder. Acta Psychiatr Scand. 2012;125(4):325–34.
55. Rytsala H, Melartin T, Leskela U, Sokero T, Lestela-Mielonen P, Isometsa E. Predictors of long-term work disability in major depressive disorder: a prospective study. Acta Psychiatr Scand. 2007;115(3):206–13.
56. Rytsala HJ, Melartin TK, Leskela US, Lestela-Mielonen PS, Sokero T, Isometsa ET. Determinants of functional disability and social adjustment in major depressive disorder: a prospective study. J Nerv Ment Dis. 2006;194(8):570–6.
57. Hays JC, Steffens DC, Flint EP, Bosworth HB, George LK. Does social support buffer functional decline in elderly patients with unipolar depression? Am J Psychiatry. 2001;158(11):1850–5.
58. Ritsner M, Gibel A, Ratner Y. Determinants of changes in perceived quality of life in the course of schizophrenia. Qual Life Res. 2006;15(3):515–26.
59. Brekke J, Kay DD, Lee KS, Green MF. Biosocial pathways to functional outcome in schizophrenia. Schizophr Res. 2005;80(2–3):213–25.
60. Koenders MA, Giltay EJ, Hoencamp E, Elzinga BM, Spinhoven P, Spijker AT. The bidirectional impact of perceived and enacted support on mood in bipolar outpatients: a two-year prospective study. Compr Psychiatry. 2015;60:59–67.
61. Daniels RE. Psychosocial predictors of symptom severity and functioning in adults with bipolar disorder. A three-month prospective study. Diss Abstr Int B Sci Eng. 2000;60(8-B):4213.
62. Johnson SL, Winett CA, Meyer B, Greenhouse WJ, Miller I. Social support and the course of bipolar disorder. J Abnorm Psychol. 1999;108(4):558–66.
63. Cohen AN, Hammen C, Henry RM, Daley SE. Effects of stress and social support on recurrence in bipolar disorder. J Affect Disord. 2004;82(1):143–7.
64. Jakubovski E, Bloch MH. Anxiety disorder-specific predictors of treatment outcome in the coordinated anxiety learning and management (CALM) trial. Psychiatr Q. 2016;87(3):445–64.
65. Shrestha S, Stanley MA, Wilson NL, Cully JA, Kunik ME, Novy DM, Rhoades HM, Amspoker AB. Predictors of change in quality of life in older adults with generalized anxiety disorder. Int Psychogeriatr. 2015;27(7):1207–15.
66. van Beljouw IM, Verhaak PF, Cuijpers P, van Marwijk HW, Penninx BW. The course of untreated anxiety and depression, and determinants of poor one-year outcome: a one-year cohort study. BMC Psychiatry. 2010;10:86.
67. Fleury MJ, Grenier G, Bamvita JM, Tremblay J, Schmitz N, Caron J. Predictors of quality of life in a longitudinal study of users with severe mental disorders. Health Qual Life Outcomes. 2013;11(1)
68. Eriksson K, Haggstrom O. Lord's paradox in a continuous setting and a regression artifact in numerical cognition research. PLoS One. 2014;9(4)
69. Studart PM, Bezerra S, Studart ABD, Galvao-de Almeida A, Miranda-Scippa A. Social support and bipolar disorder. Arch Clin Psychiatry. 2015;42(4):95–9.
70. Teo AR, Lerrigo R, Rogers MAM. The role of social isolation in social anxiety disorder: a systematic review and meta-analysis. J Anxiety Disord. 2013;27(4):353–64.
71. NHS Five Year Forward View. 2014. https://www.england.nhs.uk/wp-content/uploads/2014/10/5yfv-web.pdf. Accessed 19 Oct 2016.
72. Psychosis and schizophrenia in adults: prevention and management. National Institute for Health and Care Excellence (NICE). 2014. https://www.nice.org.uk/guidance/cg178. Accessed 19 Oct 2016.
73. Continuation and relapse prevention for adults with depression. National Institute for Health and Care Excellence (NICE). 2016. https://pathways.nice.org.uk/pathways/depression/continuation-and-relapse-prevention-for-adults-

with-depression#path=view%3A/pathways/depression/continuation-and-relapse-prevention-for-adults-with-depression.xml&content=view-index. Accessed 19 Oct 2016.

74. Mann F, Bone JK, Lloyd-Evans B, Frerichs J, Pinfold V, Ma R, Wang J, Johnson S. A life less lonely: the state of the art in interventions to reduce loneliness in people with mental health problems. Soc Psychiatry Psychiatr Epidemiol. 2017;52(6):627–38.
75. Report of the Annual Social Prescribing Network Conference. London: University of Westminster; 2016.
76. Evidence to inform the commissioning of social prescribing. York: University of York. Centre for reviews and dissemination; 2015.
77. Masi CM, Chen HY, Hawkley LC, Cacioppo JT. A meta-analysis of interventions to reduce loneliness. Personal Soc Psychol Rev. 2011;15(3):219–66.
78. Kearns A, Whitley E, Tannahill C, Ellaway A. Loneliness, social relations and health and well-being in deprived communities. Psychol Health Med. 2015; 20(3):332–44.
79. Hybels CF, Pieper CF, Blazer DG, Steffens DC. Heterogeneity in the three-year course of major depression among older adults. Int J Geriatr Psychiatr. 2016;31(7):775–82.
80. Backs-Dermott BJ, Dobson KS, Jones SL. An evaluation of an integrated model of relapse in depression. J Affect Disord. 2010;124(1–2):60–7.
81. Bosworth HB, Voils CI, Potter GG, Steffens DC. The effects of antidepressant medication adherence as well as psychosocial and clinical factors on depression outcome among older adults. Int J Geriatr Psychiatry. 2008;23(2):129–34.
82. Steffens DC, Pieper CF, Bosworth HB, MacFall JR, Provenzale JM, Payne ME, Carroll BJ, George LK, Krishnan KRR. Biological and social predictors of long-term geriatric depression outcome. Int Psychogeriatr. 2005;17(1):41–56.
83. Ezquiaga E, Garcia-Lopez A, de Dios C, Leiva A, Bravo M, Montejo J. Clinical and psychosocial factors associated with the outcome of unipolar major depression: a one year prospective study. J Affect Disord. 2004;79(1–3):63–70.
84. Gasto C, Navarro V, Catalan R, Portella MJ, Marcos T. Residual symptoms in elderly major depression remitters. Acta Psychiatr Scand. 2003;108(1):15–9.
85. Triesch SK. Interpersonal expectations and adjustment to depression. Diss Abstr Int B Sci Eng. 2002;63(3-B):1578.
86. Oxman TE, Hull JG. Social support and treatment response in older depressed primary care patients. J Gerontol B Psychol Sci Soc Sci. 2001;56(1):P35–45.
87. Brummett BH, Barefoot JC, Siegler IC, Steffens DC. Relation of subjective and received social support to clinical and self-report assessments of depressive symptoms in an elderly population. J Affect Disord. 2000;61(1–2):41–50.
88. Sherbourne CD, Hays RD, Wells KB. Personal and psychosocial risk factors for physical and mental health outcomes and course of depression among depressed patients. J Consult Clin Psychol. 1995;63(3):345–55.
89. Blazer D, Hughes DC. Subjective social support and depressive symptoms in major depression: separate phenomena or epiphenomena. J Psychiatr Res. 1991;25(4):191–203.
90. George LK, Blazer DG, Hughes DC, Fowler N. Social support and the outcome of major depression. Br J Psychiatry. 1989;154:478–85.
91. Krantz SE, Moos RH. Risk factors at intake predict nonremission among depressed patients. J Consult Clin Psychol. 1988;56(6):863–9.

4

Best practice framework for Patient and Public Involvement (PPI) in collaborative data analysis of qualitative mental health research: methodology development and refinement

Helen Jennings[1†], Mike Slade[2*†], Peter Bates[3], Emma Munday[4] and Rebecca Toney[2]

Abstract

Background: Patient and Public Involvement (PPI) in mental health research is increasing, especially in early (pre-funding) stages. PPI is less consistent in later stages, including in analysing qualitative data. The aims of this study were to develop a methodology for involving PPI co-researchers in collaboratively analysing qualitative mental health research data with academic researchers, to pilot and refine this methodology, and to create a best practice framework for collaborative data analysis (CDA) of qualitative mental health research.

Methods: In the context of the RECOLLECT Study of Recovery Colleges, a critical literature review of collaborative data analysis studies was conducted, to identify approaches and recommendations for successful CDA. A CDA methodology was developed and then piloted in RECOLLECT, followed by refinement and development of a best practice framework.

Results: From 10 included publications, four CDA approaches were identified: (1) consultation, (2) development, (3) application and (4) development and application of coding framework. Four characteristics of successful CDA were found: CDA process is co-produced; CDA process is realistic regarding time and resources; demands of the CDA process are manageable for PPI co-researchers; and group expectations and dynamics are effectively managed. A four-meeting CDA process was piloted to co-produce a coding framework based on qualitative data collected in RECOLLECT and to create a mental health service user-defined change model relevant to Recovery Colleges. Formal and informal feedback demonstrated active involvement. The CDA process involved an extra 80 person-days of time (40 from PPI co-researchers, 40 from academic researchers). The process was refined into a best practice framework comprising Preparation, CDA and Application phases.

Conclusions: This study has developed a typology of approaches to collaborative analysis of qualitative data in mental health research, identified from available evidence the characteristics of successful involvement, and developed, piloted and refined the first best practice framework for collaborative analysis of qualitative data. This framework has the potential to support meaningful PPI in data analysis in the context of qualitative mental health research studies, a previously neglected yet central part of the research cycle.

Keywords: Patient and public involvement (PPI), Mental health research, Qualitative, Collaborative data analysis, Co-production

* Correspondence: m.slade@nottingham.ac.uk
†Helen Jennings and Mike Slade contributed equally to this work.
Helen Jennings and Mike Slade are join lead authors.
[2]School of Health Sciences, Institute of Mental Health, University of Nottingham, Triumph Road, Nottingham NG7 2TU, UK
Full list of author information is available at the end of the article

Background

Patient and Public Involvement (PPI) in research is increasing. PPI can be defined as the involvement of patients, carers and the public as active partners in the design, delivery and dissemination of research to ensure that it is relevant and useful [1], or as *"research being carried out 'with' or 'by' members of the public rather than 'to', 'about' or 'for' them"* [2]. The impact of PPI on research has been investigated. A 2012 systematic review of PPI in health and social care research identified benefits as enhanced quality and appropriateness of research, development of user-focused research objectives, user-relevant research questions, user-friendly information, questionnaires and interview schedules, appropriate recruitment strategies for studies, consumer-focused interpretation of data and enhanced implementation and dissemination of study results [3]. More recent research has shown positive impacts on researchers, including their knowledge, priorities, lay communication skills and attitudes to involvement [4]. The PPI representative also benefits, e.g. through an improved life focus and relationship with their illness [1]. PPI specifically in mental health research has also shown benefits, e.g. with more PPI found in studies achieving recruitment targets [5].

The level of involvement can differ [6, 7]. Low-level involvement, called 'informed', 'consulted' or 'participation', consists of researchers asking for views which are then used to inform research decision making. Medium-level involvement, called 'involved', 'collaboration' or 'co-production', has a focus on equity within the relationship between the researcher and the PPI participant, and comprises an ongoing partnership with shared decision making. High-level involvement called 'influential', 'control' or 'service user-led', consists of people with experience of the health issue being researched having the dominant voice, delivering and managing research themselves. This framework was chosen as a pragmatic, understandable approach which is measurable [8], relates to mental health areas such as shared decision making [9] and experience of care [10], and is widely used in health research in the United Kingdom. Other frameworks for characterising involvement exist, for example at the individual level (micro level), the health-care service level (meso level), policy level (macro level) and, as in the current study, in research and education (meta level) [11]. Inclusive disability research has highlighted the importance of methods of involvement, including emancipatory research, collaboration research, and, as in this study, steering and advisory groups [12]. Involvement in research can vary across different dimensions; a recent framework published in the United Kingdom identifies six standards: inclusive opportunities, working together, support & learning, communications, impact and governance [13]. A systematic review identified types of PPI in research at the preparatory, execution and translational phases of the research cycle [14].

Applying this three-level involvement framework to clinical services, a movement towards higher levels of service user involvement in clinical practice is evident. For example, shared rather than clinician-led decision-making is now routinely recommended [15], because decision-making involvement influences recovery [16]. Just as in PPI, involvement in clinical decision-making is influenced by relational aspects, including a collaborative and trusting relationship, and access to information resources [17]. User involvement in strengthening services (e.g. in low resources settings [18]) or supporting increased participation (e.g. in in-patient settings [19]) is developing. The growth of peer support workers [20] and the development of service user-run services [21] indicates a trend towards high-level involvement in clinical services. However, the views of mental health staff (especially in-patient and less experienced staff) are more positive about patient involvement in treatment than their involvement in the planning and management of services or in professional education [22]. A systematic review concluded that organisations are still negotiating the balance between consumer leadership and traditional structures and systems [23].

Turning to PPI in research, the level of involvement may not be consistent across all parts of the research cycle. An important driver of behaviour in the scientific research community is funding, and many funders now require PPI input to proposals. For example, the leading funder of applied health research in the UK is the National Institute of Health Research (NIHR), and NIHR has a stated expectation that there will be active involvement of members of the public in the research that it funds [24]. This is operationalised through mandatory PPI sections in proposal forms for applicants to outline the extent of PPI, and through PPI representatives on funding panels. As a result, PPI in the UK has become the norm in developing health research proposals.

PPI involvement after securing funding is inconsistent. Examples of token involvement during post-funding research stages (study setup, ethical approval, data collection, data analysis, dissemination) are reported, such as more importance being given to researcher and clinician views than to PPI perspectives, and PPI processes being experienced as a tick-box exercise [25, 26]. Whilst the public voice is increasingly present in research decision-making, there is less evidence of a change in the underpinning power dynamic between the scientific research community and the public [27]. Mirroring the stage of development of involvement in clinical services (outlined earlier), the transition towards citizen science – equal partnership between scientists and citizens – is only partially complete [28].

As part of the movement towards higher levels of PPI in academic research, analysis of data is an important point of input [29]. However, service users are rarely involved in creating meaning from data [30]. This means that a valuable perspective in interpreting findings is being lost. Collaborative data analysis (CDA) of qualitative data is a recognised methodology involving a joint focus and dialogue among two or more researchers regarding a shared body of data to produce an agreed interpretation [31]. When one of the involved parties bring a PPI perspective, this can highlight taken-for-granted researcher assumptions, provide socio-cultural and political insights, and enhance the thoroughness of interpretation [32]. For example, in a study of detained psychiatric patients, mental health service user researchers coded more according to experiences and feelings, whereas university researchers coded more according to procedures and processes [33].

The Recovery Colleges Characterisation and Testing (RECOLLECT) Study is an NIHR-funded evaluation of Recovery Colleges (RCs), a new innovation which uses co-production and adult education approaches, rather than treatment, to support mental health recovery [34, 35]. RCs involve the development of a culture of 'emancipatory education' [36] with an emphasis on 'inclusivity and egalitarianism' [37]. Emerging fidelity criteria are located in counter-point to the current mental health system [38]. As part of RECOLLECT, qualitative data on mechanisms of action and outcomes were collected in three RCs. As RCs are a disruptive innovation [39] based on intentionally different values, goals and assumptions from clinical systems, there is a high risk of bias in interpreting qualitative data about them from a clinical research perspective. Therefore a collaborative data analysis approach involving people with lived experience was required to improve the quality of analysis. We refer to the (typically university-based) academic research team conducting studies (such as RECOLLECT) as the **academic researchers** (whilst recognising that academic researchers may themselves have disclosed or non-disclosed experience of mental ill-health, and noting the existence of service user-led research groups in universities) and people bringing a public or patient perspective as **PPI co-researchers** (also noting that they may have research experience).

The aims of this study were (1) to develop a methodology for involving PPI co-researchers in analysis of qualitative data; (2) to pilot and refine this methodology; and (3) to create a best practice framework for future PPI in data analysis.

Methods

The RECOLLECT Lived Experience Advisory Panel (LEAP) comprises a group of 9 people with lived experience of mental health issues, either personally or as carers. Members brought a range of research experience (from never having done research before to having collaborated on several projects), and were heterogeneous in where they lived, educational achievement and occupational background. LEAP members are referred to as the PPI co-researchers.

The RECOLLECT research team (who collected the data collaboratively analysed in Stage 2) span a range of professions (counselling, occupational therapy, psychology) and PPI experiences (PPI lead, PPI participant), and specifically include people with and without lived experience of mental health issues (directly or as a family member). The RECOLLECT research team are referred to as the academic researchers.

Ethical approval was obtained (Nottingham REC 1, 16/EM/0484) and all participants provided written informed consent.

Stage 1: Develop the CDA methodology

A critical literature review [40] was conducted by HJ, involving evaluation and synthesis of included papers. The aim of a critical review is to identify the most significant articles in a field, and it was chosen over more systematic approaches as a proportionate review approach suitable for generating a model. Databases searched were AMED, PubMed, CINAHL, MEDLINE and PsycARTICLES, with serendipitous searching [41] to identify grey literature. A scoping search indicated that terms like 'coproduction' were insignificantly specific, so search terms specifically focussed on the collaborative analysis element of coproduction were used. Inclusion criteria were (a) primary focus on qualitative collaborative data analysis; (b) published in journal or book; (c) focused on mental health research; (d) aligned with the principles of PPI and a democratic approach to public engagement [7]; and (e) published since 2007 to maximise relevance to current PPI frameworks. The initial concept search strategy comprised ("collaborative data analysis" OR "interpretation workshop" OR "participatory action research") AND ("service user" OR "public patient involvement" OR "PPI" OR "co-researcher" OR "co-investigator" OR "expert by experience" OR "client" OR "consumer" OR "survivor") AND ("mental health" OR "mental illness" OR "mental distress" OR "psychological distress") AND "qualitative". The initial search identified few papers specific to mental health, so inclusion criterion (c) was amended to include any health research, and the search strategy amended accordingly. The first author extracted data relevant to design and procedure, and characteristics of successful CDA. Findings were synthesised by the research team, and organised into methodology options and success characteristics.

Stage 2: Pilot and refine the CDA methodology

The Stage 1 synthesis was considered by academic researchers and PPI co-researchers to select a methodology for CDA in RECOLLECT, in relation to investigation about mechanisms, outcomes and change models for Recovery Colleges. Evaluation criteria were that the methodology: ensured PPI co-researcher interpretations of qualitative data collected in RECOLLECT were generated; ensured these interpretations were used to inform findings; aligned with a democratic approach to PPI [7]; were practical to apply within the constraints of a one-year study; and incorporated the design techniques that were associated with successful CDA. Decisions were amalgamated by HJ into a final synthesised methodology and procedural session plans, which were then refined by the other authors. The CDA methodology was then piloted. PPI co-researchers met with the academic researchers in four 4-h meetings, each with a minimum of 8 co-researchers present who were paid for their preparation and attendance.

The aim of this part of RECOLLECT was to develop an understanding of how RCs work (mechanisms of action) and the impact on students (outcomes). Framework analysis [42] was the underpinning methodology. Summarising the content of CDA meetings (described in Table 3): Meeting 1 ensured the ecological validity of the document analysis carried out by the academic researchers; Meeting 2 refined the preliminary, academic researcher-developed coding framework to co-produce the final coding framework; Meeting 3 created a mental health service user-led change model (organising and linking coded mechanisms of action and outcomes); and Meeting 4 enabled final verification of the change model. Each meeting was facilitated by two RECOLLECT academic researchers; one to help navigate the narrative of the discussions and the other to support group dynamics and ensure all PPI co-researchers were able to contribute. Tasks were predominantly broken down into small group or pair work initially, with all PPI co-researchers then coming together to share what they had produced. Exercises were presented both verbally and on paper, with opportunities for questions and challenge. Adequate understanding of task requirements was ascertained through check-back and observation. Insights from occupational therapy research [43, 44] were used to inform grading and adapting activities to align with an individual's capacities, in order to maximise their performance. This improves the likelihood the PPI co-researcher experience will be positive, rather than frustrating, marginalising or demoralising [45]. Exercises were paced to allow time for breaks and refreshment. Data interpretations by PPI co-researchers were captured by two academic researchers observing and writing down PPI co-researcher verbal contributions, collection of written and photographed outputs, and completion of field notes by the academic researchers.

Several strategies to enhance quality were used, such as peer examination, triangulation of researchers and PPI co-researcher perspective, triangulation of data sources (PPI, documents, qualitative interviews), and use of reflexivity in the academic researcher field notes [46]. Additionally, in the final meeting informal feedback was obtained and the Quality Involvement Questionnaire was completed by PPI co-researchers [47]. This 31-item self-report measure (each item rated 0 (low involvement) to 4) assesses perceived involvement, and has six sub-scales in two parts: Personal Factors (Your ability (range 0–28), Your potential (0–20), Your sense of being (0–20)) and Research Contexts (Research relationships (0–24), Ways of doing research (0–16) and Research structures (0–16)). Total score ranges from 0 (low involvement) to 124. As normative data are not available, it was also completed by the academic researchers to provide a comparison group.

Stage 3: Best practice framework for CDA

The most useful components of the methodology were synthesised by the academic researchers to produce best practice, based on data collected during Stage 2.

Results

Stage 1: Develop the CDA methodology

The critical review identified 10 publications for inclusion, shown in Table 1 [30–33, 48–53].

One publication was a methodology chapter [31], and the others were empirical studies using qualitative methodologies: thematic analysis [30, 33, 49, 52], qualitative content analysis [33, 48], interpretative phenomenological analysis [51], grounded theory [32] and framework analysis [48, 50, 53]. There was strong consensus across all studies that including co-researchers with lived experience in qualitative research data analysis produced richer, more in-depth and alternative understandings of the material that the academic researchers could not have developed on their own. Four methodological approaches to involving PPI co-researchers in data analysis were identified.

CDA approach 1: Consultation

In this approach the academic researchers conducted the analysis process and then presented their work to PPI co-researchers for commentary and feedback. Points of ambiguity or non-consensus identified by academic researchers were highlighted to PPI co-researchers, to achieve a PPI-informed perspective on the data. Studies using this approach tended to have people with lived experience in their research team [30, 33], so while this approach may appear the least democratic CDA approach, these studies had moved beyond the binary categorisation of researchers as academic or service users to reflect the reality of multiple aspects to identity which influence data interpretation and reflexive understanding. When used in studies with this mix of researchers in the academic team, it provides a rapid and cost-effective approach to involving a wider range of PPI perspectives.

CDA approach 2: Development

In studies using this approach [48, 51], PPI co-researchers were involved in the early stages of analysis, inductively developing themes, codes or frameworks based on small samples of transcripts. These were then deductively applied

Table 1 Included publications ($n = 10$)

Ref.	CDA approach	Qualitative design	CDA related findings
[30]	Investigates the value of multiple coding in CDA	Case study	The team were able to develop a strong consensus on the data utilising multiple perspectives
[48]	Qualitative document analysis of NIHR PPI	Case study	Involving members of the public in analysis was successful
[32]	Co-research with people with learning disabilities	Reflective report on ethnographic study	People with learning disabilities can be co-researchers with appropriate support, time and financing
[31]	Methodology chapter exploring CDA theory and application	N/A	N/A
[33]	Investigates service users interpretations of qualitative data	Secondary analysis of papers coded by PPI vs. non-PPI researchers	Service user researchers brought a different perspective, coding according to experiences and feelings, whereas university researchers coded according to processes and procedures
[49]	Process and outcomes of involving service users in data analysis.	Case study	Developed a methodology for conducting long term CDA with people with life limiting conditions
[50]	Process of involving service users in CDA	Case study	Analysed the benefits and challenges of doing CDA with people exploring involvement of patients in medication safety
[51]	Investigates the value of multiple perspectives when interpreting transcripts.	Case study	Service user researchers enhanced the breadth and depth of findings, improving overall study quality
[52]	Describes service user involvement in data analysis	Participatory study	Identified the value of the service users in sharing their perspective in CDA
[53]	Describes involving people with mental health issues in long term CDA	Case study	Described a methodology for conducting long term CDA with people with mental health issues. Found that lack of service user input in early stages of the project impacted on the extent to which co-production was achieved

by the academic researchers to the rest of the data, with resulting points of ambiguity revisited with the PPI co-researchers for clarification and commentary. Hence the focus was on PPI input to create the fundamental constructs informing how the data are understood, with the more procedural work of applying these constructs to a wider range of transcripts delegated to academic researchers. This approach fits projects with financial and time constraints, where achieving maximum PPI input with minimum expenditure is needed.

CDA approach 3: Application

In this approach, the academic researchers lead the analysis process, and then involve PPI co-researchers in applying themes, codes and frameworks to a range of transcripts, including consultation on areas of ambiguity and non-consensus [50]. PPI co-researchers do not create the constructs they are applying to the data, so (unless people with lived experience are in the academic team) this does not lead to service user input to how the data are understood.

CDA approach 4: Development and application

In studies using this approach [49, 52, 53], PPI co-researchers are given extensive training in data analysis techniques, hold multiple meetings over extensive time periods to thoroughly interrogate the data and achieve meaning at a deep, semantic level, and undertake extensive co-revision of themes, codes and frameworks as findings emerge. In essence, if the academic researchers are doing it, so are the PPI co-researchers. The process is entirely co-produced at all levels, so this approach might be termed the gold standard for PPI co-researcher involvement in CDA. In studies with long time scales and larger budgets, this is the most democratic approach to use.

Characteristics of successful CDA

Four characteristics of successful CDA were identified, shown in Table 2 with illustrative texts.

Stage 2: Pilot and refine the CDA methodology

Approaches 1 and 2 were integrated for use in RECOLLECT, as shown in Table 3. As some of the academic researchers were people with dual identities as researchers and with lived experience, concerns around tokenism in Approach 1 were less relevant. Combining this with Approach 2 allowed more meaningful involvement in understanding the data. The intention was that this combination would offer an effective way of conducting CDA within the time and resource boundaries of the study. Approach 3 was not used as it was least collaborative, and Approach 4 was not feasible in a one-year study. The authors incorporated success characteristics shown in Table 2 into planning of the CDA meetings. The CDA focus and the content of each meeting are detailed below.

The Quality Involvement Questionnaire was completed by PPI co-researchers ($n = 6$) and academic researchers ($n = 6$). Self-rated involvement was higher for PPI co-researchers for Your ability (21.2 vs. 20.5), Your potential (15.3 vs 14.2), Research relationships (22.3 vs.

Table 2 Four characteristics (with examples) of successful Collaborative Data Analysis

1. The CDA process is co-produced
   - Keep consulting; verify everything with PPI co-researchers [48]
   - Good facilitation with a supportive and valuing approach is essential. Understand the perspectives/positions of the PPI co-researchers interpreting the data. Be reflexive Be mindful of the personal investments people can hold in how topics are interpreted. [31]
   - Support PPI co-researchers to understand that while experience can be used to help interpret the data, all interpretations must have some basis in that data [50]
   - Ensure a range of perspectives amongst the PPI co-researchers interpreting the data; aim for a heterogeneous group [31, 50]
   - Listen to and explore differences of opinion. When non-consensus occurs, try to create novel synthesis to acknowledge the range of perspectives [31]
2. The CDA process is realistic within available time and resources
   - Ensure sufficient resources exist, e.g. time and money to organise and facilitate CDA. Do not underestimate this [31]
   - Keep the number of analysts relatively small [30]. Use software packages to investigate inter-coder reliability if not everyone is coding all data [31]
   - Make sure data handling and organisation is meticulous [31]
3. The demands of the CDA process are manageable for PPI co-researchers
   - Give PPI co-researchers material to read in advance [48, 49]. Make sure materials are accessible and in a range of formats where required [49, 50]
   - Provide training that ensures people can successfully complete the CDA they have been asked to do [49, 50]. Do 'warm up' activities that align with the CDA tasks people are being asked to undertake [48]. Use practical, visual aids like post-its and flip chart paper to support analysis tasks [48, 49]
   - Keep the data set relatively small and do not present people with too much raw data [30, 48]. Ensure the data analysis process is adjusted to take into account the strengths and needs of PPI co-researchers and is 'failure free' [32]. Allow ample time for analysis [30]
4. Group expectations and dynamics are effectively managed
   - Clearly set out the PPI co-researcher role and expected time commitment [31, 49, 50], and how their contributions will be valued and incorporated [31]. Clarify the division of labour (in writing if appropriate) [31, 49]
   - Be mindful of labelling: people hold multiple identities and categorisation can cause inter-group tensions. Be vigilant for power imbalances, which may occur even with the best of intentions [31]

21.0), Ways of doing research (15.7 vs. 14.3) and Research structures (13.2 vs 11.0), and higher for academic researchers for Your sense of being (18.2 vs. 17.5). Total score was 105.2 (84.8%) for PPI co-researchers and 99.2 (80.%) for academic researchers.

Informal feedback was broadly positive, with one suggestion to use more action-focussed, concrete and illustrative tasks, rather than giving too much information about theory. For example, demonstrating the use of string and self-adhesive arrows to show a causal relationship between a mechanism card and an outcome card if the PPI co-researcher believes the mechanism produces the outcome.

Stage 3: Best practice framework for CDA

Two process findings emerged from conducting the Stage 2 CDA, and from reflections from the involved academic researchers and PPI co-researchers. First, academic researcher facilitators felt that more time was needed for PPI co-researchers to complete the CDA tasks, especially regarding areas of ambiguity and achieving rationalisation and reconciliation in the analyses. Second, a balance was needed between over-planning sessions (risking stifling creativity and encouraging PPI co-researcher passivity) and carefully planning the structure and content of sessions so as to generate the deepest and most collaborative analysis. On balance, we concluded that CDA sessions need to be more structured and formalised than general PPI advisory meetings.

Based on this pilot, and for studies with limited time and financial/human resources (i.e. most funded studies, where compromises between quality and pragmatism are required), we identify a three-stage approach to CDA: Preparation, CDA and Application. Figure 1 shows a proposed best practice framework using these three stages to co-produce a qualitative coding framework.

In RECOLLECT we also used these stages to develop a service user-led model of change, developed by the PPI co-researchers and based on the co-produced coding framework. The Preparation phase was unchanged. In the CDA phase the small group work focussed on how model components (from the co-produced coding framework) relate to each other, using active and practical methods (e.g. laminated cards, sticky tape, string, self-adhesive arrows) to facilitate creativity and easy adjustments. In the Application phase a formatted version of the change model was validated with PPI co-researchers, then verified by the academic researchers with new research participants before being finalised with PPI co-researchers.

Discussion

In this study we reviewed current evidence to identify four reported approaches to CDA involving PPI co-researchers and four characteristics of successful CDA studies. We used this theory base to develop, pilot and refine a methodology, which informed our proposed best practice framework for collaborative analysis of qualitative data in mental health research.

PPI in collaborative data analysis

The National Involvement Partnership has developed the 4Pi national involvement standards: principles (respect, equality); purpose (potential and limits of change), presence (at all decision-making levels), process (engagement, communication, support, practical issues) and impact (ethos/culture, policy/practice, delivery, outputs/outcomes, diversity and equality of opportunity, PPI experience) [54]. Similarly, INVOLVE published a PPI values and principles

Table 3 Overview of RECOLLECT CDA sessions

Meeting 1 April 2017	Preparation (Approach 1) Discussion of the aims of the RECOLLECT project. Explanation of the PPI co-researcher role. Joint agreement on role expectations and ground rules (e.g. confidentiality). Identification of initial PPI suggestions about mechanisms and outcomes for RC students for inclusion as a priori codes in preliminary coding framework.
After Meeting 1	Generation of preliminary coding framework by inductive document analysis ($n = 10$) by academic researchers, incorporating meeting 1 suggestions as a priori codes. Circulation of meeting 2 documents (including preliminary coding framework) in advance
Meeting 2 July 2017	Consultation on a coding framework (Approach 1) Education around qualitative research. Reflexive exercise on what PPI co-researchers bring to the analysis. PPI co-researcher commentary on the content and language used in the preliminary coding framework, and on interpreting areas of ambiguity in data informing the preliminary coding framework
After Meeting 2	Contributions regarding content, language and interpreting areas of ambiguity incorporated into the coding framework by the academic researchers. Deductive coding of remaining documents ($n = 34$) and refinement of coding framework by academic researchers. Refined coding framework circulated to PPI co-researchers for feedback. Circulation of all meeting 3 documents in advance
Meeting 3 September 2017	User-led development of a model of change (Approach 2) Re-visiting and finalising of the refined coding framework. Education around models of change and how to create them. PPI co-researchers develop a model of change using components of the coding framework, illustrate the model with practical examples, and identify the most important components
After Meeting 3	Model of change formatted by the academic researchers. Model of change sent to PPI co-researchers for further commentary and refinement. Incorporation of feedback into the model by the academic researchers. Completion and analysis of semi-structured interviews with stakeholders ($n = 33$) by academic researchers to refine the change model. Circulation of meeting 4 documents in advance
Meeting 4 December 2017	Dissemination, reflection, group processing and celebration Final verification of the model of change. Exploring and reconciling (where possible) remaining areas of ambiguity. Completion of Involvement Questionnaire. Celebration of PPI co-researcher achievements

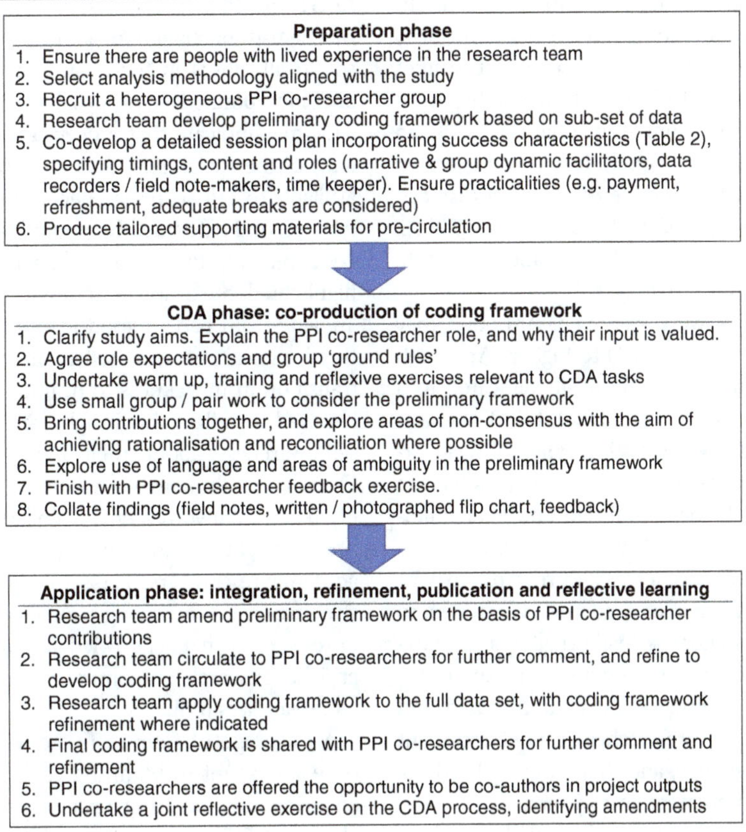

Fig. 1 Best practice framework for collaborative data analysis involving people with lived experience in coding framework co-production

framework emphasising respect, support, transparency, responsiveness, fairness of opportunity and accountability [55]. These principles informed RECOLLECT, although the aim of this study was to incorporate these principles whilst recognising the challenges of time-limited studies. If resources were less limited, desirable extensions would be involvement of PPI co-researchers in all elements of the data analysis, training and supporting PPI co-researchers to undertake the integration activities, and involvement (e.g. through online consultation) of a much larger heterogeneous and more representative PPI group. The decision to have the academic researchers develop the preliminary framework was made because the challenges of having PPI co-researchers undertake primary data coding using qualitative analysis software were deemed too complex. The potential bias introduced by this decision in the overarching interpretation could have been reduced by involving a sub-group of PPI co-researchers at the data coding stage.

The review identified only ten studies of PPI in analysis of qualitative data in mental health research. Despite the increasing PPI literature, empirical studies on involvement at this critical research stage of making sense of qualitative data were relatively few, necessitating extension of the search strategy to include non-mental health research studies. There is more published research about PPI in other research stages, such as the early stage of prioritising important research questions [56, 57]. Established methodologies now exist, such as James Lind Alliance priority setting partnerships [58]. PPI impact assessment studies consistently recommend that PPI needs to occur throughout all research stages. For example, in relation to PPI in quality improvement, guidance concludes '*To be effective, PPI should run through the full cycle of every quality improvement project, as an integral part of the fabric*' [59] (p. 26). The absence of methodologies for collaborative data analysis is an important knowledge gap.

Four approaches to CDA were identified. Although they broadly move from lower (Approach 1) to higher (Approach 4) involvement, they cannot be simplistically allocated to a level of involvement. For example, in RECOLLECT the academic researchers included people with a range of lived experience, several study applicants self-identified as having lived experience, and the PI has published and been influenced by PPI impact assessment studies [60, 61]. Similarly, the PPI group had members with a range of research experience. A particular challenge was for academic researchers to avoid viewing PPI co-researchers as 'just' bringing a lived experience perspective – the strategic essentialism issue of reifying 'people with lived experience' as an undisputed and cohesive category [62]. PPI co-researchers cannot represent the full range of lived experience, and they all bring lived experience as one identity component among many.

Both collaborating parties therefore included members with hybrid identities [63]. Given this complexity, even a consultation approach may be effective, depending on the relational context, which from a PPI perspective is central [64]. The experience of PPI co-researchers will be influenced by whether they trust the academic researchers, whether they perceive the academic researchers really do want their views, even if challenging, and whether changes happen in response to PPI input. The best practice framework adheres to democratic principles, by involving people within research related to their health needs to produce a mutually agreed interpretation of the data [27]. Collaboration was increased by the involvement of people with lived experience as academic researchers, the ongoing relationship between the academic researchers and the PPI group (allowing trusting relationships to form), and repeated contribution verification and incorporation of PPI input [2].

Evaluating the costs and benefits of CDA

Qualitative paradigms encourage researchers to focus on what being human is like, how people understand their worlds and the 'lived experience' [65]. Including PPI co-researchers in analysis supports this goal. Evidence from our pilot confirms that PPI co-researchers interpret data through an overlapping but different lens from academic researchers, so are a resource for highlighting assumptions and reducing interpretive bias [31, 32]. For example, in RECOLLECT the PPI co-researchers proposed that one particular mechanism of change (related to environment) was a precursor to all others in the change model, which was a new – and incorporated – proposal to the academic researchers. This may indicate that a deep understanding of the importance of the social, relational and environment is more easily available to PPI co-researchers than to academic researchers. As a second example, the preliminary framework included a code relating to identity change, but PPI co-researchers highlighted the implicit though unintended implication of 'moving from bad to good identity'. This may reflect encultured clinical research beliefs about improvement meaning transition from sickness to health. Again, the framework was changed to reflect this insight, and researchers also grew in self-awareness about their own values and assumptions. Overall, our findings were consistent with existing evidence [4] that PPI involvement in collaborative data analysis improves quality of the findings and beneficially impacts on academic researchers. The same finding emerges from 'inclusive research' – involving people with intellectual disabilities in research – that acknowledging differences and uniqueness enriches research outcomes and supports reflective practice by researchers [66].

An average of four to five days of academic researcher time was spent in planning each meeting, which involved ensuring that meeting tasks created a 'just right' activity challenge [37], developing training approaches that incorporated andragogic principles [67, 68], and developing supporting materials and pre-circulating these to PPI co-researchers for absorption, comment and refinement. Along with the involvement of other academic researchers ($n = 4$) and PPI co-researchers ($n = 9$) in the four whole-day meetings, overall around 20 person-days were used per meeting, i.e. around 80 person-days extra time was involved in collaborative rather than academic researcher-led data analysis. This reinforces previous warnings not to underestimate the scale of resources involved in CDA [31], and is necessary given the challenges of collaborating on complex mental health topics [69].

CDA studies identified in the review did not emphasise the importance of adjusting tasks to build on PPI co-researcher strengths and reduce the impact of needs, other than practical suggestions such as pre-circulating accessible material, allowing time for tasks, not overwhelming PPI co-researchers with data, and using aids like post-its [30, 48–50].

The goal in RECOLLECT was for the collaborative data analysis to inform the interpretation of the findings. There was little in the published literature about how to measure the extent to which this specific goal was met, beyond the recommendation of verifying findings with PPI co-researchers [48] and obtaining feedback [2, 7]. Available guidance is more general, e.g. PPI reporting guidelines [70] or ethical frameworks [25]. There is also a considerable literature on overarching frameworks for involvement in research, both relating to psychosis [71] and wider frameworks such as community-based participatory research [72], which focus more on principles and examples than on developing a best practice framework as in this study. Future research could: (a) develop a standardised measure of CDA impact (including both costs and benefits); (b) refine through piloting and then manualise the best practice framework, including resources such as relevant warm-up tasks and training exercises and potentially incorporating elements from CDA approaches 3 and 4; and (c) conduct a PPI impact assessment to evaluate the impact of CDA on study findings. This would inform decision-making in studies about whether the benefits of collaborative data outweigh the costs.

Strengths and limitations

This study has developed the first theory-based and piloted best practice framework for collaborative analysis of qualitative data. Strengths include the use of a wide range of health research evidence to inform the framework, the significant investment of human resources, the repeated respondent validation, and the collection of formal and informal feedback demonstrating active involvement by PPI co-researchers.

The findings could be strengthened by conducting a systematised rather than critical review [40], with a stronger focus on obtaining grey literature, use of broader search terms (e.g. coproduction, co-design, emancipatory research, inclusive research, partnership research) and a more formal deductive analysis approach. More consistent involvement of a sub-group of PPI co-researchers in planning the meetings would have increased co-production in the process, and might for example have led to a more structured assessment of accommodations needed by individual PPI co-researchers to allow them to fully contribute. Further piloting, especially in studies which are not as positive towards the use of lived experience as RECOLLECT, would helpfully refine and extend the best practice framework.

Conclusions

This study has developed a typology of approaches to collaborative data analysis in mental health research, identified from available evidence the characteristics of successful involvement, and developed, piloted and refined the first best practice framework for collaborative analysis of qualitative data. Involvement in analysis of findings can be viewed as a human right [73], and this framework has relevance to any qualitative research study which aims to involve people with experience of mental ill-health in interpreting findings.

Abbreviations

CDA: Collaborative data analysis; NIHR: National Institute for Health Research; PPI: Patient and Public Involvement; RC: Recovery College; RECOLLECT: Recovery Colleges Characterisation and Testing

Acknowledgements

MS is supported by the NIHR Nottingham Biomedical Research Centre. Views expressed in this publication are those of the author(s) and not necessarily those of the NHS, the National Institute for Health Research or the Department of Health.

Funding

This report is independent research funded by the National Institute for Health Research (Programme Development Grants, Recovery Colleges Characterisation and Testing (RECOLLECT), RP-DG-0615-10008) in the context of the Nottingham Biomedical Research Centre. The funders had no role in the design of the study or in collection, analysis, and interpretation of data or in writing the manuscript.

Authors' contributions

HJ, MS and RT conceived the design. HJ, MS, PB and RT planned the LEAP workshops. EM was a PPI co-researcher. HJ, MS, PB, EM and RT took part in data collection and contributed to analysis. The drafting of the paper was led by HJ and MS, with comments from PB, EM and RT. All authors read and approved the final manuscript.

Consent for publication

Not applicable.

Competing interests

The authors declare that they have no competing interests.

Author details

[1]Department of Occupational Therapy, School of Health Sciences, York St. John University, York, UK. [2]School of Health Sciences, Institute of Mental Health, University of Nottingham, Triumph Road, Nottingham NG7 2TU, UK. [3]Peter Bates Associates Ltd, Nottingham, UK. [4]RECOLLECT Lived Experience Advisory Panel, Nottingham UK.

References

1. Ashcroft J, Wykes T, Taylor J, Crowther A, Szmukler G. Impact on the individual: what do patients and carers gain, lose and expect from being involved in research? J Ment Health. 2016;25:28–35.
2. INVOLVE.: Briefing notes for researchers: involving the public in NHS, Public Health and social care research. Eastleigh: INVOLVE; 2012.
3. Brett J, Staniszewska S, Mockford C, Herron-Marx S, Hughes J, Tysall C, Suleman R. Mapping the impact of patient and public involvement on health and social care research: a systematic review. Health Expect. 2014;17:637–50.
4. Staley K. Changing what researchers 'think and do': is this how involvement impacts on research? Research for all. 2017;1:158–67.
5. Ennis L, Wykes T. Impact of patient involvement in mental health research: longitudinal study. Br J Psychiatry. 2013;203:381–6.
6. Staley K. 'Is it worth doing?' Measuring the impact of patient and public involvement in research. Research Involvement and Engagement. 2015;1:6.
7. Stacey G, Felton A, Hui A, Stickely T, Houghton P, Diamond B, Morgan J, Shutt J, Willis M. Informed, involved and influential: three is of shared decision making. Ment Health Pract. 2015;19:31–5.
8. Slade M, Jordan H, Clarke E, Williams P, Kaliniecka H, Arnold K, Fiorillo A, Giacco D, Luciano M, Égerházi A, et al. The development and evaluation of a five-language multi-perspective standardised measure: clinical decision-making involvement and satisfaction (CDIS). BMC Health Serv Res. 2014;14:323.
9. Slade M. Implementing shared decision making in routine mental health care. World Psychiatry. 2017;16:146–53.
10. Clarke E, Puschner B, Jordan H, Williams P, Konrad J, Kawohl W, Bär A, Rössler W, Del Vecchio V, Sampogna G, Nagy M, Süveges A, Krogsgaard Bording M, Slade M. Empowerment and satisfaction in a multinational study of routine clinical practice. Acta Psychiatr Scand. 2015;131:369–78.
11. Tambuyzer E, Pieters G, Van A. Patient involvement in mental health care: one size does not fit all. Health Expect. 2014;17:138.
12. Farmer M, Macleod F. Involving disabled people in social reseach. London: Office for Disability Issues; 2011.
13. National Institute for Health Research. National standards for public involvement. Southampton: NIHR; 2018.
14. Shippee D, Garces J, Lopez G, Wang Z, Elraiyah T, Nabhan M, Brito J. Patient and service user engagement in research: a systematic review and synthesized framework. Health Expect. 2015;18:1151–66.
15. National Institute for Health and Clinical Excellence. Service user experience in adult mental health: improving the experience of care for people using adult NHS mental health services. CG136. London: National Institute for Health and Clinical Excellence; 2011.
16. Loos S, Clarke E, Jordan H, Puschner B, Fiorillo A, Luciano M, Ivánka T, Magyar E, Krogsgaard-Bording M, Østermark Sørensen H, Rössler W, Kawohl W, Mayer B, Slade M, CEDAR study group. Recovery and decision-making involvement in people with severe mental illness from six countries: a prospective observational study. BMC Psychiatry. 2017;17
17. Small N, Brooks H, Grundy A, Pedley R, Gibbons C, Lovell K, Bee P. Understanding experiences of and preferences for service user and carer involvement in physical health care discussions within mental health care planning. BMC Psychiatry. 2017;17:138.
18. Samudre S, Shidhaye R, Ahuja S, Nanda S, Khan A, Evans-Lacko S, Hanlon C. Service user involvement for mental health system strengthening in India: a qualitative study. BMC Psychiatry. 2016;16:269.
19. Giacco D, Dirik A, Kaselionyte K, Priebe S. How to make carer involvement in mental health inpatient units happen: a focus group study with patients, carers and clinicians. BMC Psychiatry. 2017;17:101.
20. Pitt V, Lowe D, Hill S, Prictor M, Hetrick SE, Ryan R, Berends L. Consumer-providers of care for adult clients of statutory mental health services. Cochrane Database Syst Rev. 2013;3
21. Rose D, MacDonald D, Wilson A, Crawford M, Barnes M, Omeni E. Service user led organisations in mental health today. J Ment Health. 2016;25:254–9.
22. Kortteisto T, Laitila M, Dosent A. Attitudes of mental health professionals towards service user involvement. Scand J Caring Sci. in press;
23. Scholz B, Gordon S, Happell B. Consumers in mental health service leadership: a systematic review. Int J Ment Health Nurs. 2017;26:20–31.
24. Denegri S. Going the extra mile: improving the nation's health and wellbeing through public involvement in research. London: NIHR; 2015.
25. Pandya-Wood R, Barron D, Elliott J. A framework for public involvement at the design stage of NHS health and social care research: time to develop ethically conscious standards. Research Involvement and Engagement. 2017;3:6.
26. Boaz A, Biri D, McKevitt C. Rethinking the relationship between science and society: has there been a shift in attitudes to patient and public involvement and public engagement in science in the United Kingdom? Health Expect. 2016;19:592–601.
27. Green G. Power to the people: to what extent has public involvement in applied health research achieved this? Research Involvement and Engagement. 2016;2:28.
28. European Commission: White paper on citizen science for Europe. ec.europa.eu/futurium/en/content/white-paper-citizen-science: date of access: 29/11/2017; 2015.
29. Moss N, Daru J, Lanz D, Thangaratinam S, Khan K. Involving pregnant women, mothers and members of the public to improve the quality of women's health research. Br J Obstet Gynaecol. 2016; https://doi.org/10.1111/1471-0528.14419.
30. Sweeney A, Greenwood K, Williams S, Wykes T, Rose D. Hearing the voices of service user researchers in collaborative qualitative data analysis: the case for multiple coding. Health Expect. 2013;17:e89-e99.
31. Cornish F, Gillespie A, Zittoun T. Collaborative analysis of qualitative data. In: Flick U, editor. Handbook of qualitative data analysis. London: Sage; 2013. p. 79–93.
32. Tuffrey-Wijne I, Butler G. Co-researching with people with learning disabilities: an experience of involvement in qualitative data analysis. Health Expect. 2010;13:174–84.
33. Gillard S, Borschmann R, Turner K, Goodrich-Purnell N, Lovell K, Chambers M. 'What difference does it make?' Finding evidence of the impact of mental health service user researchers on research into the experiences of detained psychiatric patients. Health Expect. 2010;13:185–94.
34. Perkins R, Repper, J., Rinaldi, M., Brown, H.: ImROC 1. Recovery colleges. London: Centre for Mental Health; 2012.
35. Slade M, McDaid D, Shepherd G, Williams S, Repper J. ImROC briefing paper 14. Recovery: the business case. ImROC: Nottingham; 2017.
36. Kelly J, Gallagher S, McMahon J. Developing a recovery college: a preliminary exercise in establishing regional readiness and community needs. J Ment Health. 2017;26:150–5.
37. McCaig M, McNay L, Marland G, Bradstreet S, Campbell J. Establishing a recovery college in a Scottish university. Ment Health Soc Incl. 2014;18:92–7.
38. McGregor J, Repper J, Brown H. "The college is so different from anything I have done". A study of the characteristics of Nottingham recovery college. J Mental Health Training, Education and Practice. 2014;9:3–15.
39. Christensen C. The innovator's dilemma: when new technologies cause great firms to fail. In: Boston: Harvard business school; 1997.
40. Grant MJ, Booth A. A typology of reviews: an analysis of 14 review types and associated methodologies. Health Inf Libr J. 2009;26(2):91–108.
41. Aveyard H. Doing a literature review in health and social care: a practical guide. 3rd ed. London: Open University Press; 2014.
42. Gale N, Heath G, Cameron E, Rashid S, Redwood S. Using the framework method for the analysis of qualitative data in multi-disciplinary health research. BMC Med Res Methodol. 2013;13:117.
43. Chard G. Analysis of occupational performance. In: Curtin M, Molineux M, Supyk-Melson J, editors. Occupational therapy and physical dysfunction: enabling occupation. Churchill Livingstone Elsevier: Edinburgh; 2010.
44. Crepeau E, Schell, B. in Crepeau EB et al (eds) Analyzing occupations and activity. In: Willard and Spackman's Occupational Therapy 11th ed. EDN Edited by Crepeau E, Cohn, E., Schell, B. Philadelphia: Lippincott Williams & Wilkins; 2009.
45. Brett J, Staniszewska, S., Mockford, C., Seers, K., Herron-Marx, S., Bayliss, H. (2010). University of Warwick: University of Warwick.. : The PIRICOM study: a systematic review of the conceptualisation, measurement, impact and outcomes of patients and public involvement in health and social care research. Coventry: University of Warwick; 2013.

46. Krefting L. Rigor in qualitative research: the assessment of trustworthiness. Am J Occup Ther. 1991;45:214–22.
47. Morrow E, Ross F, Grocott P, Bennett J. A model and measure for quality service user involvement in health research. Int J Consum Stud. 2010;34: 532–9.
48. Baxter S, Muir D, Brereton L, Allmark C, Barber R, Harris L, Hodges B, Khan S, Baird W. Evaluating public involvement in research design and grant development: using a qualitative document analysis method to analyse an award scheme for researchers. Research Involvement and Engagement. 2016;2:13.
49. Cotterell P. Exploring the value of service user involvement in data analysis: 'our interpretation is about what lies below the surface'. Educational Action Research. 2008;16:5–17.
50. Garfield S, Jheeta, S., Husson, F., Jacklin, A., Bischler, A., Norton, C., Franklin, B.: Lay involvement in the analysis of qualitative data in health services research: a descriptive study. 2016, 2(29).
51. Mjøsund N, Eriksson M, Espnes G, Haaland-Øverby M, Jensen S, Norheim I, Kjus S, Portaasen I, Vinje H. Service user involvement enhanced the research quality in a study using interpretative phenomenological analysis – the power of multiple perspectives. J Adv Nurs. 2016;73:265–78.
52. Sixsmith J, Callender M, Hobbs G, Corr S, Huber J. Implementing the National Service Framework for long-term (neurological) conditions: service user and service provider experiences. Disabil Rehabil. 2014;36:563–72.
53. Gillard S, Simons L, Turner K, Lucock M, Edwards C. Patient and public involvement in the coproduction of knowledge. Qual Health Res. 2012;22: 1126–37.
54. National Involvement Partnership. Involvement for influence. In: London: NSUN; 2015.
55. INVOLVE: Public involvement in research: values and principles Framework Eastleigh: INVOLVE; 2015.
56. MQ: UK mental Health Research funding. London: MQ; 2015.
57. Banfield MA, Griffiths KM, Christensen HM, Barney LJ. SCOPE for research: mental health consumers' priorities for research compared with recent research in Australia. Aust N Z J Psychiatry. 2011;45(12):1078–85.
58. Crowe S, Giles C. Making patient relevant clinical research a reality. BMJ. 2016;355:i6627.
59. Healthcare Quality Improvement Partnership: Patient and public involvement in quality improvement. London: HQIP service user network; 2016.
60. Slade M, Bird V, Chandler R, Fox J, Larsen J, Tew J, Leamy M. The contribution of advisory committees and public involvement to large studies: case study. BMC Health Serv Res. 2010;10:323.
61. Slade M, Trivedi P, Chandler R, Leamy M. Developing involvement during a programme of recovery research. J Mental Health Training, Education and Practice. 2016;11:244–55.
62. Voronka J. The politics of 'people with lived experience' experiential authority and the risks of strategic essentialism. CEDAR study group. Psychiatry and Psychology. 2016;23:189–201.
63. McGivern G, Currie G, Ferlie E, Fitzgerald L, Waring J. Hybrid manager–professionals' identity work: the maintenance and hybridization of medical professionalism in managerial contexts. Public Adm. 2015;93:412–32.
64. Gamble C, Dudley L, Allam A, Bell P, Buck D, Goodare H. An evidence base to optimise methods for involving patient and public contributors in clinical trials: a mixed-methods study. Health Services and Delivery Research. 2015;3(39)
65. Smith J, Flowers P, Larkin M. Interpretative phenomenological analysis: theory, method and research. London: Sage; 2009.
66. Woelders S, Abma T, Visser T, Schipper K. The power of difference in inclusive research. Disability & Society. 2015;30:528–42.
67. Mezirow J. Transformative dimensions of adult learning. San Francisco: Jossey-Bass; 1991.
68. Honey PM, A.: The Manual of Learning Styles. Maidenhead: Peter Honey; 1986.
69. Baart I, Abma T. Patient participation in fundamental psychiatric genomics research: a Dutch case study. Health Expect. 2011;14:240–9.
70. Staniszewska S, Brett J, Simera I, Seers K, Mockford C, Goodlad S, Altman D, Moher D, Barber R, Denegri S, Entwistle A, Littlejohns P, Morris C, Suleman R, Thomas V, Tysall C. GRIPP2 reporting checklists: tools to improve reporting of patient and public involvement in research. BMJ. 2017;358: j3453.
71. Bryant W, Parsonage, J., Tibbs, A., Andrews, C., Clark, J., Franco, L.: Meeting in the mist: key considerations in a collaborative research partnership with people with mental health issues. WORK: A Journal of Prevention, Assessment, and Rehabilitation 2012, 43:23–31.
72. Lucero J, Wallerstein N, Duran B, Alegria M, Greene-Moton E, Israel B, Kastelic S, Magarati M, Oetzel J, Pearson C, Schulz A, Villegas M, White Hat E. Development of a mixed methods investigation of process and outcomes of community-based participatory research. J Mixed Methods Research. 2018;12:55–74.
73. Ollerton J, Horsfall D. Rights to research: utilising the convention on the rights of persons with disabilities as an inclusive participatory action research tool. Disability & Society. 2013;28:616–30.

5

Towards sustainable mental health promotion: trial-based health-economic evaluation of a positive psychology intervention versus usual care

Marijke Schotanus-Dijkstra[1*], Constance H. C. Drossaert[1], Marcel E. Pieterse[1], Jan A. Walburg[1], Ernst T. Bohlmeijer[1] and Filip Smit[2,3,4]

Abstract

Background: Mental well-being could be promoted and protected by positive psychology (PP) based interventions. Such interventions may be appealing for people at risk of anxiety and depressive disorders, but health-economic evaluations are scarce. The aim was to examine the cost-effectiveness of a PP intervention.

Methods: Participants with suboptimal levels of mental well-being were randomly assigned to an email guided PP-intervention ($n = 137$) or a wait-list control group ($n = 138$) with access to usual care (UC). At baseline and 6 months follow-up, data were collected on health care costs. Outcomes of interest were flourishing mental health and treatment response on anxiety and depressive symptoms.

Results: Bootstrapped mean incremental cost-effectiveness ratios were €2359 ($2899) for flourishing, €2959 ($3637) for anxiety and €2578 ($3168) for depression, suggesting appreciable health gains for low additional costs. At a willingness to pay ceiling of €10,000 ($12,290) for a treatment response, the probability that the intervention is deemed cost-effective ranged between 90 and 93%.

Conclusions: The guided PP intervention appears to be a promising strategy as seen from both a public health and a health-economic perspective, especially when there is some willingness to pay. When the PP-intervention is scaled up, then outcome monitoring is recommended to better guarantee the longer term cost-effectiveness of the intervention.

Keywords: Cost-effectiveness, Mental well-being, Guided self-help, Prevention, Positive psychology, Randomized controlled trial

Background

A new cost-effective strategy for the prevention of anxiety and depressive disorders might be to promote a flourishing mental health state in people with low or moderate levels of mental well-being [1, 2]. Earlier studies demonstrated that these people have an increased health care use[3] with concomitant health care costs and productivity losses [3–5]. Flourishing is defined as the presence of *high levels* of emotional well-being (e.g. life-satisfaction, positive affect) in combination with *high levels* of social and psychological well-being (e.g. social contribution, positive relationships, self-acceptance, purpose in life) [6, 7].

Longitudinal studies have shown that flourishing helps to protect against first-onset and recurrence of diagnosed mood and anxiety disorders [8, 9]. Other promising results stem from two of our randomized controlled trials demonstrating that individuals are able to improve their well-being up to flourishing levels using email guided bibliotherapy based on a positive

* Correspondence: m.schotanus@utwente.nl
[1]Centre for eHealth and Well-being Research, Department of Psychology, Health and Technology, University of Twente, P.O. Box 217, 7500 AE Enschede, The Netherlands
Full list of author information is available at the end of the article

psychology or related framework [10, 11]. The same studies also found beneficial effects on anxiety and depressive symptoms, suggesting that deteriorating mental health could be prevented by such self-help interventions. Self-help books are widely available and have the purpose to reach the lay public [12]. However, it is yet unknown whether positive psychology (PP) based bibliotherapy programs are cost-effective [13].

To our knowledge, only one prior study evaluated the cost-effectiveness of a positive psychology intervention, which was an online multicomponent intervention for people with mild to moderate depressive symptoms [14]. This non-guided web-based intervention contained psycho-education and practical exercises about goal setting, positive emotions, positive relations, mindfulness, optimism and mastery. Participants in the experimental condition could independently select modules and exercises to tailor the intervention to their needs. At six months follow-up, the intervention was not effective in improving the primary outcome of mental well-being, but it was effective in reducing depressive symptoms compared to a wait-list (usual care) control group. However, the online intervention was not found to be cost-effective from a societal cost-effective perspective on any outcome measure [14]. According to the authors, these somewhat disappointing findings might be partly attributed to the lack of compliance, since only 10% of the participants completed at least one module as recommended [14, 15]. Therefore, a more cost-effective self-help format for positive interventions might include some therapist involvement to increase adherence. The present economic evaluation uses our trial data of an early bibliotherapy intervention for people with suboptimal levels of mental well-being [11]. We hypothesized that this PP-based self-help intervention with some guidance over the Internet was also cost-effective relative to usual care alone.

Methods

Design and participants

The non-blinded randomized controlled trial was conducted in two parallel groups, with computerized randomization using Excel (1:1 allocation) and stratified for gender and education (low, medium, high) performed by the first author. For each group, a contact list was created in Qualtrics, making it possible to send personal emails to participants (e.g. including the result of the randomized assignment) without interference of the researcher. A sample size of 132 participants per condition was required to provide a statistical power of 80%, two-sided with α of 5% and compensating for a 25% drop-out rate, to detect a small to medium effect size (Cohen's d of 0.40) on the main outcome i.e. mental well-being (a continuous measure) [16, 17]. Although the primary outcome of the current study was the binary measure of mental well-being, a similar sample size was needed when the power calculation was adjusted to a χ^2 test and intention-to-treat data ($n = 126$ per group). Participants aged 18 years or older were recruited from the general Dutch population in January 2014 via national advertisements calling for people who were motivated to actively work on their "well-being and resilience". The participants were willing to invest an average time of 4 h per week for 9 weeks and had access to email and the Internet. Interested participants completed a contact form via a research website, and received an online informed consent procedure per email before they could access the online screening survey. Eligible participants were excluded when they were younger than 18 years of age, already possessed a flourishing mental health status as measured with the Mental Health Continuum-Short Form (MHC-SF); scoring 4 or 5 on at least one emotional well-being item together with a score of 4 or 5 on at least 6 of the 11 social and psychological well-being items [7, 18] or when they presented scores above 10 on at least one subscale of the Hospital Anxiety and Depression Scale (HADS), indicating moderate to severe anxiety or depressive symptoms [19]. Also, participants had to complete the screening and baseline questionnaire because randomization took place after baseline.

In total, 518 participants were interested in participating in the study, of which 243 participants had to be excluded [11]. The final sample of 275 participants were allocated to the intervention group ($n = 137$) or the wait-list control group ($n = 138$). The trial protocol was approved by the Ethics Committee of the University of Twente (no. 13212) and registered at The Netherlands Trial Register (NTR4297). The design of the study [20] and its main findings [11] are published elsewhere.

Interventions

Participants in the intervention group received (1) the self-help book *This is Your Life* [21], (2) a 9-week time schedule for reading the book with recommended exercises, and (3) weekly email support from a personal counselor. The book consists of eight chapters containing psycho-education, theoretical background information, and a variety of evidence-based exercises from positive psychology, but also from mindfulness and acceptance and commitment therapy. The purpose of the book is to improve an individual's capacity to savor positive emotions, discover and use character strengths, encourage flow and an optimistic attributional style, develop self-acceptance and compassion, learn to cope with adversity (resilience), and encourage to share and connect with others [20]. The chapter about discovering and using character strengths was spread out over 2 weeks in the time schedule. Participants had 8 to 12 weeks to complete the program. A full description of each chapter and recommended exercises can be found elsewhere [20].

Once a week, participants emailed their personal counselor with their experiences about the chapter and corresponding exercises. Five positive psychology students each guided 25 participants and the first author guided the remaining participants. The counselors were trained in providing email support during a study course plus a one-day workshop. In addition, they attended weekly supervision meetings. The email correspondence was aimed at increasing adherence. On average, participants reported that they had completed 6.4 (out of the 8) chapters (SD = 2.4) and had sent 6.4 extensive emails (SD = 3.62), indicating adequate adherence to the protocol [11].

Participants in the wait-list control group received the self-help book *This is Your Life* and the 9-week time schedule after completing the 6 months assessment. Participants in both conditions had unrestricted access to usual care.

Health related outcomes

The primary outcome was flourishing mental health and the secondary outcomes were anxiety and depressive symptoms. Self-reported data were obtained from online questionnaires at baseline and 6 months follow-up.

Flourishing

The 14-item MHC-SF measures mental well-being on a continuous scale but can also classify people into (1) flourishing mental health, (2) moderate mental health or (3) languishing mental health [18, 22], although we put the latter two categories together because there were few people with languishing mental health in the current sample at baseline (4.4%). In a cost-effectiveness study, hard currency (measured at the interval level) cannot be meaningfully related to health benefits that are measured at the ("elastic") ordinal measurement scale. It is economically more meaningful to relate hard currency to a binary outcome such as treatment response, where treatment response is clearly defined as reliable change [23] or as a transition from one health state (e.g. languishing or moderate mental health) to another (e.g. flourishing mental health).

The first three items of the MHC-SF measure emotional well-being (i.e. happiness, interest, life-satisfaction), the next five items measure social well-being (i.e. social contribution, social integration, social actualization, social acceptance, social coherence) and the last six items tap into psychological well-being (i.e. self-acceptance, mastery, positive relations, personal growth, autonomy, purpose in life). Each item was scored on a 6-point scale from 0 (never) to 5 (almost always). Flourishing is theoretically operationalized as scoring 4 or 5 on at least one emotional well-being item together with a score of 4 or 5 on at least 6 of the 11 remaining items, which parallels the DSM-IV approach to diagnose a major depression [7, 18, 24]. The Dutch version of the MHC-SF has shown good psychometric properties [22] and showed good internal consistency in the current study ($\alpha = 0.88$).

Anxiety and depressive symptoms

Anxiety and depressive symptoms were measured with the HADS-A and HADS-D respectively. Each subscale has 7 items with scores ranging from 0 to 3. Total summed scores range from 0 to 21, with higher scores indicating greater anxiety or depressive symptom severity. The HADS has shown good psychometric properties in the Dutch population [25, 26] and showed good internal consistency in the current sample ($\alpha = 0.76$ for both subscales). To measure treatment response on these scales, Jacobson and Truax' method [23] was applied to obtain the reliable change index to distinguish between treatment responders and non-responders. The reliable change index was calculated as $x_2 - x_1 / S_{diff}$, where x_2 is the post-test score and x_1 is the baseline score. S_{diff} is the standard error of difference between the pre- and post-test scores which is calculated as $\sqrt{(2(S_E)^2)}$, where the standard error of measurement (S_E) is calculated as $SD\sqrt{(1 - r_{xx})}$. r_{xx} is the test-retest reliability of the measure, which was 0.89 for the HADS-A and 0.86 for the HADS-D [26]. A treatment responder was estimated to be a pre-post change of at least 2.22 points on the anxiety subscale and 2.55 points on the depression subscale, taking the 95% criterion into account ($z = 1.96$).

Resource use and costing

The current study adopts a health sector perspective in accordance with national UK and US guidelines [27, 28]. Therefore, direct medical costs (health service use), direct non-medical costs (travel costs to health services) and intervention costs were included and not productivity losses. Resource use was measured with the Medical Consumption Questionnaire (MCQ) for three periods: 3 months before baseline (T0), baseline to 3 months follow-up (T1) and 3 to 6 months follow-up (T2) [29]. All costs are expressed in euros (€) for the reference year 2014. The main results are also expressed in US dollars ($). The general purchasing power parity (PPP) was used for conversion of the € to $ for 2014 (US$1.00 = NL€0.814) [30].

Direct medical and non-medical costs

Table 1 displays an overview of health service units (contacts or hours) and their standard unit cost price as reported in the Dutch guidelines for health-economic evaluations [31]. Health service costs per participant were calculated by multiplying the utilized health service units of each participant in the past 3 months with the standard unit cost price of that service. Travel costs for each health service visit were calculated by multiplying the average distance to that service according to the

Table 1 Unit cost price for direct medical and direct non-medical costs by the reference year 2014

	Direct medical costs		Direct non-medical costs	
Health service type	Unit	Unit cost price	km	Unit cost price
Family doctor – standard consult	Contact	33	1,1	3.21
Family doctor – mental health	Contact	66	1,1	3.21
Family doctor – home visit	Contact	50	NA	NA
Company doctor	Contact	33	17,6	6.34
Social worker	Contact	65	5	3.95
Regional mental health center	Contact	112	10	4.90
Regional addiction center	Contact	112	10	4.90
Independent psychologist, psychotherapist, psychiatrist	Contact	94	7	4.33
Psychologist, psychotherapist, psychiatrist in hospital[a]	Contact	91	7	4.33
Self-help group	Hour	14	7	4.33
Alternative healer[b]	Contact	55	5	3.95

[a]Unit cost price was based on a weighted mean of a general and academic hospital
[b]Unit cost price was based on own calculation as weighted average of homeopath and acupuncturist

Dutch guidelines (see Table 1) with the costs per km (€0.19). Parking costs were added to the travel costs which amounted to €3 per visit. Other costs of participants or its family members outside formal health care (e.g. informal care) which might have had a direct relation with an illness were not included in this health-economic evaluation because no severe (chronic) disorders were investigated and the sum of these costs would be limited.

Intervention costs

Each participant in the intervention group received the self-help book *This is Your Life* which was valued at €25 in 2014 as found in a large and representative online bookstore in The Netherlands. Each participant also received personal email support. Although the current study used students as counselors, in real-life health care settings these will be replaced by the family doctor's mental health nurse at €17 per consult [31]. We assume an average of nine email contacts, which puts the costs at €17*9 contacts = €153 per participant. Additional costs were incurred for recruitment, screening and training costs for the mental health nurse at €44 per participant in a real-world setting. In total, the estimated intervention costs were €222 ($273) per participant.

Analysis

Statistical analyses

Analyses of the health related outcomes were carried out in accordance with the intention-to-treat principle. Missing data on the MHC-SF, HADS-A and HADS-D at T2 were imputed using the expectation maximization (EM) algorithm in SPSS (IBM, Chicago, Ill., USA) version 22.0. The results of these health effects were also reported in our prior trial but repeated here for clarity [11].

Cost-effectiveness analyses

The Consolidated Health Economic Evaluation Reporting Standards (CHEERS) were followed [27]. Therefore, the intention-to-treat principle was also applied to the cost data and these were imputed using EM. In order to compare our results with other cost-effectiveness studies, costs were annualized by multiplying the costs of three months by 4. No discounting of costs and effects was applied because the study's follow-up did not exceed one year [27]. Furthermore, the conditions were compared as if operating under steady-state conditions. This means that it is assumed that the health care costs in the past 3 months (as well as the health gains in the past 4 weeks) as measured at the 6 month follow-up are representative for a whole year with the proviso that there were no significant baseline differences between the conditions. Therefore, only the annualized 6 months health care costs (including the intervention costs in the intervention condition) were used for calculating the incremental cost-effectiveness ratio (ICER). The ICER is calculated as $(C_1 - C_0)/(E_1 - E_0)$, where C is the average annualized per-participant health care costs in the experimental and control condition (i.e. incremental costs) and E is the proportion of flourishers or treatment responders on the HADS (i.e. incremental effects). The subscripts 1 and 0 refer to the intervention and control condition, respectively. The ICERs represent the incremental costs per additional treatment responder in the intervention as compared to the control group.

A Microsoft Excel macro was used to simulate 2500 ICERs in a non-parametric bootstrap procedure. With this resampling procedure, each estimated ICER was plotted in a cost-effectiveness plane. In this plane, the costs are presented on the x-axis and the health outcomes (i.e. flourishing, anxiety, depression) on the y-axis. When the dots are mainly plotted in the northwest (NW) quadrant (higher costs, less health) or southeast (SE) quadrant (lower costs, health gains), this means that a clear decision can be made from a cost-effective perspective; i.e. the intervention is unacceptable (dominated by usual care) in the NW quadrant and acceptable (dominant) in the SE quadrant compared to the control group. However, the northeast (NE) quadrant (higher costs, health gains) and southwest (SW) quadrant (lower costs, less health) require a more advanced decision-making to balance higher or lower costs against greater or lesser health gains, for which a cost-effectiveness acceptability curve is being used. This curve provides insight into the probability of accepting an intervention relative to a control condition. In the present study, this curve displays hypothetical willingness to pay (WTP) ceilings (€0 - €30,000) for gaining one additional treatment responder on flourishing, anxiety and depressive symptoms respectively (on the x-axis) and graphs the likelihood that the PP intervention is deemed to be of acceptable cost-effectiveness (on the y-axis).

Sensitivity analysis

The analyses were repeated for three different scenarios to examine the robustness of the results. In scenario A, the intervention costs were based on the actual number of emails sent by the personal counselor to the participant (not the assumed maximum of 9 emails) and then multiplied by the costs for consulting a family's doctor mental health nurse (€17). In scenario B, the intervention costs were raised by including the time investment of participants (valued at 3 h*9 weeks*€14) amounted to a total of €600 per participant. In scenario C, completers-only analyses were performed, using data of the 112 participants in the intervention condition and 125 participants in the control condition who completed all measurements at T2.

Results

Sample characteristics

Participants were predominantly female (85.8%), higher educated (74.5%) and in paid employment (68.4%). Mean age was 47.8 years (SD = 10.9). The mean score of the total sample for mental well-being was 2.57 (SD = 0.63), for anxiety symptoms 7.28 (SD = 2.41) and for depressive symptoms 5.80 (SD = 2.47). There were no significant between-group differences regarding participant characteristics, main outcome measures and resource costs.

Health effects

At 6 months, there were 42 participants (30.7%) with flourishing mental health in the intervention condition and 16 participants (11.6%) in the control condition ($\chi^2 = 15.01$, $df = 1$, $P = < 0.001$), as has also been reported previously [11]. The incremental effect (i.e. the proportion of flourishers in the experimental group minus the proportion of flourishers in the control group) was 0.31–0.12 = 0.19. Similar effects were found for anxiety and depressive symptoms. For the HADS-A, 57 participants (41.6%) in the intervention group met the criteria for treatment response compared to 27 participants (19.6%) in the control group ($\chi^2 = 15.74$, $df = 1$, $P = < 0.001$). For the HADS-D, these number of participants were 59 (43.1%) in the intervention group and 30 (21.7%) in the control group ($\chi^2 = 14.29$, $df = 1$, $P = < 0.001$). The incremental effects were 0.42–0.20 = 0.22 for anxiety symptoms and 0.43–0.22 = 0.21 for depressive symptoms.

Costs

At baseline, total average annualized direct medical and direct non-medical costs were €581 (SD = €1190) in the intervention condition and €675 (SD = €1246) in the control condition (Table 2). At T1, these costs were €432 (SD = €983) and €658 (SD = €1224) respectively. At T2, these costs were €506 (SD = €1001) for the guided self-help intervention and €488 (SD = €1190) for usual care. These T2 annualized costs were used for the cost-effectiveness analyses, adding the intervention costs of €222 to the intervention condition. Therefore, the annualized incremental costs at the trial's follow-up were €728–€488 = €240 ($295).

Cost-effectiveness: Flourishing

The bootstrapped mean ICER shows that additional costs of €2359 ($2899) had to be paid to improve one person from low or moderate well-being to flourishing mental health. The bootstrapped median ICER showed additional costs of €1245 ($1530; Table 3). The majority of the plotted ICERs (92%) occurred in the northeast quadrant, indicating that the intervention produced health gains at additional costs (Fig. 1). All other plotted ICERs occurred in the southeast quadrant (8%), which implies health gains at lower costs. When there is no WTP, there is a 12% probability that the guided self-help intervention is more cost-effective relative to usual care (Fig. 2). This probability increases to 93% with a WTP ceiling for a favorable treatment outcome of €10,000 ($12,290). Conversely, with a probability of 80% the WTP is approximately €8000 ($9832).

Cost-effectiveness: Anxiety and depressive symptoms

The bootstrapped mean and median ICERs for treatment response on anxiety symptoms were €2959 ($3637) and €1095 ($1346) respectively, and for depressive symptoms €2578 ($3168) and €1189 ($1461; Table 4). The distribution of the 2500 bootstrapped ICERs on the cost-effectiveness plane as well as the WTP curve show similar results as has been found for flourishing: 91 and 90% of the ICERs were plotted in the northeast quadrant for anxiety and depressive symptoms respectively. The probability of accepting the intervention in favor of

Table 2 Per participant annualized costs in Euros (€) by condition, for 3 months prior to baseline, 0–3 months during intervention (t0-t1) and 3–6 months after intervention (t1-t2)

	Baseline Mean (SD)	0–3 months Mean (SD)	3–6 months Mean (SD)
Wait-list control group (*n* = 138)			
Direct medical costs	637.16 (1185.66)	620.49 (1167.22)	462.97 (1137.84)
Direct non-medical costs	38.14 (61.87)	37.50 (59.61)	25.36 (52.71)
Intervention costs	NA	NA	NA
Total costs	675.30 (1245.89)	657.99 (1223.89)	488.33 (1189.92)
Self-help with email support (*n* = 137)			
Direct medical costs	546.83 (1128.45)	408.09 (939.50)	478.05 (956.73)
Direct non-medical costs	34.07 (63.50)	23.58 (44.69)	27.77 (45.94)
Intervention costs	NA	222	NA
Total costs	580.90 (1190.07)	653.66 (982.97)	505.82 (1001.27)[a]

[a]For further analyses, these annualized costs were included plus the intervention costs of €222. The total mean costs amounted to 727.82 (SD = 1001.27) at 6 months

usual care with no WTP was 13% for both outcomes. At a WTP of €10,000, the probability of accepting the intervention had risen to 92 and 93% respectively.

Sensitivity analyses

The results from the alternative scenarios show similar patterns for all three outcomes (see Table 3 for flourishing and Table 4 for anxiety and depression). Most mean and median bootstrapped ICERs were lowest in scenario A based on the actual intervention costs with mean ICERs between €1848 ($2271) and €2109 ($2592). Scenario B (intervention costs including the opportunity costs of the participants loss of leisure time) revealed the highest mean and median ICERs, while the completers-only analysis of scenario C was more comparable to scenario A. The percentage of ICERs on the cost-effectiveness planes for treatment response lies between 86% (scenario A) and 100% (scenario B). Furthermore, the probability of accepting the intervention over the control condition at no WTP lies between 4% (scenario B) and 18% (scenario A). In sum, these sensitivity analyses provide support for the robustness of the main analyses.

Discussion

This health-economic evaluation is the first of its kind evaluating the cost-effectiveness of bibliotherapy based

Table 3 Cost-effectiveness analysis and sensitivity analysis with flourishing as health outcome

Flourishing	Total sample	Alternative scenarios		
		A	B	C
Costs, €[a]	239	196	617	223
Effect	0.19	0.19	0.19	0.20
ICER, €[b]	1245	1058	3240	1099
Distribution on the cost-effectiveness plane				
1st quadrant (northeast)	92	86	100	89
2nd quadrant (inferior: northwest)	0	0	0	0
3rd quadrant (southwest)	0	0	0	0
4th quadrant (superior: southeast)	8	14	0	11
WTP ceiling, %				
€ 0	12	18	4	14
€ 10,000	93	92	91	93
€ 20,000	97	97	96	97
€ 30,000	100	100	100	100

Scenario A = adjustment of the per participant intervention costs, based on actual costs for counseling (the number of extensive emails sent by each participant multiplied by €17); scenario B = intervention costs raised from €222 to €600; scenario C = completers only analysis (*n* = 112 intervention group and *n* = 125 control group)

[a]Costs per 'disease-free' year (i.e. one year in flourishing mental health) at 2014 prices

[b]Bootstrapped median, which is the 50th percentile of 2500 replications of the ICER

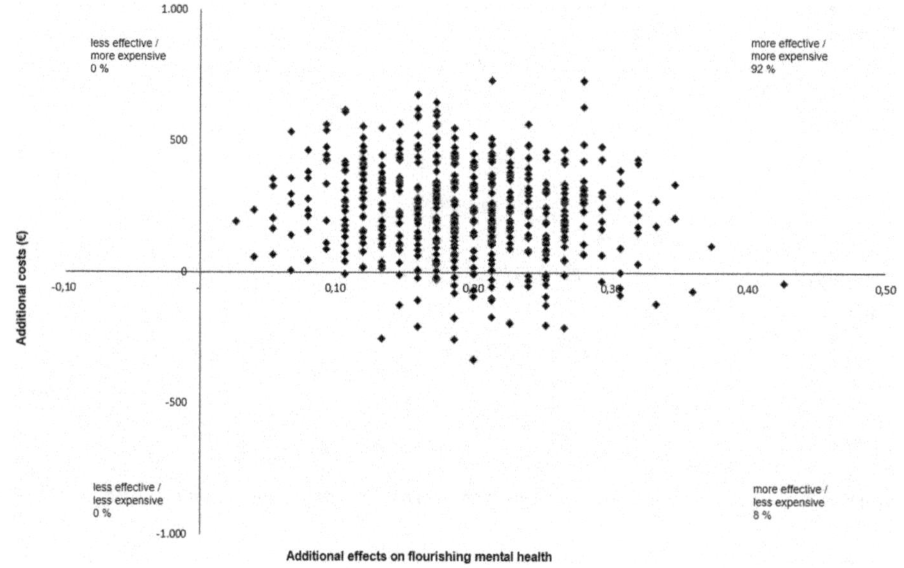

Fig. 1 Cost-effectiveness plane of 2500 bootstrapped incremental cost-effectiveness ratios (ICERs) for flourishing, primary analysis

on a positive psychology framework. Participants with low or moderate levels of mental well-being received the book *This is Your Life* with email support or were placed on a wait-list (with full access to usual care). Results demonstrated that the intervention was effective at 6 months, showing significant improvements in mental well-being (from non-flourishing to flourishing mental health) while also decreasing both anxiety and depressive symptom severity [11]. However, owing to the intervention costs, the health care costs at 6 months were higher in the intervention group than the control group. The intervention costs were varied in sensitivity analyses, but all findings pointed in the same direction: substantial health gains can be expected from the intervention against an increase in health care costs of some €883~€4534 ($1085~$5572). From a decision-making point of view it might be worthwhile to note that the probability of regarding the intervention as cost-effective exceeds 90% at a willingness to pay of €10,000 ($12,290) per treatment responder.

These findings corroborate prior findings from cost-effectiveness analyses of (guided) bibliotherapy for depression [32, 33] and binge-eating disorder [34], although these interventions were based on cognitive behavioral therapy (CBT). Economic evaluations of web-based self-help interventions (mostly CBT-based)

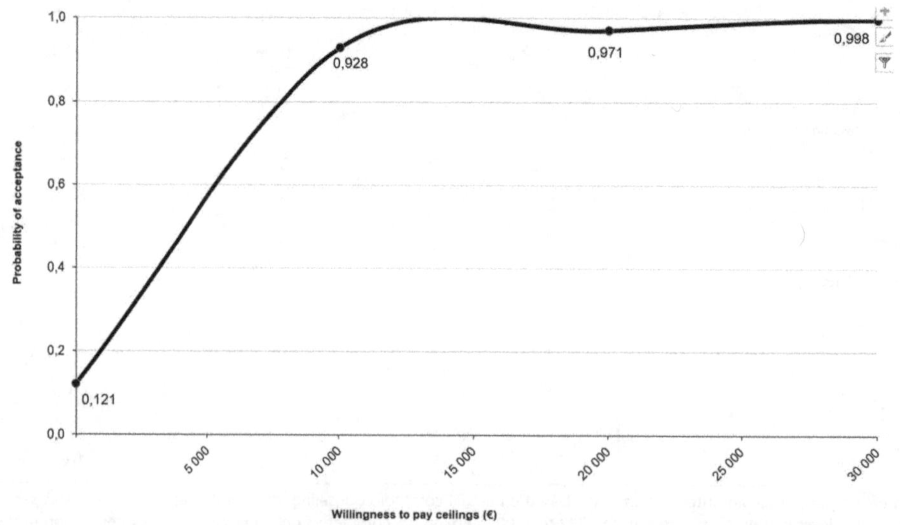

Fig. 2 Cost-effectiveness acceptability curve: bootstrapped probability ($n = 2500$) that the guided PP-based intervention is acceptable compared to care as usual given varying willingness to pay ceilings, with flourishing as health outcome

Table 4 Cost-effectiveness analysis and sensitivity analysis with anxiety and depressive symptoms as health outcomes

	Total sample		Alternative scenarios					
			A		B		C	
	Anxiety	Depression	Anxiety	Depression	Anxiety	Depression	Anxiety	Depression
Costs, €[a]	239	239	196	196	617	617	223	223
Effect	0.22	0.21	0.22	0.21	0.22	0.21	0.26	0.23
ICER, €[b]	1095	1189	883	940	2785	2897	904	968
Distribution on the cost-effectiveness plane								
1st quadrant (northeast)	91	90	86	86	100	100	89	89
2nd quadrant (inferior: northwest)	0	0	0	0	0	0	0	0
3rd quadrant (southwest)	0	0	0	0	0	0	0	0
4th quadrant (dominant: southeast)	9	10	14	14	0	0	11	11
WTP ceiling, %								
€ 0	13	13	18	18	4	4	15	15
€ 10,000	92	93	93	93	91	90	92	92
€ 20,000	97	97	97	97	97	96	97	97
€ 30,000	100	100	100	100	100	100	100	100

Scenario A = adjustment of the per participant intervention costs, based on actual costs for counseling (the number of extensive emails sent by each participant multiplied by €17); scenario B = intervention costs raised from €222 to €600; scenario C = completers only analysis ($n = 112$ intervention group and $n = 125$ control group)

[a]Costs per 'disease-free' year (i.e. one year reliable improvement in depressive symptoms) at 2014 prices

[b]Bootstrapped median, which is the 50th percentile of 2500 replications of the ICER

for mental health are more abundant [35]. To our knowledge, only one prior study evaluated the cost-effectiveness of a PP-based intervention or therapy [14]. This unguided web-based self-help intervention for people with mild to moderate depressive symptoms revealed substantially higher mean ICERs for mental well-being (€21,319) and depression (€9807) compared to the current study (€2359 and €2578 respectively). However, direct comparison of the ICERs is hindered by differences between both studies (e.g. outcome measures, societal vs. health care perspective, unguided web-based vs. guided bibliotherapy) despite some similarities in study design (e.g. recruitment strategy via newspapers in The Netherlands, mainly higher educated females and non-flourishers, a multicomponent PP structure, type of control condition). In addition, there are no known or generally accepted willingness-to-pay ceilings available for making a transition to a flourishing mental health state. Nonetheless, the cost-effectiveness acceptability curve indicates that a decision-maker has an 80% certainty that the intervention is deemed cost-effective at a WTP ceiling of roughly €8000 ($9832) and this likelihood increases to above 90% at the WTP ceiling of €10,000 ($12,290). Thus, the current study indicates that if there is a willingness to pay of at least €8000 for reaching a flourishing mental health state and avoiding anxiety and depression, guided PP-based bibliotherapy has a high likelihood to be seen as a cost-effective approach compared to usual care.

Strengths and limitations

Main strengths of the study were its well-powered and randomized controlled design, the high adherence rates and results that appeared robust under sensitivity analyses. Also, as the self-selected sample of "well-being-seekers" recruited in the general Dutch population is congruent with usual recruitment strategies for self-help interventions in The Netherlands, the sample is representative for future applications of this intervention. However, we cannot generalize to the (unselected) general population because our sample overrepresented well-educated women in their late forties with paid jobs. An important limitation of the current study relates to the lack of an active control group wherein the self-help book could have been offered without email support, as was planned [20] but not feasible [11]. Prior studies demonstrated larger effects of guided CBT-based self-help than its unguided counterpart in improving mental well-being, anxiety and depression [13, 35, 36]. Hence, we cannot rule out the influence of adding email support to the PP-based bibliotherapy. Other limitations include the relatively short follow-up of 6 months and using this time-point for the extrapolation to an entire year (i.e. assuming a steady-state of the annualized costs and effects), the use of a wait-list control group (rather than usual care alone), unblinded participants, and the absence of assessing quality-adjusted life years (QALY's) [27]. An advantage of using QALY's is that a cost-utility analysis could have been added to the analyses to obtain the costs per QALY gained which is a *generic* health-related outcome that can be used across diseases and disorders. However, a strength of the current study was to use a *specific* health-related outcome that fitted well with the target group (people with languishing or moderate mental health) and the intervention aim (to establish the transition to flourishing mental health). In addition, the MHC-SF measuring mental well-being seems more sensitive to change [22] then the EQ-5D measuring QALY's [37], although more research is needed to validate the theoretical cut-off scores for categorizing people into flourishing or not.

Public health implications

A valuable approach for public mental health seems to enhance flourishing mental health because this status has been related to reduced risk of developing anxiety and depressive symptoms and mortality [8, 9, 38, 39]. The results of the present study demonstrated that an early intervention based on PP principles has the potential to promote a flourishing mental health status and substantially reduce anxiety and depressive symptom severity at some additional costs. The intervention could offer good value for money when there is a WTP of around €8000 ($9832), which corresponds to a probability of 80% that the intervention is more cost-effective compared to usual care. Even when the intervention costs are tripled by including the time costs of the participants, the WTP for a probability of 80% falls around €8000 ($9832). The economic costs of the intervention would rise from €2359 ($2899) for one additional person to improve from suboptimal well-being to flourishing in the main analysis to €4534 ($5572) when intervention costs are tripled. However, when there is no WTP for a treatment response, there is only a 12–13% probability that the intervention is more cost-effective relative to usual care. Thus, it remains a challenge to further optimize the cost-effectiveness of PP-based self-help interventions. Perhaps this can be achieved by shortening and refining the current program and focus on its most efficacious processes: enhancing positive relations, self-compassion and optimism [40]. In addition, it remains a great challenge to reach people with a lower socio-economic status, also with PP-based interventions.

Future research should replicate our findings and examine longer-term costs and benefits of PP interventions to promote flourishing. In this regard, we recommend large-scale implementation of the guided bibliotherapy program in public mental health or primary care wherein the intervention costs and effects are carefully monitored for more than one year. It is also of utmost importance to conduct economic evaluations of a guided versus unguided PP-based intervention which could shed light on the added value of therapist involvement. Furthermore, a cost-effectiveness study wherein a self-help intervention based on CBT is compared with a self-help intervention based on PP would be interesting because a prior study found that both CBT and PP where efficacious in ameliorating mental well-being and depression, but that the PP-based intervention was significantly more preferred, thus, having an impact on a larger population [41]. Overall, a PP-based self-help intervention with some guidance over the Internet has the potential to reach large groups of people via public mental health services, primary care and as additional service in mental health institutions. Also, a PP-based self-help intervention might hold promise as a worthwhile alternative to the predominant CBT-based self-help interventions. We hope the current study inspires researchers to plan and conduct economic evaluations alongside their trials to address this gap in the mental health promotion literature [13, 42].

Conclusions

The results of this large randomized controlled trial demonstrated that a multicomponent positive psychology intervention was cost-effective on a reliable improvement in mental well-being as well as a reliable reduction in anxiety and depressive symptoms. The current study adds to prior knowledge because it is the first study worldwide demonstrating that mental health and flourishing can be substantially and cost-effectively improved via a positive psychology self-help intervention. This intervention is of great importance for public mental health and clinical practice because it has the potential to reach large groups of people through public mental health services and primary care with minimal investment.

Abbreviations

CBT: Cognitive behavioral therapy; CHEERS: Consolidated Health Economic Evaluation Reporting Standards; EM: Expectation maximization; HADS: Hospital Anxiety and Depression Scale; ICER: Incremental cost-effectiveness ratio (ICER); MCQ: Medical Consumption Questionnaire; MHC-SF: Mental Health Continuum-Short Form; PP: Positive Psychology; PPP: Purchasing power parity; QALY: Quality-adjusted life years; SPSS: Statistical Packages for Social Sciences; WTP: Willingness to pay

Authors' contributions

EB designed the study and developed the intervention. MS drafted the manuscript, coordinated the trial and analyzed the data. FS provided necessary analytical tools, supervision in analyzing the data and was a major contributor in writing the manuscript. CD, FS, MP, EB and JW provided critical revision of the article. All authors read and approved the final manuscript.

Consent for publication
Not applicable.

Competing interests
The authors declare that they have no competing interests.

Author details
[1]Centre for eHealth and Well-being Research, Department of Psychology, Health and Technology, University of Twente, P.O. Box 217, 7500 AE Enschede, The Netherlands. [2]Department of Public Mental Health, Trimbos Institute, Utrecht, The Netherlands. [3]Department of Epidemiology and Biostatistics, EMGO Institute for Health and Care Research, VU University Medical Centre, Amsterdam, The Netherlands. [4]Department of Clinical, Neuro and Developmental Psychology, EMGO Institute for Health and Care Research, VU University, Amsterdam, The Netherlands.

References
1. Forsman AK, Wahlbeck K, Aaro LE, Alonso J, Barry MM, Brunn M, Cardoso G, Cattan M, de Girolamo G, Eberhard-Gran M, et al. Research priorities for public mental health in Europe: recommendations of the ROAMER project. Eur J Pub Health. 2015;25(2):249–54.
2. Kobau R, Seligman ME, Peterson C, Diener E, Zack MM, Chapman D, Thompson W. Mental health promotion in public health: perspectives and strategies from positive psychology. Am J Public Health. 2011;101(8):e1–9.
3. Kim ES, Park N, Sun JK, Smith J, Peterson C. Life satisfaction and frequency of doctor visits. Psychosom Med. 2014;76(1):86–93.
4. Hamar B, Coberley C, Pope JE, Rula EY. Well-being improvement in a midsize employer: changes in well-being, productivity, health risk, and perceived employer support after implementation of a well-being improvement strategy. J Occup Environ Med. 2015;57(4):367–73.
5. Keyes CLM, Grzywacz JG. Health as a complete state: the added value in work performance and healthcare costs. J Occup Environ Med. 2005; 47(5):523–32.
6. Hone LC, Jarden A, Schofield GM, Duncan S. Measuring flourishing: the impact of operational definitions on the prevalence of high levels of wellbeing. Int J Wellbeing. 2014;4(1):62–90.
7. Keyes CL. Mental health in adolescence: is America's youth flourishing? Am J Orthop. 2006;76(3):395–402.
8. Keyes CLM, Dhingra SS, Simoes EJ. Change in level of positive mental health as a predictor of future risk of mental illness. Am J Public Health. 2010; 100(12):2366–71.
9. Schotanus-Dijkstra M, ten Have M, Lamers S, de Graaf R, Bohlmeijer ET. The longitudinal relationship between flourishing mental health and incident mood, anxiety and substance use disorders. Eur J Pub Health. 2017;27(3):563–8.
10. Bohlmeijer ET, Lamers SMA, Fledderus M. Flourishing in people with depressive symptomatology increases with acceptance and commitment therapy. Post-hoc analyses of a randomized controlled trial. Behav Res Ther. 2015;65:101–6.
11. Schotanus-Dijkstra M, Drossaert CHC, Pieterse ME, Boon B, Walburg JA, Bohlmeijer ET. An early intervention to promote well-being and flourishing and reduce anxiety and depression: A randomized controlled trial. Internet Interventions. 2017;9(Supplement C):15–24.
12. Schueller SM, Parks AC. The science of self-help: translating positive psychology research into increased individual happiness. Eur Psychol. 2014; 19(2):145–55.
13. Cavanagh K, Strauss C, Forder L, Jones F. Can mindfulness and acceptance be learnt by self-help?: a systematic review and meta-analysis of mindfulness and acceptance-based self-help interventions. Clin Psychol Rev. 2014;34(2):118–29.
14. Bolier L, Majo C, Smit F, Westerhof GJ, Haverman M, Walburg JA, Riper H, Bohlmeijer E. Cost-effectiveness of online positive psychology: randomized controlled trial. J Posit Psychol. 2014;9(5):460–71.
15. Bolier L, Haverman M, Kramer J, Westerhof GJ, Riper H, Walburg JA, Boon B, Bohlmeijer E. An internet-based intervention to promote mental fitness for mildly depressed adults: randomized controlled trial. J Med Internet Res. 2013;15(9):e200.
16. Bolier L, Haverman M, Westerhof GJ, Riper H, Smit F, Bohlmeijer E. Positive psychology interventions: a meta-analysis of randomized controlled studies. BMC Public Health. 2013;13:119.
17. Sin NL, Lyubomirsky S. Enhancing well-being and alleviating depressive symptoms with positive psychology interventions: a practice-friendly meta-analysis. J Clin Psychol. 2009;65(5):467–87.
18. Keyes CL, Wissing M, Potgieter JP, Temane M, Kruger A, van Rooy S. Evaluation of the mental health continuum-short form (MHC-SF) in setswana-speaking south Africans. Clin Psychol Psychother. 2008;15(3):181–92.
19. Zigmond AS, Snaith RP. The hospital anxiety and depression scale. Acta Psychiatr Scand. 1983;67(6):361–70.
20. Schotanus-Dijkstra M, Drossaert CHC, Pieterse ME, Walburg JA, Bohlmeijer ET. Efficacy of a Multicomponent Positive Psychology Self-Help Intervention: Study Protocol of a Randomized Controlled Trial. Journal of Medical Internet Research, Research Protocols. 2015;4(3):e105.
21. Bohlmeijer E, Hulsbergen M. Dit is jouw leven. Ervaar de effecten van de positieve psychologie (this is your life. Exerpience the effects of positive psychology). Uitgeverij Boom: Amsterdam, The Netherlands; 2013.
22. Lamers SMA, Westerhof GJ, Bohlmeijer ET, ten Klooster PM, Keyes CLM. Evaluating the psychometric properties of the mental health continuum-short form (MHC-SF). J Clin Psychol. 2011;67(1):99–110.
23. Jacobson NS, Truax P. Clinical significance: a statistical approach to defining meaningful change in psychotherapy research. J Consult Clin Psychol. 1991; 59(1):12–9.
24. Keyes CL. The mental health continuum: from languishing to flourishing in life. J Health Soc Behav. 2002;43(2):207–22.
25. Bjelland I, Dahl AA, Haug TT, Neckelmann D. The validity of the hospital anxiety and depression scale: an updated literature review. J Psychosom Res. 2002;52(2):69–77.
26. Spinhoven P, Ormel J, Sloekers PP, Kempen GI, Speckens AE, Van Hemert AM. A validation study of the hospital anxiety and depression scale (HADS) in different groups of Dutch subjects. Psychol Med. 1997;27(2):363–70.
27. Husereau D, Drummond M, Petrou S, Carswell C, Moher D, Greenberg D, Augustovski F, Briggs AH, Mauskopf J, Loder E, et al. Consolidated health economic evaluation reporting standards (CHEERS)--explanation and elaboration: a report of the ISPOR health economic evaluation publication guidelines good reporting practices task force. Value Health. 2013;16(2):231–50.
28. Guide to the methods of technology appraisal 2013. [https://www.nice.org.uk/article/pmg9/chapter/Foreword].
29. Bouwmans C, Hakkaart-van Roijen L, Koopmanschap M, Krol M, Severens H, Brouwer W. Medical Consumption Questionnaire. In. Rotterdam: Institute for Medical Technology Assessment, Erasmus Universiteit Rotterdam; 2013.
30. PPPs and exchange rates (http://stats.oecd.org/Index.aspx?DataSetCode=PPPGDP).
31. ZorginstituutNederland. Kostenhandleiding: Methodologie van kostenonderzoek en referentieprijzen voor economische evaluaties in de gezondheidszorg. In. Diemen: Zorginstituut Nederland; 2015.
32. Smit F, Willemse G, Koopmanschap M, Onrust S, Cuijpers P, Beekman A. Cost-effectiveness of preventing depression in primary care patients: Randomised trial. Br J Psychiatry. 2006;188(APR.):330–336.
33. Vos T, Corry J, Haby MM, Carter R, Andrews G. Cost-effectiveness of cognitive-behavioural therapy and drug interventions for major depression. Aust N Z J Psychiatry. 2005;39(8):683–92.
34. Lynch FL, Striegel-Moore RH, Dickerson JF, Perrin N, Debar L, Wilson GT, Kraemer HC. Cost-effectiveness of guided self-help treatment for recurrent binge eating. J Consult Clin Psychol. 2010;78(3):322–33.
35. Donker T, Blankers M, Hedman E, Ljotsson B, Petrie K, Christensen H. Economic evaluations of internet interventions for mental health: a systematic review. Psychol Med. 2015;45(16):3357–76.
36. Beshai S, Wallace LM, McDougall KH, Waldmann K, Stea JN. Reduced contact cognitive-behavioral interventions for adult depression: a review. The Journal of Psychology. 2016;150(2):252–79.
37. Payakachat N, Ali MM, Tilford JM. Can the EQ-5D detect meaningful change? A Systematic Review Pharmacoeconomics. 2015;33(11):1137–54.
38. Keyes CL, Eisenberg D, Perry GS, Dube SR, Kroenke K, Dhingra SS. The relationship of level of positive mental health with current mental disorders

in predicting suicidal behavior and academic impairment in college students. J Am Coll Heal. 2012;60(2):126–33.
39. Keyes CL, Simoes EJ. To flourish or not: positive mental health and all-cause mortality. Am J Public Health. 2012;102(11):2164–72.
40. Schotanus-Dijkstra M, Pieterse ME, Drossaert CHC, Walburg JA, Bohlmeijer ET. Possible mechanisms in a multicomponent positive psychology self-help intervention to improve mental well-being, anxiety and depression: A multiple mediation model. In press.
41. Parks AC, Szanto RK. Assessing the efficacy and effectiveness of a positive psychology-based self-help book. Terapia psicológica. 2013;31:141–9.
42. Lewis C, Pearce J, Bisson JI. Efficacy, cost-effectiveness and acceptability of self-help interventions for anxiety disorders: systematic review. Br J Psychiatry. 2012;200(1):15–21.

6

Attachment, mentalisation and expressed emotion in carers of people with long-term mental health difficulties

Mary Gemma Cherry[1*], Peter James Taylor[1,2], Stephen Lloyd Brown[3] and William Sellwood[4]

Abstract

Background: Expressed emotion (EE) is a global index of familial emotional climate, which is comprised of emotional over-involvement (EOI) and critical comments (CC)/hostility. Although EE is an established predictor of negative outcomes for both people with long-term mental health difficulties and their family carers, its psychological underpinnings remain relatively poorly understood. This paper examined associations between attachment, mentalisation ability and aspects of EE.

Methods: Carers of people with long-term mental health difficulties ($n = 106$) completed measures of adult attachment (the Experiences in Close Relationships-Short Form questionnaire), mentalisation (the Reading the Mind in the Eyes Test and the Emotional Self-Efficacy Scale) and EE (the Family Questionnaire). Data were analysed using hierarchical multiple regression.

Results: Attachment avoidance and facets of mentalisation were directly and uniquely positively associated with CC/hostility, with attachment avoidance and other-directed emotional self-efficacy (one facet of mentalisation) each significantly predicting CC/hostility scores after controlling for the effects of EOI and demographic variables. However, no associations were observed between EOI, attachment anxiety and mentalisation. Furthermore, no indirect effects from attachment to EE via mentalisation was found.

Conclusions: Although it would be premature to propose firm clinical implications based on these findings, data indicate that it may be beneficial for clinicians to consider attachment and mentalisation in their conceptualisation of carers' criticism and hostility. However, further research is needed to clarify the magnitude of these associations and their direction of effect before firm conclusions can be drawn.

Keywords: Attachment, Mentalisation, Expressed emotion, Carers, Cross-sectional, Quantitative, Criticism, Hostility, Emotional over-involvement

Background

Approximately six and a half million people in the United Kingdom (UK) provide unpaid care to others, typically family members or close friends, with this number projected to rise to nine million by 2037 [1]. Of these, approximately 13% (equivalent to one in 10 people in the UK) provide care to someone with a long-term mental health difficulty, saving the UK economy an estimated 17 billion per year [2]. Caring for someone with a long-term mental health difficulty can be a challenging and emotional experience, with carers often displaying higher levels of anxiety, depression, and general psychological distress than members of the general population [3, 4]. As such, a strong moral and financial argument can be made for developing effective, flexible and inclusive services and interventions which support carers in their roles and safeguard their wellbeing, and the wellbeing of those to whom they provide care [5].

Over the last 60 years, increasing research attention has been paid to the potential influence of family environment on care outcomes, particularly the role of 'expressed emotion' (EE). The term 'expressed emotion' encompasses

* Correspondence: gcherry@liv.ac.uk
[1]Division of Clinical Psychology, University of Liverpool, Whelan Building, Quadrangle, Brownlow Hill, Liverpool L69 3GB, UK
Full list of author information is available at the end of the article

particular attitudes, emotions and behaviours expressed by family carers towards the person (s) to whom they provide care [6]. Key components include emotional over-involvement (EOI), critical comments (CC), and hostility [6]. Emotional over-involvement is characterised by overly self-sacrificing and/or intrusive behaviours and exaggerated emotional responses, whereas the term 'CC/hostility' is commonly used to refer to critical, negative or blaming attitudes or statements towards service-users [6].

Expressed emotion is a complex concept which can evoke in family carers immense guilt and shame [7], which in turn can influence EE behaviours [8]. Whilst not pathological in itself, EE is a consistent and reliable predictor of relapse across a range of mental health difficulties [9–11]. However, the psychological processes associated with EE require further understanding [6]. The majority of existing research in this area has investigated the utility of an attribution-based framework [3, 6], which postulates that EE results from carers' appraisals of, and beliefs about, the controllability, stability and internality/externality of service-users' mental health difficulties, rather than the specific symptomatology displayed. However, although this model has received empirical support, particularly regarding the hypothesised associations between attributions and CC/hostility [6], inconsistent findings regarding the relationship between carers' attributions and their EOI suggest that it does not adequately account for the psychological processes underlying EOI [6].

More recently, EE has begun to be seen as a developmentally-based process of adaptation to, and coping with, illness-based separation and loss, which has led to increasing recognition of the potential application of attachment theory, and the related theory of mentalisation, to understanding individual differences in carers' EE [7, 12]. Attachment theory is a way of understanding psychosocial development, which posits that individuals form enduring patterns of interpersonal behaviour through internalisation of interactions with their primary carer (s) in infancy [13]. These patterns are represented cognitively in the form of a stable internal working model (IWM) of attachment, which subsequently influences behaviour in close relationships throughout the lifespan, particularly those in which an individual is required to give or receive care [13]. Carers' attachment may therefore aid or impede their ability to provide effective and attuned care [14, 15].

Carers high on attachment anxiety (characterised by habitual preoccupation and over-involvement in close relationships combined with fear of abandonment) may engage in emotionally over-involved behaviours in an attempt to facilitate interpersonal closeness [16]. Alternatively, if carers high on attachment anxiety perceive their relative to be unavailable or rejecting, they may defend against the associated painful feelings of self-blame by externalising blame onto others in the form of criticism or hostility [17]. In contrast, carers high on attachment avoidance (characterised by difficulty in trusting others, devaluation of close relationships and avoidance of intimacy) may engage in regulatory, anger-driven behaviour such as criticism and hostility in an attempt to avoid and/or cope with the discomfort associated with the caring role [18, 19].

Attachment theory may therefore provide a theoretical framework for understanding individual differences in carers' EE [20]. It is generally accepted that attachment representations are relatively stable across an individual's lifespan [21]. Although there is evidence to support the notion that attachment representations can be modified during psychological therapy, such change is likely to require substantial time, effort and commitment [22]. A developmental and malleable factor related to attachment style, which is also likely to be an important contributor to the development and maintenance of EE but which can be easily modified, is an individual's ability to mentalise [23].

The term 'mentalisation' shares conceptual overlap with constructs such as theory of mind, emotional self-efficacy and reflective functioning [23], and can be broadly defined as the process by which an individual is able to use learned self-other representations to attend to the implicit and explicit subjective mental states and mental processes of self and others [24]. Mentalisation develops partly as a function of attachment [24]; reflective, sensitive and attuned early caregiving (i.e. relationships low in attachment avoidance and attachment anxiety) is hypothesised to facilitate well-developed mentalisation, whilst poorly attuned or neglectful early caregiving is theorised to lead to impaired mentalisation [23].

Well-developed mentalisation may help to facilitate accurate evaluation and regulation of one's own and others' thoughts, feelings and behaviours, and thus discourage emotionally over-involved, critical or hostile caregiving. Conversely, less well-developed mentalisation may contribute to high EE by limiting carers' awareness of both the amount of support needed by the service-user *and* the impact of their behaviours on the service-user [24]. Mentalisation theory may therefore also form a theoretical framework for the study of individual differences in carers' EE.

Given that mentalisation is amenable to therapeutic intervention [23], consideration of the potential effect of mentalisation on the hypothesised associations between attachment and EE may have greater clinical implications than consideration of attachment alone. However, the relationships between attachment, mentalisation and components of EE in carers of people with long-term mental health difficulties have yet to be studied. This study tested a mediational model suggesting that adult attachment dimensions differentially influence aspects of EE through their effects on mentalisation (Fig. 1; [14, 15, 17]). It is

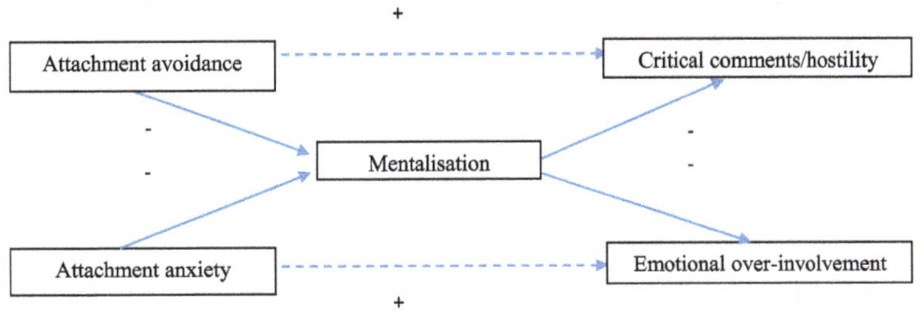

Fig. 1 Figurative summary of mediational hypotheses

hoped that a better understanding of the relationships between these constructs will contribute to improved outcomes for both individuals with long-term mental health difficulties and their carers. Specifically the following hypothesises were explored:

1. Attachment avoidance and attachment anxiety would be positively related to CC/hostility and EOI respectively;
2. Mentalisation would be negatively related to attachment avoidance, attachment anxiety, CC/hostility and EOI;
3. Mentalisation would partially mediate the effect of attachment anxiety and attachment avoidance on EOI and CC/hostility respectively.

Methods

Research design

This study used a cross-sectional design with a convenience sample, using multiple self-report measures.

Participant characteristics

Family carers of people with long-term mental health difficulties participated in this study. Inclusion criteria were that participants completed at least one of the study's measures, and self-certified as fulfilling the inclusion criteria outlined in the participant information sheet. Specifically, participants were required to: a) be 18 years of age or over; b) provide at least 10 h of face-to-face care per week to a relative with a non-organic long-term mental health difficulty for at least 6 months; c) understand English sufficiently to provide informed consent to participate. 'Long-term mental health difficulty' was defined in the participant information sheet as a severe and enduring mental health difficulty, present for at least 6 months, which impairs psychological well-being and social, occupational and/or interpersonal functioning [25]. Specific mental health diagnoses were not specified as inclusion/exclusion criteria as EE influences outcome across a range of diagnoses [9]. Carers of people with organic mental health difficulties, such as learning disabilities, dementia or acquired brain injuries, were excluded.

The final sample comprised 106 carers. Participants were primarily White British ($n = 77$; 72.64%) and female ($n = 86$; 81.13%), with a mean age of 47.13 ($SD = 13.49$, range 22–87). Participants cared for relatives aged between 18 and 92 ($M = 42.76$, $SD = 17.64$), and had done so for an average of 11.46 years ($SD = 9.66$, range 1–45). Participants reported caring for individuals with a range of mental health difficulties, of which the most common were affective disorders ($n = 79$, 74.53%). Amount of care provided ranged from less than 15 h ($n = 18$, 16.98%) to over 75 h ($n = 29$, 27.36%) per week. Half of the sample ($n = 52$, 49.06%) reported caring for individuals with additional physical health, substance misuse, and/or attentional/neurological additional difficulties. Table 1 displays demographic information for the final sample.

Measures and covariates

Demographic information

A 15-item self-report measure was used to gather relevant demographic information, including information pertaining to the nature and duration of the caring role.

Expressed emotion

Expressed emotion was assessed using the 20-item Family Questionnaire [26]. This measure was chosen because it is the only self-report measure of EE with consistently comparable sensitivity and specificity to the Camberwell Family Interview (CFI), the 'gold-standard' measure of EE [26]. Participants rate the extent to which they identify with a range of statements concerning the family environment (e.g., "It's hard for us to agree on things") using a 4-point Likert scale. Responses produce two subscale scores: EOI and CC/hostility. Each range from 0 to 40, with low scores representing low EOI and/or CC/hostility. Participants can also be dichotomised into high or low EOI and/or CC/hostility categories based on cut-off scores of 27 and 23 respectively. The FQ demonstrates good 2-week test-retest reliability and strong internal consistency (all Cronbach's $\alpha > .79$) [26], with categories correlating highly with those from the CFI [27]. Cronbach's α for the EOI and CC/hostility subscales in this sample were .80 and .69 respectively.

Table 1 Demographic data ($n = 106$)

Demographic Variable	*n* (%) unless otherwise stated	
	Carers	Service-users
Age (years), *M* (*SD*), range	47.13 (13.49), 22-87[a]	42.76 (17.64), 18–92[b]
Gender		
Male	19 (17.92)	57 (53.77)
Female	86 (81.13)	44 (41.51)
Not stated	1 (0.94)	5 (4.72)
Ethnicity		
Caucasian	94 (88.68)	96 (90.57)
South Asian	4 (3.77)	3 (2.83)
Other Asian background	1 (0.94)	2 (1.89)
Mixed background	1 (0.94)	1 (0.94)
Other	4 (3.77)	3 (2.83)
Not stated	2 (1.89)	1 (0.94)
Employment status		
Employed	63 (59.43)	22 (20.75)
Not currently in paid employment	15 (14.15)	47 (44.34)
Student	2 (1.89)	8 (7.55)
Retired	15 (14.15)	17 (16.04)
Other	10 (9.43)	8 (7.55)
Not stated	1 (0.94)	4 (3.77)
Relationship to service-user[e]		
Partner/spouse	35 (33.02)	n/a
Parent	8 (7.55)	n/a
Child	13 (12.26)	n/a
Other	5 (4.72)	n/a
Not stated	45 (42.45)	n/a
Weekly care provision (hours)		
10–14	18 (16.98)	n/a
15–29	21 (19.81)	n/a
30–44	17 (16.04)	n/a
45–59	2 (1.89)	n/a
60–74	5 (4.72)	n/a
≥75	29 (27.36)	n/a
Not stated	14 (13.21)	n/a
Duration of caregiving (years), *M* (*SD*), range	11.46 (9.66), 1-45[c]	n/a
Duration of difficulties (years), *M* (*SD*), range	n/a	12.76 (10.91). 1-50[d]
Diagnosis, *n* (%)		
Affective disorder only	n/a	56 (52.83)
ED only	n/a	6 (5.66)
SSD only	n/a	16 (15.09)
PD only	n/a	2 (1.89)
Affective disorder and SSD	n/a	8 (7.55)
Affective disorder and PD	n/a	5 (4.72)
Affective disorder and ED	n/a	10 (9.43)
Not stated	n/a	3 (2.83)
Additional comorbid difficulties, *n* (%)	n/a	
None	n/a	48 (45.28)
Physical health difficulties	n/a	44 (41.51)
Substance misuse difficulties	n/a	1 (0.94)
Attentional/neurological difficulties	n/a	4 (3.77)
Physical health and attentional/neurological difficulties	n/a	1 (0.94)
Substance misuse and attentional/neurological difficulties	n/a	2 (1.89)
Not stated	n/a	6 (5.66)

Note: all information provided by carers
ED eating disorders, *M* mean, *n/a* not applicable, *PD* personality disorders, *SD* standard deviation, *SSD* schizophrenia spectrum disorders
[a] $n = 105$
[b] $n = 104$
[c] $n = 105$
[d] $n = 101$
[e] relationship data were not available for 45 participants due to an online data collection error

Attachment

Adult attachment was assessed using the 12-item Experiences in Close Relationships: Short Form (ECR-SF) questionnaire [28]. This was selected because it has favourable psychometric properties, is short in length and allows for precise and psychometrically-robust assessment of attachment [29]. Participants rate the extent to which each item describes their feelings about close relationships in general (e.g. "My desire to be very close sometimes scares people away") using a 7-point Likert scale. Responses produce two subscale scores, attachment avoidance and attachment anxiety, which correspond to the two-dimensional model of adult attachment [29]. Each range from six to 42, with low scores indicating low attachment avoidance and/or attachment anxiety. The ECR-SF demonstrates acceptable construct validity with the original ECR, and displays good internal consistency and 6-month test-retest reliability (all Cronbach's $\alpha > .78$) [28]. Cronbach's α for the attachment avoidance and attachment anxiety subscales in this sample were .74 and .73 respectively.

Mentalisation

The Reading the Mind in the Eyes Test: Revised Version (RMET) [30] and the Emotional Self-Efficacy Scale (ESES) [31] were selected to assess different aspects of mentalisation: theory of mind (ToM) and emotional self-efficacy respectively.

The reading the mind in the eyes test Originally developed as a tool to discriminate adults with Asperger syndrome or high-functioning autism from controls, the RMET [30] is now widely used to assess ToM (the ability to conceive of and determine others' mental states). It was chosen for use in this study because it is the only validated test of the extent to which individuals can identify external aspects of emotion in others that demonstrates no correlation with general intelligence [32]. Participants are presented with 36 photographs of the facial region around the eyes and are asked to choose one of four single-word descriptors of possible mental states. Scores range from zero to 36, with higher scores indicating greater ToM ability. Variable psychometric properties have been reported for the RMET; some studies have shown uni-dimensionality with good internal consistency and test-retest reliability (Cronbach's $\alpha > .80$), whilst others have found multiple factors to underlie the construct [33]. The Cronbach's α for current sample was .58.

The emotional self-efficacy scale Emotional self-efficacy was assessed using the 32-item self-report ESES. This measure was chosen because it is formulated against an established model of mentalisation (emotional intelligence) and allows for reliable and valid assessment of an important facet of mentalisation: self-perceived emotional competency in relation to self and others [34]. Participants rate their confidence in carrying out the function described by each item on a 5-point Likert scale. When scored using Dacre Pool and Qualter's [34] revised scoring system, responses produce four subscale scores: 1) Using and Managing One's Own Emotions; 2) Identifying and Understanding One's Own Emotions; 3) Dealing with Others' Emotions; and 4) Perceiving Others' Emotions through Body Language and Facial Expressions [31]. This four-factor structure has been supported, with each factor demonstrating good internal consistency (Cronbach's $\alpha > .80$) [34]. Cronbach's α for the four subscales in the current sample were .92, .89, .90 and .83 respectively.

Procedure

Potential participants were invited to read the participant information sheet and complete a consent form and the study measures either online, via the Qualtrics platform (www.qualtrics.com), or by completing and returning a questionnaire pack using the stamped addressed envelope provided.[1] Participation took approximately 20 min, and was voluntary. As an incentive, participants were offered entry into a prize draw for one of three £50 UK high street vouchers upon completion; contact details were stored separately from other data to protect participants' anonymity.

Advertisements containing a link to complete the study online were placed on social media and UK mental health charities' websites, Facebook pages and Twitter feeds. Twenty questionnaire packs were distributed to potential participants directly by carer support coordinators working for specialist local independent sector carer support organisations within the UK. A further ten packs were given to potential participants by the author directly, during her attendance at 4 monthly carer meetings in the North West of England (informal fora for carers to meet and share their experiences).

Seven questionnaire packs were returned, and a further 273 people consented to participate online ($N = 280$), of which 108 (38.57%) fulfilled the eligibility criteria. Two were excluded (one showed little variance in their responses and one participated twice), resulting in a final sample size of 106 (37.86%; Fig. 2).

Sample size, power and precision

A priori power calculations indicated that, in order to adequately detect a medium effect size ($f^2 = .15$) with a.80 power level and a standard α level of.05 [35], a minimum of 104 participants were required for the most complex planned analysis: a multiple linear regression containing three control variables and the combined effect of seven predictor variables [36].

Data analysis

All statistical analyses were conducted using the Statistical Package for the Social Sciences (SPSS) 22.0.1 [37]. Raw data were first screened for inputting errors and summed scale scores were calculated where appropriate. Scales with more than 10% of items missing were excluded from analyses ($n = 2$). As Little's test suggested that missing data were missing completely at random ($\chi^2 = 238.21$, $df = 342$, $p > .05$) [38], listwise deletion was employed throughout subsequent analyses. Independent sample *t*-tests, Mann Whitney *U* tests, chi-squared tests, Analysis of Variances (ANOVAs) and correlational analyses were used as appropriate for initial data exploration, including assessment of multicollinearity between independent variables. The hypothesised associations among key variables were initially tested using correlational analyses. A series of hierarchical multiple regression analyses were then conducted to examine the hypotheses that attachment and mentalisation would each be predictive of facets of EE. Finally, potential mediation of any relationships between attachment and EE variables by mentalisation variables was tested using bias-corrected and accelerated bootstrapping over 5000 resamples with sample replacement [39].

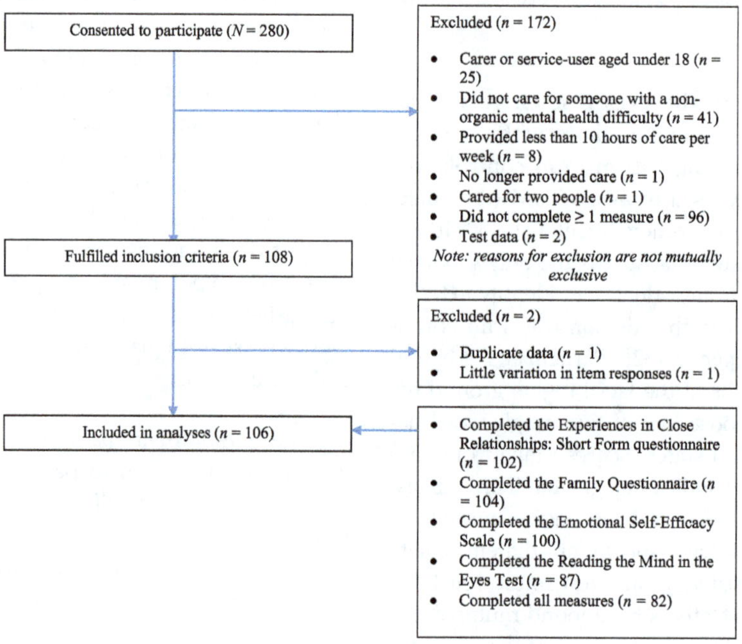

Fig. 2 Flowchart of participant inclusion

Results

Initial data exploration

Table 2 displays descriptive statistics and zero-order correlations for key variables. Service-users' age was significantly negatively correlated with CC/hostility (r = –.28, p < .01). Furthermore, females scored significantly higher than males on total EE (M = 58.61, SD = 8.34 and M = 51.37, SD = 6.35 respectively, t(101) = – 3.56, p < .01), EOI (M = 28.79, SD = 4.91 and M = 24.68, SD = 4.58 respectively, t(101) = – 4.10, p < .01) and CC/hostility (M = 29.82, SD = 4.21 and M = 26.68, SD = 3.85 respectively, t(101) = – 3.14, p < .01). All Cohen's d values exceeded.80, indicating a large effect size (Cohen, 1988). No other significant differences were noted between key variables as a function of any of the demographic variables measured (all p values > .05). As expected, both FQ and ESES subscale scores were significantly inter-correlated. However, no significant associations were noted between RMET scores and ESES subscale scores (all p values > .05).

Preliminary hypothesis testing

As shown in Table 2, attachment avoidance was significantly positively correlated with total EE and CC/hostility scores, and significantly negatively correlated with RMET scores. Furthermore, CC/hostility was significantly negatively correlated with RMET scores and borderline significantly positively correlated with E3 scores (p = .06). Neither EOI nor attachment anxiety were significantly correlated with any other variable.

Primary hypothesis testing

As EOI was not significantly correlated with any of the independent variables, no further analyses were conducted with EOI as a dependent variable. However, given the significant associations between CC/hostility and the independent variables noted above, a series of hierarchical multiple regression analyses were conducted to examine the hypotheses that attachment avoidance and mentalisation would each be predictive of CC/hostility scores. Given the results of the preliminary analyses, and the strong positively correlation noted among EOI and CC/hostility (r = .63), gender, EOI and service-users' age were entered as control variables into Step 1. The independent variables were then entered into Step 2 (Table 3). The fit of data within the assumptions of multiple linear regression was assessed by examining the distribution and heteroscedasticity of regression residuals; no violations were identified. Predictor variables had variance inflation factor (VIF) factors of > .10 and Tolerance values of < 10, indicating no violation of multicollinearity assumptions. One outlier was identified (standardised residual of > 3.3). However, this was not removed and results remained the same with or without its inclusion (Cook's distance > 1; Mahalanobis distance < critical χ^2 value).

The control variables (EOI, service-user age, carer's age) collectively predicted a significant proportion (42%) of the variance in CC/hostility (Table 3; adjusted R^2 = .42, F(3, 81) = 20.77, p < .01, f^2 = 0.72). Inclusion of the independent variables accounted for a further 12% of the variance in CC/hostility (adjusted R^2 = .54, F(10, 81) = 10.51, p < .01,

Table 2 Descriptive and bivariate statistics

Variable		*M* (*SD*), range	1	2	3	4	5	6	7	8	9	10
1	Total EE	57.19 (8.45), 38–75	–									
2	EOI	28.00 (5.07), 17–38	.92**	–								
3	CC/hostility	29.19 (4.31), 20–38	.89**	.63**	–							
4	Attachment avoidance	19.80 (7.01), 6–40	.33**	.22	.40**	–						
5	Attachment anxiety	21.70 (7.29), 6–36	.16	.11	.17	.15	–					
6	RMET	25.09 (3.96), 13–34	−.20	−.15	−.23*	−.31**	−.02	–				
7	E1	30.42 (8.96), 10–50	−.03	−.07	.02	−.03	−.12	.03	–			
8	E2	20.56 (5.51), 6–30	.11	.11	.09	−.09	−.09	.18	.67**	–		
9	E3	27.41 (6.85), 8–40	.09	.03	.21	.04	−.10	−.05	.75**	.58**	–	
10	E4	9.88 (3.19), 3–15	.10	.02	.14	−.01	−.03	−.02	.70**	.67**	.73**	–

Note: $n = 82$ (correlational analyses); italicised values indicate Pearson's product-moment correlation coefficient; non-italicised values indicate Spearman's Rho values

CC critical comments, *E1* Using and managing your own emotions subscale, *E2* Identifying and understanding your own emotions subscale, *E3* Dealing with emotions in others subscale, *E4* Perceiving emotion through facial expression and body language subscale, *ECR:SF* Experiences in Close Relationships: Short Form, *EE* Expressed Emotion, *EOI* emotional over-involvement, *ESES* Emotional Self-Efficacy Scale, *FQ* Family Questionnaire, *M* mean, *RMET* Reading the Mind in the Eyes Test, *SD* standard deviation

* = significant at $p < .05$; ** = significant at $p < .01$

$f^2 = 1.17$), with service-users' age ($\beta = -.24$, $p < .01$), EOI ($\beta = .51$, $p < .01$), attachment avoidance ($\beta = .20$, $p < .01$) and the 'Dealing with Others' Emotions' subscale of the ESES ($\beta = .28$, $p < .05$) each making significant contributions to the final model. Similar findings emerged when a trimmed model (Model 2; Table 3) was estimated; the model explained a significant proportion of the variance in CC/hostility (adjusted $R^2 = .43$, $F(4, 93) = 18.22$, $p < .01$, $f^2 = 0.75$), with EOI ($\beta = .54$, $p < .01$), with attachment avoidance ($\beta = .20$, $p < .01$) and the 'Dealing with Others' Emotions' subscale of the ESES ($\beta = .18$, $p < .05$) each significantly contributing. Attachment avoidance and the 'Dealing with Others' Emotions' subscale of the ESES remained significant predictors of CC/hostility when the control variables were removed ($\beta = .30$, $p < .01$ and $\beta = .22$, $p < .05$, respectively), and collectively accounted for 12% of the variance in CC/hostility scores (adjusted $R^2 = .12$, $F(2, 95) = 7.33$, $p < .01$, $f^2 = 0.14$).

Table 3 Hierarchical multiple linear regression models showing predictors of CC/Hostility

	Variable	Cumulative			Simultaneous		
		R^2	ΔR^2	*F* change	B	β	95% CI for B
Model 1: Demographic Characteristics, Attachment and Mentalisation as Predictors of CC/Hostility ($n = 82$)							
Step 1	Carers' gender	.44	.42	*F* (3, 81) = 20.77**	−.58	−.06	−2.18 to 1.03
	Service-users' age				−.05	−.24**	−.09 to −.01
	EOI				.41	.51**	.27 to.54
Step 2	Attachment anxiety	.60	.54	*F* (10, 81) = 10.51**	.02	.03	−.07 to.10
	Attachment avoidance				.11	.20**	.02 to.21
	RMET				−.10	−.09	−.28 to.08
	E1				−.12	−.26	−.24 to.00
	E2				−.05	−.07	−.22 to.12
	E3				.16	.28*	.01 to.32
	E4				.27	.22	−.08 to.61
Model 2: Service-Users' Age, EOI, Attachment Avoidance and Understanding Others' Emotions as Predictors of CC/Hostility ($n = 94$)							
Step 1	Service-users' age	.38	.37	*F* (2, 93) = 27.74**	−.04	−.16	−.08 to.00
	EOI				.45	.54**	.31 to.59
Step 2	Attachment avoidance	.45	.43	*F* (4, 93) = 18.22**	.12	.20**	.03 to.22
	E3				.11	.18*	.02 to.21

Note: * $p < .05$; ** $p < .01$; *CC* critical comments, *CI* confident interval, *E1* Using and managing your own emotions subscale, *E2* Identifying and understanding your own emotions subscale, *E3* Dealing with emotions in others subscale, *E4* Perceiving emotion through facial expression and body language subscale, *EOI* emotional over-involvement, *RMET* Reading the Mind in the Eyes Test

A post-hoc sensitivity analysis was conducted in which EOI was removed from the model. The final model explained a significant proportion of the variance in CC/hostility (adjusted $R^2 = .46$, $F(4, 93) = 6.08$, $p < .01$). Attachment avoidance remained a significant predictor of CC/hostility ($\beta = .28$, $p < .01$), but the 'Dealing with Others' Emotions' subscale of the ESES became non-significant, though a trend was still apparent ($\beta = .15$, $p = .10$).

Potential mediation of any relationships between attachment and EE variables by mentalisation variables

Table 4 shows the total indirect effect attributable to the five mentalisation variables. No evidence of indirect effects was found. To avoid Type 1 errors, we did not examine the mediating effects of the five mentalisation variables separately.

Discussion

This study is the first investigation known to us of the relationships among attachment, mentalisation, EOI and CC/hostility in carers of people with long-term mental health difficulties. A key contribution of the current study is the finding that, in a carer population, both attachment avoidance and facets of mentalisation were directly, and independently, positively associated with self-reported CC/hostility even after controlling for EOI. However, data indicated no support for the hypothesised relationships between attachment anxiety, mentalisation and EOI. Furthermore, there was no support for the hypothesis that adult attachment dimensions would differentially influence aspects of EE through their effects on mentalisation ability.

As predicted, avoidantly attached carers were less able to detect external explicit aspects of others' emotional states (i.e. have less well-developed mentalisation) and were more likely to report engaging in critical or hostile caregiving behaviours than their counterparts [18, 24]. This supports the notion that carers high on attachment anxiety may behave in a critical or hostile way in an attempt to regulate their discomfort with the close caregiving role [13]. However, the hypothesis that facets of mentalisation would be negatively associated with CC/hostility was only partially supported. As expected, a significant negative correlation was noted between RMET and CC/hostility scores. However, RMET scores did not significantly predict CC/hostility scores after controlling for the effects of EOI, gender, and service-users' age, thereby militating against considering mentalisation, as assessed using the RMET, as a significant contributor to CC/hostility. Furthermore, ESES 'Dealing with Others' Emotions' subscale scores significantly and independently positively predicted CC/hostility scores when EOI was controlled for in a regression model, indicating that carers' self-perceived competency in dealing with others' emotions is likely to be related to CC/hostility. This was not expected, but it is plausible that this may reflect a tendency for carers high on other-directed emotional self-efficacy to inaccurately, yet confidently, assume they understand service-users' symptoms (e.g. "I understand why she is behaving in that way; I know she is staying in bed because she is lazy"). Consistent with the thesis of Barrowclough and Hooley's [6] attributional model, this hypothesis may help to account for the observed positive associations noted between ESES 'Dealing with Others' Emotions' subscale scores and CC/hostility (e.g. "I'm being critical because she needs reprimanding and encouraging"). However, it must be stated that this suggestion remains conjectural at present, and should be treated with caution, particularly given that E3 became non-significant when EOI was removed from the model.

Collectively, findings with respect to CC/hostility tentatively suggest that both attachment avoidance and facets of mentalisation may each be important therapeutic factors to consider with respect to CC/hostility, and to a roughly equal extent. Although there is a paucity of empirical data against which to compare these findings, data are consistent with attachment and mentalisation theories [13, 23], and provide support for conceptualising EE, and particularly CC/hostility, as a developmental and interpersonal process. However, it would be premature to draw firm conclusions regarding the relationships between attachment, mentalisation and CC/hostility without further research, particularly in light of the null findings with respect to the hypothesised mediation pathways, the unexpected findings with respect to other-focused emotional self-efficacy and the results of the sensitivity analysis.

No associations were observed among EOI, attachment anxiety and mentalisation, thereby refuting the hypothesis that whilst anxiously attached carers may engage in

Table 4 Bootstrapping estimates of the total indirect effects of mentalisation variables on the relationships between attachment variables and expressed emotion variables

	Corrected estimate	SE	Lower 95%	Higher 95%
Anxious Attachment - EOI	.0076[a]	.0479	−.0918	.1095
Anxious Attachment - CC/Hostility	−.0168	.0401	−.1016	.0574
Avoidant Attachment - EOI	.0213	.0330	−.0517	.0819
Avoidant Attachment - CC/Hostility	.0213	.0230	−.0493	.0831

[a] Figures are unstandardized beta estimates

emotionally over-involved strategies in order to elicit proximity, love and support from their relative [17], mentalisation would partially mediate this relationship by facilitating sensitive and reflective caregiving [24]. As participants' ECR:SF, RMET, ESES and FQ scores were broadly comparable with previously published literature [26, 28, 30, 34], it is unlikely, although possible, that these null findings are reflective of the participant group studied. Instead, it is possible that if associations do exist among attachment, mentalisation and EOI, then a larger sample size may be required in order for these to be detected [40].

This study has several limitations that may have influenced the generalisability of findings. First, whilst comparable with other studies using a carer population [41, 42], the current sample size rendered structural equation modelling unfeasible and resulted in one regression analysis being underpowered, therefore increasing the risk of Type II errors. Second, the paucity of available relationship data limited the potential for subgroup analyses, which may have provided further clarity on the relationships between variables. Third, the lack of conceptual clarity regarding the most effective way to operationalise and measure mentalisation means that the measures of mentalisation utilised in this study, although broad ranging, may not have fully encompassed the construct [32]. Furthermore, the low internal consistency of the RMET may have influenced the findings [43]. Fifth, diagnoses were neither confirmed nor disconfirmed, which may limit the comparability of the findings with other studies. Similarly, no measure of patient functioning was included. This was because the aim of the study was to investigate the associations among attachment, mentalisation and EE across a broad range of caring relationships; strict inclusion criteria and highly controlled conditions, removed from routine clinical practice, were therefore not felt appropriate. However, this resulted in a heterogeneous sample. Further sources of heterogeneity lie in the extent of co-morbid disorders and the levels of face-to-face contact. Clearly multiple morbidities imply greater care requirements and the impact of EE has been known to be moderated by contact times [44, 45]. Sixth, although the study follows mostly a trait logic in hypothesising relationships between attachment, mentalisation and EE, theories of attachment and mentalisation emphasise that, whilst dispositional, both attachment styles and mentalisation ability are differentially expressed according to contextual demand [23, 32, 46]. Seventh, we did not control for potentially confounding factors of the tested associations, such as severity of service users' symptoms, whether carers and service users live together, and duration and frequency of care provision. Finally, the study's cross-sectional nature meant that it was not possible to imply causality or direction from the findings, nor was it possible to explore changes in the observed variables or relationships over time. Furthermore, the use of self-report measures increases the risk of social desirability bias, which should be taken into account when interpreting the results.

Future studies may wish to militate against these limitations by recruiting large and representative samples of carers from clinical and non-clinical populations. Future research should aim to clarify the nature of the relationship (s) between attachment, mentalisation and EE, together with potential mediating and moderating factors such as relationship to the care recipient, illness type and severity and weekly time spent caring. Of particular interest may be the potential influence of the interaction between carers' and service-users'/families' attachment, given that attachment and mentalisation are interpersonal processes [47]. It may also be beneficial to consider the potential role of guilt and/or shame, given their relational nature and empirical links to both attachment [17] and EE [8]. Finally, mixed inter and intra-individual approaches which enable researchers to examine behaviour over a range of contexts, thus elucidating both stability and situational variability of carer-patient interactions, are recommended for future investigation. Telling family members that the care they give is high in expressed emotion, in some senses toxic to the person they care for, is clearly insensitive and may heighten the problem because of guilt and shame [8]. The research presented here, one way of re-conceptualising carer behaviours, may enable a more sensitive understanding of carers' experiences, which may ultimately allow for increasingly effective support to be developed for them and the relatives they care for.

Conclusions

Despite its limitations, the findings of this study extend current knowledge of the associations between attachment, mentalisation and EE in carers of people with long-term mental health difficulties. Specifically, the findings that carers' attachment avoidance and specific aspects of mentalisation are each associated with levels of criticism and hostility indicate that it may be beneficial for clinicians to consider attachment and mentalisation in their conceptualisations of carers' criticism and hostility [48]. However, it would be premature to recommend specific FIs, such as those which explicitly take into account attachment perspectives [47] and mentalisation [23], without further research to clarify the nature of the relationships between attachment, mentalisation and EE, together with their mechanisms of action.

Endnotes

[1]This approach was chosen because it was felt that participants may feel more comfortable disclosing feelings about close relationships in an anonymous, self-report context

Abbreviations

ANOVA: Analysis of variance; CC: Critical comments; CFI: Camberwell Family Interview; ECR:SF: Experiences in Close Relationships: Short Form questionnaire; EE: Expressed emotion; EOI: Emotional over-involvement; ESES: Emotional self-efficacy scale; FI: Family intervention; FQ: Family questionnaire; IWM: Internal working model; RMET: Reading the mind in the eyes questionnaire; SPSS: Statistical package for the social sciences; ToM: Theory of mind; UK: United Kingdom; VIF: Variance inflation factor

Authors' contributions

MGC conceived the study, collected and analysed data and drafted the first draft of this manuscript. PJT, SLB and WS contributed to study design and data analysis and drafting the paper. All authors read and approved the final manuscript.

Consent for publication

Not applicable.

Competing interests

The authors declare that they have no competing interests.

Author details

[1]Division of Clinical Psychology, University of Liverpool, Whelan Building, Quadrangle, Brownlow Hill, Liverpool L69 3GB, UK. [2]Division of Psychology & Mental Health, University of Manchester, Zochonis building, Manchester M13 9PL, UK. [3]Department of Psychological Sciences, University of Liverpool, Whelan Building, Quadrangle, Brownlow Hill, Liverpool L69 3GB, UK. [4]Division of Health Research, University of Lancaster, Furness Building, Bailrigg, Lancaster LA1 4YW, UK.

References

1. Carers UK. Facts about carers: Policy Briefing. UK: Carers; 2014.
2. Yeandle S, Buckner L. Valuing Carers 2015- the rising value of carers' support. UK: Carers; 2015.
3. Kuipers E, Onwumere J, Bebbington P. Cognitive model of caregiving in psychosis. Br J Psychiatry. 2010;196(4):259–65.
4. Perlick D, Miklowitz D, Link B, Struening E, Kaczynski R, Gonzalez J, Manning L, Wolff N, Rosenheck R. Perceived stigma and depression among caregivers of patients with bipolar disorder. Br J Psychiatry. 2007;190:535–6.
5. Department of Health: Carers strategy: Second national action plan 2014–2016.; 2014.
6. Barrowclough C, Hooley J. Attributions and expressed emotion: a review. Clin Psychol Rev. 2003;23:849–80.
7. Patterson P. Attachment, loss and expressed emotion. In: Gumley A, Gillham A, Taylor K, Schwannauer M, editors. Psychosis and Emotion: the role of emotions in understanding psychosis, therapy and recovery. UK: Routledge; 2013.
8. Cherry M, Taylor P, Brown S, Rigby J, Sellwood W. Guilt, shame and expressed emotion in carers of people with long-term mental health difficulties: a systematic review. Psychiatry Res. 2017;249:139–51.
9. Butzlaff R, Hooley J. Expressed emotion and psychiatric relapse: a methodological study. Arch Gen Psychiatry. 1998;55(6):547–52.
10. Haidl T, Rosen M, Schultze-Lutter F, Nieman D, Eggers S, Heinimaa M, Juckel G, Heinz A, Morrison A, Linszen D, et al. Expressed emotion as a predictor of the first psychotic episode - results of the European prediction of psychosis study. Schizophr Res. 2018;S0920-9964(18):30171–3.
11. Weintraub M, Hall D, Carbonella J, Weisman de Mamani A, Hooley J. Integrity of literature on expressed emotion and relapse in patients with schizophrenia verified by a p-curve analysis. Fam Process. 2017;56(2):436–44.
12. Patterson P, Birchwood M, Cochrane R. Expressed emotion as an adaptation to loss: prospective study in first-episode psychosi. Br J Psychiatry. 2005; 187(48):s59–64.
13. Bowlby J. Attachment and loss: volume II. Separation: anxiety and anger. London: Penguin Books; 1973.
14. Diamond D, Doane J. Disturbed attachment and negative affective style: an intergenerational spiral. Br J Psychiatry. 1994;164:770–81.
15. Paley G, Shapiro D, Worrall-Davies A. Familial origins of expressed emotion in relatives of people with schizophrenia. J Ment Health. 2000;9:655–63.
16. Bartholomew K, Shaver P. Methods of assessing adult attachment: do they converge? In: Simpson J, Rholes W, editors. Attachment theory and close relationships. New York: Guildford Press; 1998.
17. Mikulincer M, Shaver P. Attachment theory and emotions in close relationships: exploring the attachment-related dynamics of emotional reactions to relational events. Pers Relat. 2005;12(2):149–68.
18. Mikulincer M, Gillath O, Haleevy V, Avihou N, Avidan S, Eshkoli N. Attachment theory and reactions to others' needs: evidence that activation of the sense of attachment security promotes empathic responses. J Pers Soc Psychol. 2001;83:881–95.
19. Campbell L, Simpson J, Kashy D, Rholes W. Attachment orientations, dependence, and behavior in a stressful situation: an application of the actor-partner interdependence model. J Soc Pers Relat. 2001;18:821–43.
20. Chen C. The relationship between attachment quality and expressed emotion among adult children caring for parents with dementia. USA: University of North Carolina; 2007.
21. Fraley C. Attachment stability from infancy to adulthood: meta-analysis and dynamic modeling of developmental mechanisms. Personal Soc Psychol Rev. 2002;6(2):123–51.
22. Taylor P, Rietzschel J, Danquah A, Berry K. Changes in attachment representations during psychological therapy. Psychother Res. 2015;25(2):222–38.
23. Bateman A, Fonagy P. Mentalization-based treatment for personality disorder: a practical guide. Oxford: Oxford University Press; 2016.
24. Fonagy P, Gergely G, Jurist E. Affect regulation, mentalization and the development of the self. New York: Karnac Books; 2003.
25. How common are mental health problems? [http://www.mind.org.uk/information-support/types-of-mental-health-problems/statistics-and-facts-about-mental-health/how-common-are-mental-health-problems/]. Accessed Aug 2018.
26. Weidermann G, Rayki O, Feinstein E, Hahlweg K. The family questionnaire: development and validation of a new self-report scale for assessing expressed emotion. Psychiatry Res. 2002;109:265–79.
27. Vaughn C, Leff J. The measurement of expressed emotion in the families of psychiatric patients. Br J Soc Clin Psychol. 1976;15:157–65.
28. Wei M, Russell D, Mallinckrodt B, Vogel D. The experiences in close relationships scale (ECR)- short form: reliability, validity, and factor structure. J Pers Assess. 2007;88:187–204.
29. Bartholomew K, Horowitz L. Attachment styles among young adults: a test of a four-category model. J Pers Soc Psychol. 1991;61:226–44.
30. Baron-Cohen S, Wheelwright S, Hill J, Raste Y, Plumb I. The "reading the mind in the eyes" test revised version: a study with normal adults, and adults with Asperger syndrome or high-functioning autism. J Child Psychol Psychiatry. 2001;42:241–51.
31. Kirk B, Schutte N, Hine D. Development and preliminary validation of an emotional self-efficacy scale. Personal Individ Differ. 2008;45:432–6.
32. Newbury-Helps J. Are difficulties in mentalizing associated with severity of antisocial personality disorder? London: University College London; 2011.
33. Olderbak S, Wilhelm O, Olaru G, Geiger M, Brenneman M, Roberts R. A psychometric analysis of the reading the mind in the eyes test: toward a brief form for research and applied settings. Front Psychol. 2015;6:1503.
34. Dacre Pool L, Qualter P. The dimensional structure of the emotional self-efficacy scale (ESES). Aust J Psychol. 2012;64(3):147–54.
35. Fritz C, Morris P, Richler J. Effect size estimates: current use, calculations, and interpretation. J Exp Psychol Gen. 2012;141:2–18.
36. Faul F, Erdefelder E, Lang A, Buchner A. G*power 3: a flexible statistical power analysis program for the social, behavioral, and biomedical sciences. Behav Res Methods. 2007;39:175–91.
37. IBM Corp: IBM SPSS Statistics for Windows. Version 210. Armonk: IBM Corp; Released 2012.
38. Little R, Rubin D. Statistical analysis with missing data. New York: Wiley; 1987.
39. Preacher K, Hayes A. Asymptotic and resampling strategies for assessing and comparing indirect effects in multiple mediator models. Behav Res Methods. 2008;40:879–91.
40. Burbach F. Towards a systemic understanding of family emotional atmosphere and outcome after psychosis. In: Gumley A, Gillham A, Taylor K, Schwannauer M, editors. Psychosis and Emotion: the role of emotions in understanding psychosis, therapy and recovery. UK: Routledge; 2013.

41. Brookfield K. Factors associated with carers' emotional over-involvement (EOI) in long-term mental health difficulties. UK: University of Liverpool; 2010.
42. McMurrich SL, Johnson SL. The role of depression, shame-proneness, and guilt-proneness in predicting criticism of relatives towards people with bipolar disorder. Behav Ther. 2009;40(4):315–24.
43. Field A. Discovering statistics using IBM SPSS statistics. 4th ed. London: Sage Publications; 2013.
44. Vaughn C, Leff J. The influence of family and social factors on the course of psychiatric illness: a comparison of schizophrenic and depressed neurotic patients. Br J Psychiatry. 1976;129:125–37.
45. Bebbington P, Kuipers L. The predictive utility of expressed emotion in schizophrenia: an aggregate analysis. Psychol Med. 1994;24:707–18.
46. Fraley R, Roberts B. Patterns of continuity: a dynamic model for conceptualizing the stability of individual differences in psychological constructs across the life course. Psychol Rev. 2005;112(1):60–74.
47. Crittenden P, Dallos R, Landini A. Attachment and family therapy. New York: McGraw-Hill; 2014.
48. Byng-Hall J. The crucial roles of attachment in family therapy. J Fam Ther. 2008;30(2):129–46.

7

A qualitative study on the stigma experienced by people with mental health problems and epilepsy in the Philippines

Chika Tanaka[1*], Maria Teresa Reyes Tuliao[2], Eizaburo Tanaka[3], Tadashi Yamashita[4] and Hiroya Matsuo[1]

Abstract

Background: Stigma towards people with mental health problems (PMHP) is known to have substantial negative impacts on their lives. More in-depth exploration of the stigma and discrimination experienced by PMHP in low- and middle-income countries is needed. Previous research suggests that negative attitudes towards PMHP are widespread among the Filipino general public. However, no study has investigated PMHP's own experiences of being stigmatised in the Philippines.

Methods: A qualitative study was conducted on the stigma experienced by PMHP (including people with epilepsy) and its related factors in the Philippines, employing the constructivist grounded theory approach. We analysed data on 39 PMHP collected through interviews with PMHP, their carers, and community health volunteers who know them well.

Results: The findings highlight the culturally and socio-economically specific contexts, consequences, and impact modifiers of experiences of stigma. Participants emphasised that PMHP face stigma because of the cultural traits such as the perception of mental health problem as a disease of the family and the tendency to be overly optimistic about the severity of the mental health problem and its impact on their life. Further, stigma was experienced under conditions where mental health care was not readily available and people in the local community could not resolve the PMHP's mental health crisis. Stigma experiences reduced social networks and opportunities for PMHP, threatened the economic survival of their entire family, and exacerbated their mental health problems. An individual's reaction to negative experiences can be fatalistic in nature (e.g. believing in it is God's will). This fatalism can help PMHP to remain hopeful. In addition, traditional communal unity alleviated some of the social exclusion associated with stigma.

Conclusions: The study indicates that existing stigma-reduction strategies might have limitations in their effectiveness across cultural settings. Therefore, we propose context-specific practical implications (e.g. emphasis on environmental factors as a cause of mental health problems, messages to increase understanding not only of the possibility of recovery but also of challenges PMHP face) for the Philippines.

Keywords: Stigma, Discrimination, Mental illness, The Philippines, Qualitative

Background

Stigma and discrimination against people with mental health problems (PMHP) are a global public health issue [1–3] and can have substantial negative impacts on all aspects of a person's life, from employment and housing to social and family life [4–7]. Public stigma, the general public's reaction towards a stigmatised group, can be conceptualised as having three distinct elements [8]. First, a negative belief about a stigmatised group is seen as stereotype. Second, an emotional reaction to the stereotype is seen as prejudice. Third, a behavioural manifestation of the prejudice is discrimination. Historically, research on stigma related to mental health has been conducted mainly on stereotypes, prejudices, and intentions to discriminate that are held by the general public with regard to PMHP. Such research revealed that the general public frequently label PMHP as dangerous, blameworthy, incompetent and weak, which is often accompanied with emotions of fear and anger and can lead to

* Correspondence: chika128@gmail.com
[1]Graduate School of Health Sciences, Kobe University, 701, 2-6-2, Yamamoto-dori, Chuo-ku, Kobe, Hyogo 650-0003, Japan
Full list of author information is available at the end of the article

behavioural intention of avoidance, punishment, and coercion [9–12]. Further, the literature shows that internalisation of public stigma or self-stigma is also frequent among PMHP, which reduces self-esteem, causes social isolation, and inhibits help-seeking behaviour [6, 13–15].

Recent research has more often investigated levels of discrimination using direct reports from PMHP. The results of such research suggest that discrimination against PMHP is a universal phenomenon around the world [2, 3, 16]; however, PMHP's experiences of discrimination and its related factors might differ in high-income countries (HICs) versus low- and middle- income countries (LMICs). Some studies suggest that PMHP experience a lower level of stigma in LMICs [17], such as India [18], China [19], and Nigeria [20], compared with HICs. The reasons for the more positive acceptance of PMHP in those settings have been considered to be a more supportive environment with social cohesion as well as more social role options that PMHP are able to fulfil [21, 22]. At the same time, there is also accumulating evidence revealing that in LMICs, experiences of stigma, discrimination and human rights abuses related to mental health problems are common and severe [23–27]. The stigmatisation in LMICs has been attributed to the combined effects of socioeconomic and ethno-cultural characteristics of the setting [28]. For example, the economic situation of widespread poverty may contribute to further marginalisation of PMHP who are not able to financially contribute to society [29]. Moreover, the cultural value of collectivism may results in discrimination towards PMHP especially with regarding to marriage and childrearing, since a person's mental health problem is often seen as the family's mental health problem [30]. Overall, practices and outcomes of stigma differ across cultures and socioeconomic backgrounds [29, 31, 32], and meaningful comparison across cultural settings may not be achievable with cross-cultural measures [33]. In consideration of this, researchers have called for an in-depth qualitative exploration of the experiences of stigma among PMHP in LMICs settings, where about 85% of the world's population live [21].

PMHP in the Philippines, a lower-middle income country in Asia, might experience a significant level of stigma and discrimination. Filipino immigrants believed that personal characteristics (i.e. self-centeredness and "soul weakness") resulted in mental health problems [34, 35], which have been shown to be related to blaming PMHP and discriminatory behaviour in other settings [36]. Also, a multi-country survey revealed that, among 16 countries surveyed, the Philippines had the second highest proportion of citizens who agreed that PMHP should not be hired for a job even if they are qualified [37]. Further, some studies that involved interviews with Filipino immigrants living in Australia and the United States and that sampled from the general population revealed that a fear of being labelled as 'crazy' and spoiling their family's reputation made Filipinos hesitate to seek help from mental health professionals [35, 38, 39]. Although these previous studies provide some knowledge regarding public stigma in the Filipino context, all of them looked at stereotypes, prejudices and intentions to discriminate held by the general public towards PMHP. To our knowledge, there is no study investigating PMHP's own experiences of being stigmatised and discriminated against and the related factors in the Philippines.

To fill the gaps in the literature, we conducted a qualitative study on the factors related to experiences of stigma as well as the experiences itself of PMHP in the Philippines, using interviews with PMHP and people who know them well. Revealing the existence, types, and sources of stigma experienced by PMHP in the Philippines can contribute to the stigma research in Asian LMIC settings. Further, exploring the experiences of stigma and its related factors can provide fundamental knowledge for the design of an effective stigma reduction program in the Filipino setting.

Methods

The current research utilised the principles of constructivist grounded theory, which is deemed suitable for revealing the social phenomenon of PMHP's experiences of stigma [40] in the Filipino context. The constructivist grounded theory assumes a relativist ontology (accepting that multiple realities exist) and a subjectivist epistemology (involving a co-construction of meaning through interaction between the researcher and participant) [41]. It provides a means of studying power, inequality, and marginality [42].

Setting

Our study was conducted in Muntinlupa, the southernmost city in the Philippines' National Capital Region. The city has a population of 481,461 as of 2016. The majority comprises Tagalog ethnic groups and professes Christian, primarily Roman Catholic, faith. Households below the food threshold, the minimum income required to meet basic food needs, account for 21.5% of the total in the city [43]. The majority of citizens cannot afford private medical services, which cost five times more than the public medical services [44]. With respect to public psychiatric service, the city has one outpatient and no in-patient facility. The nearest public in-patient psychiatric facility is located about 23 km away.

Main data collection

Participants

We collected data on PMHP from three different sources of information: PMHP themselves, their carers, and community health volunteers who knew them well. The eligibility criteria for PMHP were 1) having a mental health problem, listed in the Diagnostic and Statistical Manual of Mental Disorders 5 (DSM-5), or epilepsy, and 2) currently not using residential care. Epilepsy was included for several reasons. First, people with epilepsy are known to suffer stigma and discrimination [45, 46]. Second, the condition has a long history of being classified as a psychiatric problem [47]. Third, even with the present-day efforts promoting mental health in LMICs, epilepsy is often treated together with mental health issues [48]. Last, pilot interviews revealed that local lay people do not clearly differentiate epilepsy from mental health problems.

For the recruitment, we approached 42 PMHP in person; one of them declined to participate owing to time constraints. Thus, we obtained informed consent from 41 PMHP. Among them, two PMHP were excluded because they were confirmed to have only physical health problems and no mental health problems as listed in DSM-5. Consequently, we used data of 39 PMHP for our analysis. The profiles of the final sample are shown in Table 1. In 20 of the PMHP, we interviewed the PMHP and their main carer, usually a parent or sibling. In the remaining 19 PMHP, only a main carer was interviewed, as the 19 PMHP had communication difficulties that hindered them from answering interview questions. Additionally, in 11 PMHP, we conducted interviews with a community health volunteer who was in charge of the district in which the PMHP lived.

Recruitment

We aimed to include a wide variation in the characteristics of the PMHP, namely, gender, age, marital status, educational attainment, employment status, religion, type of mental health problem, and history of using health and welfare services. To achieve this, the participants were recruited by purposive sampling in cooperation with two different collaborating stakeholders. First, as stigma was considered to inhibit Filipino people from seeking professional help for their mental condition [35, 49], we recruited the majority of PMHP ($n = 36$) in cooperation with community health volunteers, which enabled us to recruit PMHP regardless of their history of receiving health care. The community health volunteers had good knowledge of the profiles of the residents of the district under their charge and covered all the areas of the city. Second, we recruited a small number of PMHP ($n = 3$) with common mental health problems (e.g. anxiety and depressive problems) from the outpatient clinical practice of a psychiatrist, as the community health volunteers did not identify any people with these types of problems.

To check the eligibility of those who had never been diagnosed by a specialist as having a mental health problem, a research member, ET, carefully reviewed the data

Table 1 Profiles of people with mental health problems

	n	$N = 39$ (%)
Sex		
Male	26	(66.7)
Female	13	(33.3)
Age range		
0–19 years	11	(28.2)
20–39 years	18	(46.2)
40–59 years	8	(20.5)
60–69 years	2	(5.1)
Highest educational attainment		
No formal education	4	(10.3)
Primary school or lower	16	(41.0)
High school or higher	17	(43.6)
Still in full-time education	2	(5.1)
Employment status		
Out of work[a]	34	(87.2)
Employed for wages	4	(10.3)
Self-employed	1	(2.6)
Marital status		
Single[b]	32	(82.1)
Married/ Domestic partnership	5	(12.8)
Widowed/ Separated	2	(5.1)
Religion		
Roman Catholic	28	(71.8)
Iglesia ni Cristo	3	(7.7)
Protestant	3	(7.7)
Islam	1	(2.6)
Other Christian	4	(10.3)
Classification of mental health problems		
Neurodevelopmental	13	(33.3)
Schizophrenia Spectrum and Other Psychotic	10	(25.6)
Substance-related and Addictive	8	(20.5)
Epilepsy	2	(5.1)
Anxiety	2	(5.1)
Trauma and Stressor-related	1	(2.6)
Depressive	1	(2.6)
Sleep -Wake	1	(2.6)
Data deficient	1	(2.6)
Lifetime mental health or welfare service use		
Yes	26	(66.7)
No	13	(33.3)
Current mental health or welfare service use		
Yes	12	(30.8)
No	27	(69.2)

[a]Children under 15 years old, the legal working age, ($n = 3$) are included
[b]Children under 18 years old, the legal marriage age, ($n = 8$) are included

of the individual participants, including interview recordings, transcriptions, and field notes, and then provided informed presumption if the participants had a mental health problem or not. ET also assessed which chapter, the broadest classification in DSM-5, the participant most fitted. ET has clinical experience as a psychiatrist in Japan for over 15 years.

Interview procedures

Data on the PMHP were collected through semi-structured in-depth interviews. Prior to the beginning of data collection, an interview guide was developed, referring to previous research [18, 50], and then modified based on six pilot interviews in the setting. The interview guide had a series of open questions on three major topics: onset of mental health problems and coping behaviours, experiences of being treated negatively owing to the problem and its consequences, and activities PMHP gave up because of how others might respond to their health problem. The interview guides for interviews with PMHP and for interviews with carers and community health volunteers can be accessed in Additional files 1 and 2, respectively. Consistent with the grounded theory methods, we used the interview guide as a flexible tool that could be revised as the analysis progressed. The carers and community health volunteers were not asked about their own experiences of stigma as a carer or person working in mental health. Instead, we asked them about the PMHP's experiences regarding the same topics, based on their observations. Demographic data of the PMHP were also obtained at the beginning of the interview.

The first author, CT (female, a Japanese public health nurse), conducted all of the data collection between January and March 2017. During the interview, Tagalog or English was used as preferred by the participants. When Tagalog was chosen, the interviews were interpreted by one of two health workers who had lived in the city for more than 30 years and were fluent in both Tagalog and English. After explaining the study and gaining informed consent, the interviews were conducted in their home, a health centre, or the city hospital, depending on the participants' preference. Wherever possible, we conducted interviews in a space where there was no one but the interviewee, interviewer, and interpreter around. However, five PMHP were not willing to be interviewed alone. In which case, a family member was in the same place and assisted the interview. All the interviews were digitally recorded with interviewees' permission and lasted between 19 and 53 min; the median length was 29 min. The participants received 100 Philippine pesos (1.9 US dollars) as acknowledgement for their participation.

Supplementary data collection

We included data of interviews with seven health workers into our analysis to gain a wider perspective on the stigma experienced by PMHP. CT conducted the interviews during her one-month participant observation at health services provided by the city government. During the observation, CT discussed the role of stigma and its impact on PMHP with more than 85 health and welfare workers. We analysed seven interviews with those who shared episodes on PMHP with whom they were in direct contact as a part of their duty at work. The interviewees were three community health volunteers, two nurses, one doctor, and one rehabilitation program officer. Notes were taken during the interviews and six out of seven interviews were audiotaped with their permission.

Analyses

All of the recordings were transcribed verbatim by two trained transcribers. Tagalog recordings were simultaneously translated into English by the transcribers fluent in English and Tagalog. An independent research assistant randomly selected 10% of the English transcripts and checked their accuracy by matching them with the Tagalog and English recordings. During this checking process, no significant errors were found thus the transcripts were quality assured.

Data analysis started as soon as the initial data were collected. We set aside theoretical ideas from the existing literature; instead, we remained open to exploring the theoretical possibilities we could discern from the data. After reading each of the transcripts at least twice, CT and ET independently conducted the initial coding. Simple codes were created to describe the phenomenon in each segment of data, using the qualitative data analysis software, Nvivo Version 11.4.1 (QSR International, 2016). The initial codes with identical meanings were merged through discussion, whereas those with different meanings were left unchanged to increase the variety in the interpretation of the data. We used data from interviews with cares, health volunteers, health and welfare workers to increase variety of data on stigma experienced by PMHP and gain comprehensive understanding of its context. Thus, when accounts showed some discrepancy between a person with mental health problem and his/her carer or a person who knew him/her well, we used the data from both accounts for our analysis.

The authors gradually moved on to the focus coding, in which the initial codes were concentrated on or collapsed into categories that make analytical sense, and then tested these against extensive data. The interpersonal interaction between people with and without mental health problems was treated as the central phenomenon of our interest. To explore comprehensively PMHP's experiences of stigma, we decided to treat any "uncomfortable treatments from others" reported as stigma experience, regardless of the actors' motivation. We constantly compared data on similarities and differences within a participant as well as across participants to examine the categories and develop links among them. CT led the preliminary focus coding. Subsequently, discussions were held between CT, ET, and HM, in which we reviewed the developed categories and links to determine if they were grounded in data and sufficiently explained the phenomenon.

After analysing the data of the 35 PMHP, a tentative model that explains the relations between categories was developed. We then collected and analysed data on four additional PMHP. Through discussion, the full research team determined that the categories and themes were sufficiently relevant and that the model held true for these additional PMHP. We then concluded that the model was theoretically saturated.

Results

Analyses revealed four interrelated themes surrounding stigma experienced by PMHP: (1) the context affecting stigma experience, (2) stigma experience, (3) impact modifier of the stigma experience, and (4) consequence of the stigma experience. Figure 1 shows the relationship among the themes.

Context affecting stigma experience

We identified two contextual categories that changed how others treated PMHP in a negative way.

Public belief about mental health problems

Public beliefs surrounding mental health issues are a contextual category of stigma experienced by PMHP in the Philippines. It consists of three themes: familial problems, unrealistic pessimism and optimism about severity, and oversimplified chronic course.

Familial problems

Community health volunteers and health workers observed that families of PMHP and people in the local community do not provide appropriate support for PMHP because they perceive mental affliction as a family problem and indicative of so-called "bad blood". The belief that mental health problems can be transmitted among relatives pushed families of PMHP to deny the existence of mental health issues and people in the community to distance themselves from PMHP. A nurse shared an episode of a male patient with depression:

> *His family could not accept the idea that one of their relatives is actually depressed. (...) It's because in our culture, when it comes to mental illness, it tends to be a family affair. People think if one of you has a history of mental illness, there is a chance that almost all of you already have that as well. We care about how others think about our family more than anything else. And other people feel that it is not their place to intervene in some family matters. (Interview 48, Nurse, Female)*

In particular, marrying age PMHP faced stigma because of the belief in heredity. People in the community often believe that PMHP have mental health problems in their family's blood and are afraid of developing those problems in their kinship via marriage.

> *I had one neighbour that I reported to the barangay [district government] because she mocked me. She was saying that I had mental illness in our blood and no one dare marry me and get in trouble. (Interview 51, PMHP, Male)*

Unrealistic pessimism and optimism about severity

PMHP experienced stigma when others were overly pessimistic about the severity of a mental health problem. Participants often criticised those who believe that mental health problems generally cause severe functional impairments. This belief has resulted in unfair treatment towards PMHP in the Philippines.

> *[Researcher: What is the biggest challenge for the [social inclusion] program?] Finding a job. It's very difficult. The community people don't believe they*

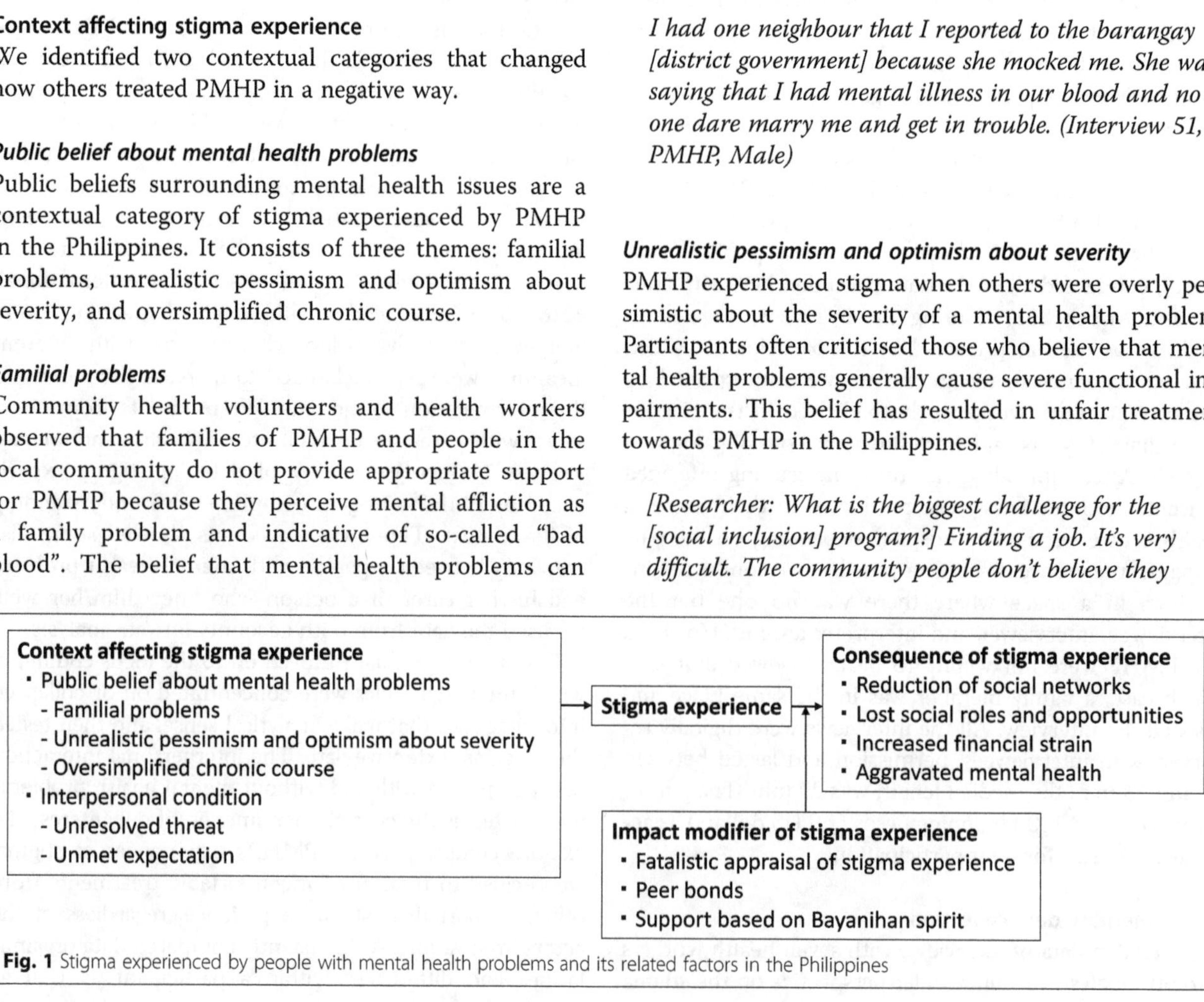

Fig. 1 Stigma experienced by people with mental health problems and its related factors in the Philippines

> *[PMHP] are functional and don't hire them. (...) So now some barangays [district governments] have started to hire them. We hope people see them working hard and start to trust them. (Interview 27, Rehabilitation program officer, Male)*

Meanwhile, unrealistic optimism about its severity also caused stigma. The commonly held belief is that individuals are able to overcome any psychological suffering by themselves, and as a result, it will not become a serious problem. It was common for PMHP to be doubted or withheld empathy in such a culture that emphasises resilience and humour under stressful situations.

> *Filipinos are proud of being resilient. We find something funny in any difficult situation. But when you have this illness, that kind of thinking gives you a huge pressure. (...) One day, I opened up about my mental illness to my friends, but they all had the same reaction. They laughed at me and didn't take it seriously. (Interview 71, PMHP, Female)*

Oversimplified chronic course

The *oversimplified chronic course* of mental health problems emerged as one of the causes of stigma. People without any experience of a mental health problem often misunderstand the repetitive relapse and remission in the course of a mental health problem. They tend to apply an acute illness model and expect a complete cure in the short term. However, as the symptoms are prolonged, they begin to mistrust the PMHP's account.

> *After one month of no work, I was able to work and sleep. But in February, it came back. I couldn't sleep for several days. (...) My supervisors were thinking that I should be working a night shift duty, but I told them that I would have to take sick leave. But because it was the same reason for my previous absent, they are already thinking that I am making up stories. (Interview 30, PMHP, Male)*

Interpersonal condition

Interpersonal condition was identified as a direct trigger of stigma experience. It consists of two themes: unresolved threat and unmet expectation.

Unresolved threat

Unresolved threat is a condition where PMHP are at risk of hurting themselves or others owing to their mental health problems, with the people in contact with the PMHP failing to manage such risks. Under such conditions, PMHP often experience physical violence, being avoided, and being restricted by others. Although the PMHP, their families, and community health volunteers attributed the threats to PMHP's personal factors, such as personality and outwardly noticeable symptoms, they also emphasised the culpability of people in the local community for their lack of understanding and skills in interacting with PMHP. When others became familiar with PMHP, they successfully managed those threats and prevented PMHP from experiencing stigma. The mother of a boy with a neurodevelopmental problem told us:

> *My son easily becomes violent. For example, when someone takes and plays with his toy. The neighbours don't understand why he is angry and they bully him. But there are also some playmates who fully understand him. When they know that my son is about to be angry, they immediately keep distance from him. And after a while, my son calms down and they start playing around together. (Interview 4, Mother of a boy with a mental health problem)*

Unmet expectation

Unmet expectation was another context of stigma. In this context, there is a gap between PMHP's abilities and other people's expectations of them. Some PMHP reported suffering from stigma when others' expectations were too high for their situation. People in this cultural setting tend to value strong bonds and reciprocity among families and neighbours. PMHP sometimes were unable to perform in accordance with this value owing to their mental health conditions. Violation of this value was judged as morally wrong.

> *They [the neighbours] say I should help my mum by doing washing, cleaning, and taking care of my brother, even when I say I feel weak or don't know how to. (Interview 5, PMHP, Female)*

> *She is big but still doesn't help her mother. That's why the neighbours don't like her. They say she is not a good daughter. (Interview 18, Community health volunteer, Female)*

Meanwhile, some other PMHP experienced stigma when others underestimated PMHP's abilities. Families often criticised other people that looked only at PMHP's disabilities but not at their abilities.

> *When someone in our neighbourhood was trying to talk to my sister and she did not respond back, they started bullying her and calling her crazy. [Researcher: How do you think we can change such situation?] I think proper communication towards her would be the*

best since she's really a good listener. The problem is that other people don't know she actually understands things really well. (Interview 8, Sister of a woman with a mental health problem)

Stigma experience

Although we frequently found that PMHP were positively treated by others because of their mental health problems, we also discovered that almost all the PMHP participants were faced with negative treatment from others. PMHP experienced *psychological abuse* (e.g. being verbally insulted, laughed at, stared at, gossiped about, doubted), *physical violence* (e.g. being hit, stones being thrown at them), being *restricted* (e.g. being told not to go outside alone, tied with a rope to a pillar), not being *supported* (e.g. lack of understanding and sympathy), being *taken advantage of* (e.g. being cheated out of money and belongings), being *neglected* (e.g. privacy not being protected, medical care not being provided), and being *rejected* (e.g. not being associated with, not being hired). Families were an important source of stigma in terms of prominence as stigma from families was often repetitive (e.g. frequently being slapped) and prolonged (e.g. being locked up in a room for several months). PMHP also experienced stigma frequently from their neighbours, and sometimes from school friends, co-workers and employers. People who were involved with PMHP as a part of their duty at work (i.e. health workers and public safety officers) were a source of stigma as well. For complete information on the stigma experience by source, please see Table 2.

Impact modifier of stigma experience

Even if the nature of stigma experiences were similar, the extent and degree of its influence on PMHP's life varied depending on *impact modifier of stigma experience*. PMHP had three impact modifiers consisting of internal (i.e. fatalistic appraisal) and external (i.e. peer bonds, community unity) factors.

Fatalistic appraisal of stigma experience

Fatalistic appraisal of stigma experience offered PMHP and their families a strategy to cope with the emotional pain caused by stigma experience. People in the setting generally believed that God predetermined life events in the past, present and future. Some PMHP and their family accepted unfair treatments from others as "fate." They were able to remain hopeful because they believed that God would help them if they had faith in God.

Sometimes people say he is crazy. [Researcher: What do you do in response to that?] Nothing. People say

Table 2 Stigma experience by type and source and its examples[a]

Psychological abuse	
Family	My other siblings say that she's crazy. (Interview 70, Sister of PMHP)
Friends	Her classmates were bullying her (Interview 21, Mother of PMHP)
Neighbours	They [neighbours] say bad things to me like "abnoy" ["abnormal" in Tagalog]. (Interview 55, PMHP)
Coworkers, Employers	I don't like them [coworkers] gossiping about me. (Interview 32, PMHP)
Health care providers	They told me that I was lazy. (Interview 42, PMHP)
Strangers on the street	When a vehicle stopped and the driver stared at her I got mad. (Interview 38, Father of PMHP)
Physical violence	
Family	He [Father] sometimes slaps him. (Interview 15, Mother of PMHP)
Friends	My high school friends started throwing stones at me and saying I'm crazy (Interview 6, PMHP)
Neighbours	When my neighbour hit him I needed to bring him to the hospital (Interview 1, Mother of PMHP)
Public safety officers	They [public safety officers] hit me and I was very scared. (Interview 58, PMHP)
Restricted	
Family	We tied him down with a rope because he would always wander around. (Interview 43, Mother of PMHP)
Not supported	
Family	Her brothers don't understand her. (Interview 8, Sister of PMHP)
Friends	No one really understands me, even my friends. (Interview 60, PMHP)
Coworkers, Employers	They [coworkers] usually laugh because they don't know it's hard having this problem. (Interview 12, PMHP)
Taken advantage of	
Neighbours	He usually rents a bike in our neighbour for five pesos, but sometimes he'll pay with twenty pesos and they won't give him the change. (Interview 7, Mother of PMHP)
Neglected	
Family	We had to let him live with us because his parents abandoned him when he was little. (Interview 44, Aunt of PMHP)
Health care providers	When we visited the hospital, we saw that she was naked and she was already held with other mental patients in the room. There were no assessments done for her [for urinary tract infection]. (Interview 38, Father of PMHP)
Rejected	
Family	My brother says to "keep her out of the home." (Interview 63, Sister of PMHP)
Friends	[Researcher: Did he have many friends?] Yes, before. But now, they avoid him. (Interview 65, Mother of PMHP)
Coworkers, Employers	I kept failing to find a job. That's why I need to hide it [mental health problem]. (Interview 16, PMHP)

[a]A listed source with an example of a particular type of stigma experience indicates that at least one incidence of that type was reported by the participant

> *what they want to say. We just say "God is good." As long as we believe in Him, it will be alright. (Interview 23, Sister of a man with a mental health problem)*

Peer bonds

Peer bonds, the emotional bonds with other people with similar mental health problems, empowered PMHP to change their stigmatised situation in a positive way. Stigma experience could marginalise them in the community, but when they were together with peers who understood not only their health condition but also their lowered social status, they were empowered and motivated to change the situation for themselves and their peers.

> *[Researcher: What are the barriers to your recovery?] The different perceptions of people towards us [she and other people with mental health problems]. It is so discouraging for us. And we are the only ones who can understand each other very well. We are like brothers and sisters already. Nevertheless, we make sure that the reason we join the [rehabilitation] program is not only for ourselves but to show them that we can change ourselves for the better. If we will be given a chance to work again, we will make 100 percent effort to get things done accordingly. (Interview 34, PMHP, Female)*

Support based on Bayanihan spirit

Support based on Bayanihan spirit, a traditional concept of community unity, relieved the negative impacts of stigma on PMHP. It was not rare that community people gave food or rented a house free to PMHP and their family who had little income. Helping one another in a time of need was inherent in their lives, called Bayanihan in Tagalog. For example, a homeless woman with schizophrenia told us that she had felt hopeless because she had been bullied at school and was in a materially deprived circumstance. However, she was now enjoying her life and managing to make a living because some of her neighbours treated her as a valued community member (e.g. regularly invited her to a local dancing event) and occasionally gave her food. A community health volunteer explained why she had good relationships with the community as follows:

> *That is natural here. When your family member is sick, neighbours and friends are there to pay for medicines, bring food, help with housework, and take care of small kids. We call it Bayanihan. (Interview 3, Community health volunteer, Female)*

Consequence of stigma experience

Stigma experience was found to bring about a substantial negative impact on PMHP's social networks, roles, opportunities, and mental health.

Reduction of social networks

Stigma experience reduced PMHP's social networks, which led to them spending their days isolated at home without any interaction with people outside of their immediate family. This was due not only to the direct influence of experiences of stigma (i.e. being *physically restrained*, being *avoided by others*) but also the indirect influence of changes in three aspects: PMHP's behaviour, restriction by families, and relationships with others. First, after being negatively treated, PMHP tended to "close off to everybody" and distanced themselves from others.

> *Going out is sometimes like an obstacle. (...) After that [hearing my friends gossiping about me], I have been afraid of people's judgments. (Interview 62, PMHP, Female)*

Second, families started to restrict PMHP's behaviour to protect them from further stigma experiences.

> *We do not allow him to go out. We are afraid that something like that [neighbours calling him crazy] might happen to him again or someone might abduct him. (Interview 9, Sister of a man with a mental health problem)*

Third, stigma experiences provoked conflicts, from a quarrel to a physical fight, and worsened the relationship between PMHP and others. The conflicting relationships produced a further stigmatising attitude towards PMHP.

> *He got into a fight with his playmates because they said bad words to him. (...) Many of our neighbours told me that he should be in a cell. They told me that they knew a policeman who could put him in jail. (Interview 1, Mother of a man with metal health problem)*

Lost social roles and opportunities

As a result of stigma experience, PMHP *lost social roles and opportunities*, such as being employed, going to school, having a romantic partner, getting married, parenting, helping with household chores and the family business, taking care of younger siblings and joining religious activities.

> *She was a member of the choir in church. She likes singing and has a good voice. And plenty of friends visited her in the past and they went to church together. But no more. Nobody visits her, and she quit attending it. (Interview 10, Mother of a woman with a mental health problem)*

Increased financial strain

Lost social roles and opportunities increased financial strain, which negatively affected the families as well as PMHP themselves. In this setting, PMHP and their families lived in communities where many people find it difficult to make a living. The cost of transportation to medical facilities and treatment fees put them in a further difficult situation economically. In such conditions, entire families often suffered from the financial strain that was due to stigma to the degree that they could not afford basic items including food and clothing.

> *If only I could find a good job like when I was well. Even though we do not have enough money to buy things, my family really makes an effort to find ways that we can buy those medicines. (Interview 20, PMHP, Male)*

Aggravated mental health

The participants reported that the stigma experiences *aggravated mental health* in PMHP. The memory of negative treatment from others often stuck in their mind and its influence lasted for a long time. A 32-year-old woman with anxiety problem explained how the experience of being bullied when she was a teenager influenced her current condition:

> *It triggers my anxiety. When I remember their facial expressions, even now, I feel overwhelmed and breathless (Interview 39, PMHP, Female).*

The experience of stigma also affected the mental health condition of PMHP by preventing them from seeking help. Some PMHP and their families choose to keep their mental health status a secret. However, families have limited capacities to take care of a person with a mental health problem, especially in the case of someone with severe symptoms. In the worst case in terms of the influence of stigma on PMHP's mental health, a community health volunteer reported that the parents of a daughter with a mental health problem locked her up in her room and took care of her without seeking professional help. However, her condition kept deteriorating and eventually she committed suicide inside her room.

Discussion

To our knowledge, this is the first study to document the stigma experienced by PMHP in the Philippines. This study adds to the understanding of discrimination in LMIC settings and its related contextual factors in the Philippines.

First, our results showed that PMHP in the Philippines experienced stigma, which brought about negative impacts on PMHP's social networks, roles and opportunities, financial burden, and mental health. Although stigma types, sources, and areas of impact were generally consistent with the existing literature in this field [4, 6, 51], we found that experiences of stigma threatened the economic survival of the entire family of PMHP and increased the mental health crisis in the LMIC context, given the minimal welfare and mental health care provisions. Several studies with participants recruited from clinical settings have shown that PMHP in LMICs suffered less from stigma [2, 18–20]. In this study, we involved PMHP without psychiatric service use, which prevented us from overlooking the stigma experienced by the poorest and most marginalised PMHP. Our findings might better reflect the reality in LMIC settings, where it is estimated that more than 70% of PMHP receive no treatment for their mental health conditions [52].

Second, we found that pessimistic and over-optimistic reactions to a mental health problem are among the important contexts of experiences of stigma in the Philippines. Historically, stigma research has mainly focused on the pessimistic view on the prognosis and its negative effects [10, 53–56]. Meanwhile, when the over-optimistic view on the outcome of mental health problems has been documented among Filipino immigrants, it was only recognised as a barrier to help-seeking [35, 39]. Our qualitative exploration's original finding is that the over-optimistic belief among the community regarding the severity of mental health problems results in PMHP's receiving inappropriate or negative treatment. This is an important finding for the Philippines, because resilience and optimism under difficult situations are among the well-known cultural traits of Filipinos [57, 58]. Stigma resulting from optimism might be prevalent in the Philippines; a prior study showed that among the 16 countries, the Philippines posted the highest proportion of respondents who agreed that mental illness would improve on its own [59].

Third, the results indicated that mental health problems were perceived as problems of the family and discouraged people from accepting mental health problems. The finding is consistent with psychiatrists' clinical experiences with Filipino patients [60, 61]. We also found that a belief in transmissibility among relatives led to PMHP experiencing reduced marriage opportunities. Previous studies conducted on Chinese descent groups [62–64] showed that the threat of genetic contamination was related to endorsement of reproductive restriction. We propose that it might hold true in the Filipino context, meaning that the threat to family lineage through genetic contamination via marriage accounts for some of the discrimination experienced by PMHP.

Fourth, we revealed a context-specific impact modifier of stigma experiences, namely, *fatalistic appraisal of stigma experience*. Existing studies have discussed that Filipinos typically attribute illness to "the will of God" [39, 49, 65]. A new finding of this study is that negative treatments from others were also attributed to fate. Globally, it is known that fatalistic appraisal of negative events inhibits active coping and worsens health [66, 67]. However, we found that fatalism offered a spiritual coping strategy and shielded PMHP from the adverse effects of stigma in the Catholic dominant setting of the Philippines. These findings are consistent with the literature that have showed that fatalism facilitates adjustment to negative life events [49, 68, 69]. Moreover, *support based on Bayanihan spirit* was another culturally relevant impact modifier. The origin of the Bayanihan spirit is traced back to the country's tradition wherein towns' people cooperate to carry a family's entire house on their shoulders to a new location. It is considered a core essence of the Filipino culture. Our finding supports the arguments by Lasalvia [21] and Mascayano et al. [29] that communal network, which tends to be better maintained in LMICs, is among the existing strengths to reduce the negative effects of stigma.

Lastly, the research method of obtaining perspectives from multiple participants who witnessed and experienced stigma allowed us to reveal that the interpersonal conditions (i.e. *unresolved threat* and *unmet expectations*) preceded stigma experiences. Consistent with previous research from India [24] and Indonesia [70], in the setting where mental health care is not readily available at a local level, people in the community needed to cope with the possible danger of PMHP to self or others and can violate PMHP's human rights. Similar to the results of prior qualitative analyses of interviews with PMHP and their families [18, 71], the expectations of others in contrast to PMHP's actual capabilities caused negative reactions from others. Those interpersonal conditions might be a more important determinant of stigma experiences than PMHP's personal factors, considering the previous studies showing individual variables (e.g. employment status, symptom, and treatment experiences) accounted for only less than 30% of total variance of experienced stigma [2, 3].

Practical implications

Our results suggest that mental health care must have the objective of the reduction of stigma towards PMHP. The Department of Health and Local Government Units are required by the Mental Health Act [72], established in 2018 as the first law of its kind in the Philippines, to initiate and sustain nationwide campaigns to raise the level of awareness on the protection and promotion of mental health and rights. In conducting stigma reduction campaigns, they should: 1) target families of PMHP, community people, health workers, and public safety officers; 2) avoid genetic explanations for mental health problems and emphasise the role of environmental and social factors as its cause; 3) increase public understanding of not only the possibility of recovery but also the challenges that PMHP face; and 4) improve families' and community members' skills in assessing and coping with possible danger posed by PMHP to self or others [73–76]. These interventions might be more effective when they utilise the existing communal network and increase social contact between PMHP and others [77, 78] We also propose that mental health and welfare services for PMHP should: 1) be community-based and support PMHP in meeting expectations that are meaningful for themselves and others; 2) provide opportunities for PMHP to share their experiences with peers to empower them [79–81]; and 3) prevent PMHP from internalising experiences of stigma with acknowledgement of fatalistic appraisal of them as a coping strategy. Lastly, to mitigate the adverse influences of stigma, it is necessary to change the structure of health care and welfare service provision for PMHP (e.g. inclusive education, welfare benefits, and job schemes). It is also essential to provide effective and accessible mental health care.

Study limitations

We were unable to recruit people with common mental health problems who were not using psychiatric services. In fact, community health volunteers do not recognise any people having common mental health problems. This may reflect stigma-related situations where local people do not recognise the manifestation of symptoms of those problems as a health issue, or where people with those problems hide their conditions. Additionally, cultural and language barriers may have played a part in data collection and interpretation. However, we also encountered a number of situations where the interviewee provided the data collector, who was from another cultural background, with further explanations, especially on their culture. Further, some interviews were too short to be considered an in-depth interview. Also, we needed to rely in part on data from narratives of people who know PMHP well, instead of from PMHP themselves. These were because the interviewer had difficulty encouraging some participants, especially PMHP, to talk about sensitive topics. Thus, there might be experiences and related themes that we could not explore. Lastly, we conducted the study in one city; thus, the results may not be generalisable to another part of the Philippines (e.g. rural and Muslim-dominant areas).

Conclusions

Our findings highlight that PMHP in the Philippines experience substantial discrimination and its adverse effects are severe to the degree that it threatens the financial survival of the entire family. Culture-bound beliefs and social structure (e.g. perceiving mental health problems as a familial problems, traditional communal unity) played important roles in shaping and modifying stigma experiences. More research is needed to develop stigma reduction interventions utilising these findings and to evaluate their effectiveness.

Abbreviations

DSM: The Diagnostic and Statistical Manual of Mental Disorders; HICs: High-income countries; LMICs: Low- and middle-income countries; PMHP: People with mental health problems

Acknowledgments

We are grateful to the interviewees for their participation. We would like to thank Dr. Magdalena C. Meana, Dr. Ma. Luisa Babaran-Echavez, and barangay health workers for their assistance with data collection.

Authors' contributions

CT had a major role in the conception of the study, undertook the data collection, carried out the data analysis, and had a major role in writing the manuscript. MT contributed to the design of the study, assisted the data collection and interpretation, and supervised writing the manuscript. ET assisted data collection, conducted data analysis, and revised the manuscript. YT assisted data collection and revised the manuscript. HM supervised the design of the study, had a role in data analysis, and revised the manuscript. All authors read and approved the final manuscript.

Consent for publication

Participants were informed that the information they shared in the interviews would be published in anonymised form. Written informed consent for publication was obtained.

Competing interests

The authors declare that they have no competing interest.

Author details

[1]Graduate School of Health Sciences, Kobe University, 701, 2-6-2, Yamamoto-dori, Chuo-ku, Kobe, Hyogo 650-0003, Japan. [2]City Health Office, City Government of Muntinlupa, Muntinlupa, Philippines. [3]Hyogo Institute for Traumatic Stress, Kobe, Japan. [4]Kobe City College of Nursing, Kobe, Japan.

References

1. Seeman N, Tang S, Brown AD, Ing A. World survey of mental illness stigma. J Affect Disord. 2016;190:115–121. Available from: https://doi.org/10.1016/j.jad.2015.10.011 Elsevier.
2. Lasalvia A, Zoppei S, Van Bortel T, Bonetto C, Cristofalo D, Wahlbeck K, et al. Global pattern of experienced and anticipated discrimination reported by people with major depressive disorder: a cross-sectional survey. Lancet. 2013;381:55–62. Available from: https://doi.org/10.1016/S0140-6736(12)61379-8 Elsevier Ltd
3. Thornicroft G, Brohan E, Rose D, Sartorius N, Leese M. Global pattern of experienced and anticipated discrimination against people with schizophrenia: a cross-sectional survey. Lancet; 2009;373:408–415. Available from: https://doi.org/10.1016/S0140-6736(08)61817-6. Elsevier Ltd
4. Sharac J, McCrone P, Clement S, Thornicroft G. The economic impact of mental health stigma and discrimination: a systematic review. Epidemiol Psichiatr Soc. 2010;19:223. Available from: https://www.ncbi.nlm.nih.gov/pubmed/21261218.
5. Clement S, Schauman O, Graham T, Maggioni F, Evans-Lacko S, Bezborodovs N, et al. What is the impact of mental health-related stigma on help-seeking? A systematic review of quantitative and qualitative studies. Psychol Med. 2015;45:11–27 Available from: http://www.ncbi.nlm.nih.gov/pubmed/24569086.
6. Livingston JD, Boyd JE. Correlates and consequences of internalized stigma for people living with mental illness: a systematic review and meta-analysis. Soc Sci Med. 2010;71:2150–2161. Available from: https://doi.org/10.1016/j.socscimed.2010.09.030 Elsevier Ltd
7. Link BG, Phelan JC. Conceptualising stigma. Annu Rev Sociol. 2001 [cited 2018 Jul 3];27:363–385. Available from: https://www.annualreviews.org/doi/pdf/10.1146/annurev.soc.27.1.363
8. Corrigan PW. Mental health stigma as social attribution: implications for research methods and attitude change. Clin Psychol Sci Pract. 2006;7:48–67 Available from: http://doi.wiley.com/10.1093/clipsy.7.1.48.
9. Mannarini S, Boffo M. Anxiety, bulimia, drug and alcohol addiction, depression, and schizophrenia: what do you think about their aetiology, dangerousness, social distance, and treatment? A latent class analysis approach. Soc Psychiatry Psychiatr Epidemiol. 2015;50:27–37.
10. McGinty EE, Goldman HH, Pescosolido B, Barry CL. Portraying mental illness and drug addiction as treatable health conditions: effects of a randomized experiment on stigma and discrimination. Soc Sci Med; 2015;126:73–85. Available from: https://doi.org/10.1016/j.socscimed.2014.12.010. Elsevier Ltd
11. Angermeyer MC, Dietrich S. Public beliefs about and attitudes towards people with mental illness: a review of population studies. Acta Psychiatr Scand. 2006;113:163–79.
12. Corrigan PW, Markowitz FE, Watson A, Rowan D, Kubiak MA. An attribution model of public discrimination towards persons with mental illness. J Health Soc Behav. 2003;44:162–79.
13. Corrigan P, Watson A. The paradox of self-stigma and mental illness. Clin Psychol Sci Pract. 2002;9:35–53 Available from: https://onlinelibrary.wiley.com/doi/10.1093/clipsy.9.1.35.
14. Evans-Lacko S, Brohan E, Mojtabai R, Thornicroft G. Association between public views of mental illness and self-stigma among individuals with mental illness in 14 European countries. Psychol Med. 2012;42:1741–52.
15. Mccann TV, Renzaho A, Mugavin J, Lubman DI. Stigma of mental illness and substance misuse in sub-Saharan African migrants: a qualitative study. Int J Ment Health Nurs. 2017;27:956–65.
16. Camden Schizoph E, Corker EA, Beldie A, Brain C, Jakovljevic M, Jarema M, et al. Experience of stigma and discrimination reported by people experiencing the first episode of schizophrenia and those with a first episode of depression: The FEDORA project Anamaria Vasilache 2 , Margda Waern 3,4 , Norman Sartorius 10 , Graham Thornicroft 1 and the FEDORA study group. Int J Soc Psychiatry. 2015 [cited 2018 Jul 3];61:438–445. Available from: http://journals.sagepub.com/doi/pdf/10.1177/0020764014551941
17. Lasalvia A, Van Bortel T, Bonetto C, Jayaram G, Van Weeghel J, Zoppei S, et al. Cross-national variations in reported discrimination among people treated for major depression worldwide : the ASPEN / INDIGO international study. Br J Psychiatry. 2015;207:507–14.
18. Koschorke M, Padmavati R, Kumar S, Cohen A, Weiss HA, Chatterjee S, et al. Experiences of stigma and discrimination of people with schizophrenia in India. Soc Sci Med; 2014;123:149–159. Available from: https://doi.org/10.1016/j.socscimed.2014.10.035. Elsevier Ltd
19. Lv Y, Wolf A, Wang X. Experienced stigma and self-stigma in Chinese patients with schizophrenia. Gen Hosp Psychiatry. 2013;35:83–8. Available from: https://doi.org/10.1016/j.genhosppsych.2012.07.007 Elsevier Inc.
20. Oshodi YO, Abdulmalik J, Ola B, James BO, Bonetto C, Cristofalo D, et al. Pattern of experienced and anticipated discrimination among people with depression in Nigeria: a cross-sectional study. Soc Psychiatry Psychiatr Epidemiol. 2014;49:259–66.
21. Lasalvia A. Tackling the mental illness stigma in low- and middle-income countries: lessons learned from high-income countries and mistakes to avoid. Epidemiol Psychiatr Sci. 2015;24:395–8 Available from: https://www.cambridge.org/core/journals/epidemiology-and-psychiatric-sciences/article/tackling-the-mental-illness-stigma-in-low-and-middleincome-countries-lessonslearned-from-highincome-countries-and-mistakes-to-avoid/83D63EA7FD15A3A3F2F9085E7E1700A2.
22. Rosen A. Destigmatizing day-to-day practices: what developed countries can learn from developing countries. World Psychiatry. 2006;5:21–24. https://www.ncbi.nlm.nih.gov/pmc/articles/PMC1472257/.
23. Alonso J, Buron A, Bruffaerts R, He Y, Posada-Villa J, Lepine JP, et al. Association of perceived stigma and mood and anxiety disorders: results from the world mental health surveys. Acta Psychiatr Scand. 2008;118:305–14.
24. Mathias K, Kermode M, San Sebastian M, Koschorke M, Goicolea I. Under the banyan tree--exclusion and inclusion of people with mental disorders in rural North India. BMC Public Health. 2015;15:–446 Available from: https://bmcpublichealth.biomedcentral.com/articles/10.1186/s12889-015-1778-2.
25. Maramis A, Van Tuan N, Minas H. Mental health in Southeast Asia. Lancet. 2011;377:700–2.

26. Minas H, Diatri H. Pasung: Physical restraint and confinement of the mentally ill in the community. Int J Ment Health Syst. 2008;2 Available from: https://www.ncbi.nlm.nih.gov/pmc/articles/PMC2442049/.
27. Tawiah PE, Adongo PB, Aikins M. Mental Health-Related Stigma and Discrimination in Ghana: Experience of Patients and Their Caregivers. Ghana Med J. 2015 [cited 2018 Jul 3];49:30–6. Available from: http://www.ncbi.nlm.nih.gov/pubmed/26339082.
28. Lauber C, Rössler W. Stigma towards people with mental illness in developing countries in Asia. Int Rev Psychiatry [Internet]. 2007;19:157–78 Available from: https://www.ncbi.nlm.nih.gov/pubmed/17464793.
29. Mascayano F, Armijo JE, Yang LH. Addressing stigma relating to mental illness in low- and middle-income countries. Front Psychiatry. 2015;6:1–4.
30. Abdullah T, Brown TL. Mental illness stigma and ethnocultural beliefs, values, and norms. Clin Psychol Rev. 2011;31:934–48.
31. Semrau M, Evans-Lacko S, Koschorke M, Ashenafi L, Thornicroft *G. stugma* and discrimination related to mental illness in low- and middle-income countries. Epidemiol. Psychiatr. Sci. [Internet]. 2015;24:382–94. Available from: https://www.ncbi.nlm.nih.gov/pubmed/25937022.
32. Yang LH, Kleinman A, Link BG, Phelan JC, Lee S, Good B. Culture and stigma: adding moral experience to stigma theory. Soc Sci Med. 2007;64:1524–35.
33. Yang LH, Thornicroft G, Alvarado R, Vega E, Link BG. Recent advances in cross-cultural measurement in psychiatric epidemiology: utilizing "what matters most" to identify culture-specific aspects of stigma. Int. J. Epidemiol. [internet]. 2014;43:494–510. Available from. https://www.ncbi.nlm.nih.gov/pubmed/24639447.
34. Edman JL, Johnson RC. Filipino American and Caucasian American beliefs about the causes and treatment of mental problems. Cultur Divers Ethnic Minor Psychol. 1999;5:380–6.
35. Thompson S, Hartel G, Manderson L, Woelz-Stirling N, Kelaher M. The mental health status of Filipinas in Queensland. Aust N Z J Psychiatry. 2002; 36:674–80.
36. Corrigan PW, Rowan D, Green A, Lundin R, River P, Uphoff-Wasowski K, et al. Challenging two mental illness Stigmas : personal responsibility and dangerousness. Schizophr Bull. 2002;28:293–310.
37. Pescosolido BA, Medina TR, Martin JK, Long JS. The "Backbone" of Stigma: Identifying the Global Core of Public Prejudice Associated With Mental Illness. Am. J. Public Health [Internet]. 2013;103:853–60. Available from: https://www.ncbi.nlm.nih.gov/pubmed/23488508.
38. Gong F, Gage SJL, Tacata LA. Helpseeking behavior among Filipino Americans: a cultural analysis of face and language. J Community Psychol. 2003;31:469–88.
39. Javier JR, Supan J, Lansang A, Beyer W, Kubicek K, Palinkas LA. Preventing Filipino mental health disparities: perspectives from adolescents, caregivers, providers, and advocates. Asian Am J Psychol [Internet]. 2014;5:316–24 Available from: https://www.ncbi.nlm.nih.gov/pmc/articles/PMC4319658/.
40. Charmaz K. Constructing Grounded Theory. 2nd ed. SAGE Publications Ltd; 2014.
41. Charmaz K. Grounded theory methods in social justice research. In: Denzin NK, Lincoln YS, editors. SAGE Handb. Qual. Res. SAGE; 2011. p. 359–380.
42. Charmaz K. The Power of Constructivist Grounded Theory for Critical Inquiry. Qual. Inq. [Internet]. 2017;23:34–45. Available from: http://journals.sagepub.com/doi/10.1177/1077800416657105
43. City Government of Muntinlupa. POVERTY AND EMPLOYMENT STATISTICS [Internet]. 2017 [cited 2017 Jun 30].
44. Philippine Statistics Authority. Philippines National Demographic and Health Survey 2013. 2013 [cited 2017 Jun 30]. Available from: https://dhsprogram.com/pubs/pdf/FR294/FR294.pdf.
45. Boling W, Means M, Fletcher A. Quality of Life and Stigma in Epilepsy, Perspectives from Selected Regions of Asia and Sub-Saharan Africa. Brain Sci. [Internet]. Multidisciplinary Digital Publishing Institute (MDPI); 2018 [cited 2018 Jun 27];8. Available from: http://www.ncbi.nlm.nih.gov/pubmed/29614761.
46. Herrmann LK, Welter E, Berg AT, Perzynski AT, Van Doren JR, Sajatovic M. Epilepsy misconceptions and stigma reduction: Current status in Western countries. Epilepsy Behav. [Internet]. 2016 [cited 2018 Jun 27];60:165–73. Available from: http://www.ncbi.nlm.nih.gov/pubmed/27208826.
47. Koch-Stoecker S. Neuropsychiatric issues in epilepsy. In: Matsuura M, Inoue Y, editors. Neuropsychiatr. issues epilepsy [Internet]. John Libbey Eurotext; 2010 [cited 2018 Jun 27]. p. 233. Available from: https://books.google.co.jp/books?id=FQXhAAAAQBAJ&pg=PA174&lpg=PA174&dq=epilepsy+Emil+Kraepelin&source=bl&ots=r35Oh0rwjA&sig=lZa-67-5hrTVkzSl4HEloGkaobQ&hl=en&sa=X&ved=0ahUKEwjd26SwkvPbAhWEnZQKHUvrDZsQ6AEIsAEwEw#v=onepage&q=epilepsyAQ28EmilKraepelin&f=false.
48. World Health Organization. mhGAP Training Manuals - for the mhGAP Intervention Guide for mental, neurological and substance use disorders in non-specialized health settings, version 2.0 [Internet]. WHO. World Health Organization; 2017 [cited 2018 Jun 27]. Available from: http://www.who.int/mental_health/mhgap/training_manuals/en/
49. Tuliao AP. Mental health help seeking among Filipinos: a review of the literature. Asia Pacific J Couns Psychother [Internet]. 2014;5:124–36 Available from: http://www.tandfonline.com/doi/abs/10.1080/21507686.2014.913641.
50. Yang LH, Valencia E, Alvarado R, Link B, Huynh N, Nguyen K, et al. A theoretical and empirical framework for constructing culture-specific stigma instruments for Chile. Cad. saude coletiva [Internet]. 2013;21:71–9. Available from: /pmc/articles/PMC3753780/?report=abstract.
51. Hamilton S, Pinfold V, Cotney J, Couperthwaite L, Matthews J, Barret K, et al. Qualitative analysis of mental health service users' reported experiences of discrimination. Acta Psychiatr Scand. 2016;134:14–22.
52. Demyttenaere K, Bruffaerts R, Posada-Villa J, Gasquet I, Kovess V, Lepine JP, et al. Prevalence, severity, and unmet need for treatment of mental disorders in the World Health Organization world mental health surveys. JAMA [internet]. 2004;291:2581–90. Available from. http://www.ncbi.nlm.nih.gov/pubmed/15173149.
53. Wig NN, Suleiman MA, Routledge R, Murthy RS, Ladrido-Ignacio L, Ibrahim HH, et al. Community reactions to mental disorders. A key informant study in three developing countries. Acta Psychiatr. Scand. [Internet]. 1980;61:111–26. Available from: https://www.ncbi.nlm.nih.gov/pubmed/7361584.
54. Ando S, Yamaguchi S, Aoki Y, Thornicroft G. Review of mental-health-related stigma in Japan. Psychiatry Clin Neurosci. 2013;67:471–82.
55. van Boekel LC, Brouwers EP, van Weeghel J, Garretsen HF. Comparing stigmatising attitudes towards people with substance use disorders between the general public, GPs, mental health and addiction specialists and clients. Int J Soc Psychiatry [Internet]. 2014;61:539–49 Available from: http://isp.sagepub.com/cgi/doi/10.1177/0020764014562051.
56. Clement S, Jarrett M, Henderson C, Thornicroft G. Messages to use in population-level campaigns to reduce mental health-related stigma: consensus development study. Epidemiol Psichiatr Soc. 2010;19:72–9.
57. Dy MB. Values in Philippine culture and education. Washington, DC: CRVP; 1994.
58. Social Weather Stations. Social Weather Station Survey. [Internet]. 2017 [cited 2017 Nov 9]. Available from: https://www.sws.org.ph/swsmain/artcldisppage/?artcsyscode=ART-20170816103037
59. Pescosolido BA, Martin JK, Olafsdottir S, Long JS, Medina TR, Martin JK. The theory of industrial society and cultural schemata: does the "cultural myth of stigma" underlie the WHO schizophrenia paradox? Am J Sociol. 2015;121: 783–825.
60. Araneta EG. Psychiatric Care of Pilipino Americans. In: Gaw AC, editor. Cult. Ethn. Ment. Illn. Washington, DC: American Psychiatric Press; 1993. p. 377–412.
61. Sanchez F, Gaw A. Mental health Care of Filipino Americans. Psychiatr Serv [Internet] 2007;58:810–815. Available from: https://www.ncbi.nlm.nih.gov/pubmed/17535941
62. Wonpat-Borja AJ, Yang LH, Link BG, Phelan JC. Eugenics, genetics, and mental illness stigma in Chinese Americans. Soc Psychiatry Psychiatr Epidemiol. 2012;47:145–56.
63. Yang LH, Purdie-Vaughns V, Kotabe H, Link BG, Saw A, Wong G, et al. Culture, threat, and mental illness stigma: identifying culture-specific threat among Chinese-American groups. Soc. Sci. Med. [internet]. Elsevier Ltd. 2013;88:56–67 Available from: https://doi.org/10.1016/j.socscimed.2013.03.036.
64. Yang LH, Kleinman A. "Face" and the embodiment of stigma in China: the cases of schizophrenia and AIDS. Soc Sci Med. 2008;67:398–408.
65. Abad PJB, Tan ML, Baluyot MMP, Villa AQ, Talapian GL, Reyes ME, et al. Cultural beliefs on disease causation in the Philippines: challenge and implications in genetic counseling. J Community Genet. 2014;5:399–407.
66. De Los Monteros KE, Gallo LC. The relevance of fatalism in the study of Latinas' cancer screening behavior: a systematic review of the literature. Int J Behav Med. 2011;18:310–8.
67. Roberts RE, Roberts CR, Chen IG. Fatalism and risk of adolescent depression. Psychiatry [internet]. 2000;63:239–52. Available from. http://www.ncbi.nlm.nih.gov/pubmed/11125670.

68. Cheng H, Sit JWH, Twinn SF, Cheng KKF, Thorne S. Coping with breast Cancer survivorship in Chinese women the role of fatalism or fatalistic voluntarism. Cancer Nurs. 2013;36:236–44.
69. Gonzalez P, Nuñez A, Wang-Letzkus M, Lim J-W, Flores KF, Nápoles AM. Coping with breast cancer: reflections from Chinese American, Korean American, and Mexican American women. Heal Psychol [Internet] 2016;35: 19–28. Available from: https://www.ncbi.nlm.nih.gov/pubmed/26389720.
70. Nurjannah I ,Mills J PT& UK. Human rights of the mentally ill in Indonesia. Int Nurs Rev. 2015;62:153–61.
71. Habtamu K, Alem A, Hanlon C. Conceptualizing and contextualizing functioning in people with severe mental disorders in rural Ethiopia: a qualitative study. BMC psychiatry [internet]. 2015;15:34. Available from: https://bmcpsychiatry.biomedcentral.com/articles/10.1186/s12888-015-0418-9.
72. An act establishing a national mental health policy for the purpose of enhancing the delivery of integrated mental health services, promoting and protecting the rights of persons utilizing psychiatric, neurologic and psychosocial health services, APPROPRI [Internet]. Republic of the Philippines; 2018. Available from: http://www.officialgazette.gov.ph/2018/06/20/republic-act-no-11036/
73. Kitchener B, Jorm A. Mental health first aid training for the public: evaluation of effects on knowledge, attitudes and helping behavior. BMC Psychiatry [Internet]. 2002;2:10. Available from: http://www.biomedcentral.com/1471-244X/2/10
74. Morgan AJ, Ross A, Reavley NJ. Systematic review and meta-analysis of Mental Health First Aid training: Effects on knowledge, stigma, and helping behaviour. Doran CM, editor. PLoS One [Internet]. 2018 [cited 2018 Jun 28];13:e0197102. Available from: https://journals.plos.org/plosone/article?id=10.1371/journal.pone.0197102.
75. Bond KS, Jorm AF, Kitchener BA, Reavley NJ. Mental health first aid training for Australian medical and nursing students: an evaluation study. BMC Psychol. [Internet]. 2015 [cited 2018 Jun 28];3:11. Available from: http://www.ncbi.nlm.nih.gov/pubmed/25914827.
76. Jorm AF, Kitchener BA, Fischer J-A, Cvetkovski S. Mental Health First Aid Training by e-Learning: A Randomized Controlled Trial. Aust. New Zeal. J. Psychiatry [Internet]. 2010 [cited 2018 Jun 28];44:1072–81. Available from: http://www.ncbi.nlm.nih.gov/pubmed/21070103.
77. Corrigan PW, Morris SB, Michaels PJ, Rafacz JDRN. Challenging the public stigma of mental illness: a meta-analysis of outcome studies. Psychiatr. Serv. [Internet]. 2012;63:963–73 Available from: https://www.ncbi.nlm.nih.gov/pubmed/23032675.
78. Corrigan PW, Michaels PJ, Vega E, Gause M, Larson J, Krzyzanowski R, et al. Key ingredients to contact-based stigma change: A cross-validation. Psychiatr. Rehabil. J. [Internet]. 2014 [cited 2018 Jun 28];37:62–4. Available from: http://www.ncbi.nlm.nih.gov/pubmed/24417232.
79. Corrigan PW, Larson JE, Michaels PJ, Buchholz BA, Del Rossi R, Fontecchio MJ, et al. Diminishing the self-stigma of mental illness by coming out proud. Psychiatry Res. 2015;229:148–54.
80. Rüsch N, Abbruzzese E, Hagedorn E, Hartenhauer D, Kaufmann I, Curschellas J, et al. Efficacy of Coming Out Proud to reduce stigma's impact among people with mental illness: pilot randomised controlled trial. Br. J. Psychiatry [Internet]. 2014 [cited 2018 Jun 28];204:391–7. Available from: http://www.ncbi.nlm.nih.gov/pubmed/24434073.
81. Corrigan PW, Rüsch N, Scior K. Adapting disclosure programs to reduce the stigma of mental illness. Psychiatr. Serv. [internet]. 2018 [cited 2018 Jun 28];appi.Ps.2017004. Available from: http://www.ncbi.nlm.nih.gov/pubmed/29606076.

8

Mechanisms associated with maternal adverse childhood experiences on offspring's mental health in Nairobi informal settlements: a mediational model testing approach

Manasi Kumar[1,2*], Beatrice Amugune[3], Beatrice Madeghe[4], Grace Nduku Wambua[5], Judith Osok[1], Anastasia Polkonikova-Wamoto[1], David Bukusi[6], Fred Were[7] and Keng-Yen Huang[8]

Abstract

Background: Adverse childhood experiences (ACEs) is a significant public health and social welfare problem in low-and middle income countries (LMICs). However, most ACEs research is based on developed countries, and little is known about mechanisms of early ACEs on adulthood health and offspring's wellbeing for populations in LMICs. This area is needed to guide social welfare policy and intervention service planning. This study addresses these research gaps by examining patterns of ACEs and understanding the role of ACEs on adulthood health (i.e., physical, mental health, experience of underage pregnancy) and offspring's mental health in Kenya. The study was guided by an Integrated Family Stress and Adverse Childhood Experiences Mediation Framework.

Methods: Three hundred ninety four mothers from two informal communities in Kariobangi and Kangemi in Nairobi were included in this study. The Adverse Childhood Experiences International Questionnaire (ACE-IQ), the Kessler Psychological Distress Scale (K10), Overall Health and Quality of Life items, and Child Behavior Checklist were used to study research questions. Data was gathered through a one-time interview with mothers. Structural Equational Modeling (SEM) was applied for mediational mechanism testing.

Results: Among 13 ACE areas, most mothers experienced multiple adversity during their childhood (Mean (SD) = 4.93 (2.52)), with household member treated violently (75%) as the most common ACE. SEM results showedthat all domains of ACEs were associated with some aspects of maternal health, and all three domains of maternal health (maternal mental health, physical health, and adolescent pregnancy) were significantly associated with development of offspring's mental health problems.

Conclusion: ACEs are highly prevalent in Kenyan informal settlements. Consistent with cross cultural literature on family stress model, maternal ACEs are robust predictors for poor child mental health. Preventive interventions for child mental health need to address maternal adverse childhood traumatic experiences as well as their current health in order to effectively promote child mental health.

Keywords: Maternal mental health, Adverse childhood experiences, Family stress model, Internalizing problems, Externalizing problems, Urban poverty

* Correspondence: m.kumar@ucl.ac.uk
[1]Department of Psychiatry, University of Nairobi, Nairobi, Kenya
[2]Research Department of Clinical Health and Educational Psychology, University College London, London, UK
Full list of author information is available at the end of the article

Background

In Kenya, it is estimated that 60 to 80% of urban residents live in informal settlements with slum like conditions [1]. More than half of the estimated population of 46 million Kenyans are young people under 18 of years of age [2]. A large number of those grow up experiencing poverty, poor health, nutrition, and deficient care [3] According to World Bank, 36.1% of the Kenyan population lives below the poverty line [4]. This population comprises of 52.3% in the rural and 34.8% of urban dwellers living in poverty [1]. Between 60 and 70% of Nairobi city's population live in congested informal settlements, commonly referred to as slums, without proper access to sanitation, clean water, health care and other social services [5].

Adversity and stressful environment can lead to parental depression, which has a detrimental impact on parenting, family functioning, parent-child relationships, and offspring's physical, social and behavioral health, and cognitive functioning [6]. According to findings of the National survey on violence against children, (KVACS, 2010), child abuse and neglect are common adversity events experienced by many Kenyan caregivers during their childhood. KVACS report on adults further indicates that during childhood, 32% of females and 18% of males experience sexual violence, 66% of females and 73% of males' experienced physical violence, 26% of females and 32% of males experience any violence as a child and 13% of females and 9% of males experienced all three types of violence during childhood [7]. Similarly, Mbagaya, Oburu & Bakermans-Kranenburg [8] reported 59% of child physical abuse (without differentiation of its severity in Kenya), and most violence against children was perpetuated by parents or close relatives [7].

There is paucity of new data to authoritatively evaluate long term impacts of ACEs on adulthood wellbeing and offspring's health and development in Kenya. This knowledge gap also exists for other Sub-Saharan African (SSA) countries. In SSA context, it is likely that the effects of poverty and limited resources would exacerbate the impact of adverse childhood experiences on adulthood and their offspring's health. This study aims to address these gaps by examining the relationship between adverse childhood experiences and their offspring's mental health.

Our integrated conceptual framework

This study was guided by the integration of the Family Stress Model [9–12] and the adverse childhood experiences (ACE) framework, proposed by the Centre for Disease Control/World Health Organization [13, 14] which posits that the level of parental and environmental-related stress influences family functioning and child outcomes. The Family Stress model specifically focuses on the current experience of severe economic pressures and other stressors that tend to undermine parents' mental health, family functioning and subsequent child adjustment [15]. The ACE framework focuses on how early experience of neglect, psychological distress and violence related stressors impacts on an individual's health-risk behaviors and adulthood chronic disease development. This framework focuses more on the impact on the individual's long-term outcomes, and less on their impact on the offspring. There are a couple of empirical findings about ACE which are worth noting here. *ACEs are common across cultures and social class contexts* with higher vulnerability to some groups such as those in economic hardships or refugee contexts. *ACEs form into clusters* therefore when analyzing their impact and addressing these it is important to see their *cumulative impact* than individual impact. What is of most relevance is that *ACEs have strongly demonstrated a dose-response relationship* with adult psychopathology as well as with other health conditions [16]. Some studies have argued that whilst ACEs were significantly predictive of all adult mental health outcomes beyond demographic and socioeconomic characteristics; social disadvantage continues to be identified as being a unique contributing factor and therefore merits continued examination of ACEs integrated within a social disadvantage framework [17, 18]. This study utilizes an integrated ACEs and family stress model, that allows us to examine impact of ACEs on adolescent health-risky behaviors (i.e., adolescent pregnancy) and adulthood health (i.e., physical and mental health), and influence of these current family contexts on offspring's health and development.

Objectives and associated hypotheses

Guided by the integrated ACEs and Family Stress framework, this study included four research objectives.

1. Describe patterns of ACEs in 13 areas among Kenyan mothers from two vulnerable communities located within Nairobi informal settlements in Kenya.
   We hypothesize high level of ACEs would be found in women who live in informal settlements.
2. Examine whether mothers' ACEs associated with adverse health outcomes in adulthood (including physical health, mental health, and adolescent pregnancy).
   We hypothesize ACEs experienced in maternal caregivers' childhood would negatively associated with their adulthood functioning.
3. Examine whether ACEs related to offspring's mental health problems.
   We hypothesize maternal ACE exposure would be significant predictors of greater offspring internalizing and externalizing problems.

Methods

Participants

The original sample included 431 parents (415 mothers and 16 fathers). Parents/primary caregivers who had 2–16 years old children and seeking maternal and child health services at Kariobangi and Kangemi public health centers were eligible to the study. Parents in this study were defined as biological birth parents. Parents who were psychologically unstable were ineligible for the study. For the purpose of this study, we further limited our participants to mothers ($n = 415$) and focused on the psychopathology mechanism testing in the family context where mothers are the primary caregivers. We excluded fathers given the small sample size ($n = 16$). Among the eligible mothers, 394 (95%) had data for all study variables. They were considered as the final analytical sample for this study.

The original study sample size was estimated based on the anticipated small to moderate effect $f^2 = .04$ to .10 (or $R^2 = 4–16\%$), 10 observed variables (8 independent variables, 2 dependent variables), with power level .80, and probability level .05 of a SEM model. We anticipate a minimum sample size of 160–380 would be required [19].

Setting and data collection procedure

Participants were recruited between Oct 2015 to April 2016 from two maternal and child health (MCH) centers from two underserved informal settlement communities of Nairobi. We chose these health service settings because families of young children tend to utilize preventive or treatment services from these providers. Eligible parents (describe above) were approached to obtain oral or written informed consent. For parents who were literate, the consent information was shared verbally, and a written consent form (with written information about the study) was given at the time of obtaining consent. A signed consent form was documented for parents who agreed to participate. For parents who were illiterate, an oral consent was obtained, and a literate witness (e.g., an adult who parents trusted) signed the consent form on their behalf, which was then documented. Consent and interviews were conducted in Kiswahili (99%; as it is the most common local language in Kenya) or English (1%, the official language in Kenya education system) based on parents' preference.

After consent, parents were scheduled for an interview at the MCH center by a trained bachelor or masters-level social science researcher. Participating parents were asked questions related to their childhood experience, their current health and wellbeing, and their child's health. For families with more than one child (age range 2–16 years), only one child was targeted. Children did not directly participate in the study activities, and they were not the subjects of this study. The study procedures and method of consent was approved by the Institutional Review Board of the Kenyatta National Hospital/University of Nairobi (IRB number: KNH/UoN-ERC Ref. P520/08/2015). To comply with ethical guidelines, participants who identified with a high depression score (cut-off of 10 or more based on our interview questionnaire Kessler Psychological Distress Scale; described below) or requested for other mental health services (due to stress or anxiety) during the data collection interview were referred to the Mental Health Clinic or provided with some onsite psychosocial support.

Measures

All study measures, except CBCL and parental health, have been used in Kenyan context, and are available in Kiswahili. To validate CBCL and parental health, a formal translation process was undertaken with permission from the test-developer Achenbach. The Kiswahili version of questionnaires was translated and back-translated, and a team review approach was used to resolve any discrepancies between the versions. Scale reliability (assessed using internal consistency Cronbach's Alpha/α) and validity for all study measures based on current study sample are reported below, which demonstrated all study measures to be reliable and valid with our study Kenya sample.

Adverse childhood experiences

Was assessed using *The Adverse Childhood Experiences International Questionnaire (ACE-IQ)* [20]. ACE-IQ assesses adult caregivers' experiences of childhood adversities such as child maltreatment and other traumatic stressors. Caregivers were asked to rate the frequency (never to many times/always) of their childhood experiences on 29 items, which were then categorized and converted to yes/no binary score in 13 areas. These binary scores were used to estimate prevalence of ACEs in diverse areas. To capture dose/level of the ACEs, summary scores (sum score) in 5 domains as well as a total score (sum of 13 areas) were also created. These include *Neglect domain* (2 ACE areas), *Family Psychological Distress domain* (4 ACE areas), *Home Violence domain* (3 ACE areas), *Sexual violence* (1 ACE area), and *Community Violence domain* (3 ACE areas) (see Table 1 for ACE areas and domains). These summary scores were used for subsequent psychopathology analyses. Inter-correlations (r) among four ACE domain scores were raged from .16–.26 ($p < .001$).

Maternal Physical and Mental Health

Three self-report measures were used to assess maternal physical and mental health. The *Kessler Psychological Distress Scale* (K10; 10 items, $\alpha = .94$ based on the current study sample) [21] assessed anxiety and depressive symptoms that mothers experienced. Mothers rated

Table 1 Caregivers' Adverse Childhood Experiences

ACE (Yes/No in 13 areas)	Examples (number of items)	Prevalence
Neglect		%
1 Physical neglect	1. Caregiver not give you enough food or sending you to school even it could easily been done; too drunk/ intoxicated by drugs to take care of you (any 3 items)	38.5
2 Emotion neglect	2. Caregiver not understand your problems/worries, knowing what you were doing with your free time (any 2 items)	42.6
Psychological Distress of Family Members		
3 One or no parents, parental separation or divorce	1. Parents ever separated/divorced, or father/mother/guardian die (any 2 items)	53.8
4 Alcohol/drug abuser in the household	2. Live with a household member who was a problem drinker, alcoholic, or misused street/prescription drugs (1 item)	44.1
5 Someone chronically depressed, mentally ill	3. Live with a household member who was depressed, mentally ill, or suicidal (1 item)	21.7
6 Incarcerated household member	4. Live with a household member who ever sent to jail or prison (1 item)	19.6
Violence at Home		
7 Household member treated violently	1. See or hear a parent/household member being yelled at/screamed at/sworn at/ insulted or humiliated; being slapped/kicked/punched/beaten up; or being hit/cut with an object (any 3 items)	74.8
8 Emotion abuse	2. You being yelled/screamed/sworn/insulted or humiliated, or being threaten/abandon, thrown out by parents/guardian (any 2 items)	38.0
9 Physical abuse	3. You being spanked/ slapped/kicked/ punched/beaten up; or being hit/cut with an object by parents/guardian (any 2 items)	39.2
Violence in Community		
10 Bullying many time	1. Being bullied (1 item)	22.4
11 Community violence	2. See or hear someone being beaten up, stabbed, short, or being threatened with a knife or gun in real life (any 3 items)	44.6
12 Collective violence	3. Force to go and live in other place; family member or friend killed or beaten up by soldiers, police, gangs, or militia (any 4 items)	39.6
Sexual violence		
13 Contact sexual abuse	1. Someone touch/fondle you, make you touch their body, attempt oral/anal/vaginal intercourse with you, or actually have intercourse with you in a sexual way when you did not want them to (any 4 item)	16.0
Nnumber of ACE Risk By Domain		Mean (SD)
Neglect (score 0–2)	• Physical + Emotional Neglect	0.81 (0.72)
Psychological distress of family members (score 0–4)	• One or no parent + substance abuse + mental ill + incarcerated household member	1.38 (1.09)
Violence at home (score 0–3)	• Emotion abuse + physical abuse + household member treated violently	1.52 (1.04)
Violence in community (score 0–3)	• Bullying + community + collective violence	1.06 (0.90)
Total # ACE risk (0–13)	13 areas in ACEs	4.93 (2.52)

10 symptom items on a 5-point scale (1 = none of the time; 5 = all of the time). A total score was created for 10 symptom items. Based on the recommendation, a clinical cut-off score of 25 was also used to estimate prevalence for mental disorder Individuals with a score of 25 or above would suggest a high likelihood of having a mental disorder. The scale has demonstrated to have good predictive validity using Structured Clinical Interview for DSM-IV (SCID) [22]. *Parental health* was assessed based on mother perception of overall health and quality of life (2 items; $\alpha = .70$ for the study sample) on a 5-point scale (1 = poor, 2 = fair, 3 = good, 4 = very good, 5 = excellent) [23]). A mean score ≤ 2 indicates poor health. *Adolescent pregnancy status* (1 = give birth to the first child at age 18 or younger, 0 = give birth to the first child ≥19 years) was also used to estimate

adolescent risky health behavior. Inter-correlation (*r*) between maternal mental health (K10) and maternal health were 0.34, and between adolescent pregnancy and mental health were 0.16 (all with $ps < .05$), suggesting sound validity of the measures for our Kenyan sample.

Child Mental Health

CBCL was used to assess child internalizing and externalizing problems on a 3-point scale (0 = not true, 2 = very or often true). Internalizing disorders present with an inward directed emotional and behavioral distress such as depression and externalizing disorders present with a propensity towards expressing distress outwards such as conduct disorder. Two CBCL age versions and 3 norm samples were used to score standardized T scores (1.5–5 version, 6–18 version for 6–11 years old and for 11–18 years old [24]. The research team carried out a formal translation of the 6–18 years with permission from the CBCL author Thomas Achenbach. Scale reliability were adequate for both internalizing problem ($\alpha = .76–.85$ based on our Kenyan 3 age-group samples) and externalizing problem ($\alpha = .87–.89$ based on the current Kenyan samples).

Demographics and Covariates

To consider potential confounders, maternal age, education status (1 = secondary or higher, 0 = primary or less), marital status (1 = married/living with the partner, 0 = divorced/single/ widowed) and employed status (1 = employed/self-employed, 0 = unemployed/homemaker) were included. Food insecurity (using Household Hunger Scale; 3 items; if any item was rated as yes was considered as food insecure [25] was also included as a demographic indicator.

Data analysis

To study *prevalence and patterns of ACEs*, a series of descriptive analyses were conducted. To study the *association between ACEs and maternal health* (physical, mental health, and adolescent pregnancy) *and child mental health* (i.e., externalizing such as aggression and conduct disorders and internalizing problems such as depression, anxiety and somatic complaints), a series of univariate logistic regression analyses were conducted. We examined impacts of 13 categories of ACEs separately to understand unique contribution to maternal and child health. In addition, to study "dose/level" of ACEs, we also examined four domains and total number of ACEs as predictors. To study *the mediational mechanism (ACEs → maternal health → child mental health),* we applied structural equation modeling (SEM), allowing for (a) meditational links from ACE domains to maternal health to child mental health, (b) variables within each domain (i.e., ACEs, maternal health, child mental health) to be correlated; and (c) adjusting for potential confounders (i.e., maternal age, education status, marital status, and employed status). The SEM model was tested using MPLUS 7] and used weighted least square mean and variance (MLSMV) estimation method. To judge the closeness of fit of the hypothesized association model, three indices were used [23]: chi square ($\chi^2 > .05$), root mean square error of approximation (RMSEA < .08), and comparative fit index (CFI > .95).

Results

Socio-demographic characteristics

Our sample comprises of 394 biological mothers with mean age of 31.56 years (SD = 7.06 years, 52% were < 30 years). About one half of the mothers (52%) in our sample were employed or categorized themselves as self-employed, 70% had educational attainment of primary school or less, 66% were married or living with partner, 32% had her 1st child at or before age 18 (or 60% at or before age 20). Most families (98%) were Christian, 63% experiencing food insecurity, and on average, had 2.84 children (SD = 1.33) and 4.82 (SD = 1.56) household members at home. Target children were on average 6.78 years old (SD = 3.04 years, 41% 1.5–5 years, 53% 6–11 years, and 6% 12–18 years), and 45% were boys.

Adverse childhood experiences (ACEs) of mothers

Table 1 shows prevalence of adverse childhood experiences in 13 areas, and total numbers of ACE by domains and in all 13 areas. The average number of ACEs experienced by mothers was 4.93 (SD = 2.52). Among the 13 ACE areas, the categories of household member treated violently (75%), presence of one or no parents, parental separation or divorce or living with one or no parents (54%), community violence (45%) living with alcohol/ drug abuser (44%), and emotion neglect (43%), and collective violence experience (40%) were the most common childhood adversity experiences.

Association between maternal ACEs and maternal and child health

We first examined patterns of mental health of our study caregivers and their children. For maternal health, 33% of mothers had moderate to severe mental disorder indication based on K10 (using the clinical cut-off 25). Another striking finding was that 32% had their first child at the age of 18 years or before, and 42% reported being in poor or fair health. With regards to the offspring, 15.6 and 10.2% were at-risk for internalizing and externalizing problems (T score ≥ 60), respectively. For the purpose of the analysis, we also used T-score cutoff of 50 (above norm mean) (24), which resulted in 44% of children with the internalizing score above mean standardized T score, and 31% with the externalizing score above mean standardized T score.

Next, we examined the associations between ACEs and maternal and offspring's health using logistic regression analyses. Univariate un-adjusted associations are reported in Table 2.

As hypothesized, all total number of risk in 5 ACE domains and across all ACE risks were associated with poor maternal mental health and early motherhood (being adolescent mothers). The odds for poor maternal health increase as number of ACEs increase. In addition, the most consistent ACE predictor for poor maternal health was emotional abuse and physical neglect. For child mental health, maternal experience of physical neglect, emotion abuse, and physical abuse during their childhood were most consistent predictors for poor offspring's mental health. In addition, two ACE domains which were, *violence at home and violence in community,* and total number of ACE risks were significantly associated with poor child mental health (on both externalizing and internalizing problems).

Mediational mechanisms

To examine whether the influence of ACEs on offspring's mental health is mediated by caregivers' health, adjusted SEM was carried out. Four demographic covariates (i.e., maternal age, education status, marital and employed status) were considered to adjust for potential confounders The overall χ^2 statistics based on the original theoretical model showed a reasonable fit in the SEM, χ^2 (10) = 59.69, p = <.001, RMSEA = .113 and CFI = .95. To improve the model fit, we add additional three paths (i.e., psychological distress of family member ➔ internalizing problem; violence at home ➔ externalizing and internalizing problems) guided by modification indexes suggested in the MPLUS. After including

Table 2 Associations between ACEs and Maternal and Offspring's Health

ACE (Yes/No in 13 areas)	Child Health				Maternal Health					
	At-risk for Child Externalizing Problems		At-Risk for Child Internalizing Problems		At-Risk for Maternal Mental Disorder		Adolescent Pregnancy		Poor Maternal Physical Health	
	OR	p	OR	p	OR	p	OR	p	OR	p
Neglect										
Physical neglect	1.56	.040	1.92	.002	3.33	<.001	1.83	.006	1.63	.017
Emotion neglect	0.65	.054	0.92	.685	1.22	.343	2.03	.001	1.36	.129
Psychological Distress of Family Members										
One or no parents, parental separation or divorce	1.07	.742	1.36	.128	1.17	.470	1.55	.045	1.01	.968
Alcohol/drug abuser in the household	1.03	.910	1.21	.338	1.37	.141	1.32	.205	1.15	.502
Someone chronically depressed, mentally ill	0.67	.147	0.66	.091	1.65	.042	1.18	.530	1.00	.983
Incarcerated household member	1.33	.275	1.17	.521	1.69	.040	1.14	.626	.913	.720
Violence at Home										
Household member treated violently	1.26	.357	1.85	.009	1.27	.334	1.18	.508	.840	.444
Emotion abuse	1.89	.003	4.14	<.001	2.36	<.001	2.34	<.001	1.49	.051
Physical abuse	2.32	<.001	3.37	<.001	1.81	.005	1.30	.232	1.15	.487
Violence in Community										
Bullying many time	1.44	.148	1.22	.411	1.95	.005	1.72	.029	2.00	.004
Community violence	1.68	.015	1.46	.061	1.14	.547	1.29	.241	1.07	.727
Collective violence	1.01	.951	1.18	.418	2.39	<.001	1.25	.306	1.08	.715
Sexual violence										
Contact sexual abuse	1.50	.145	1.49	.142	1.42	.205	1.93	.017	1.37	.243
Number of ACE Risk By Domain (Score Range)										
Neglect (0–2)	1.29	.065	1.01	.951	1.92	<.001	1.86	<.001	1.45	.008
Psychological distress of family members (0–4)	1.09	.373	1.02	.826	1.28	.010	1.22	.045	1.01	.923
Violence at home (0–3)	2.05	<.001	1.45	<.001	1.45	<.001	1.33	.008	1.09	.358
Violence in community (0–3)	1.23	.061	1.27	.044	1.55	<.001	1.30	.027	1.21	.084
Total # ACE risk (0–13)	1.21	<.001	1.11	.013	1.26	<.001	1.20	<.001	1.08	.051

Note. Analyses were based on univariate logistic regression

additional three paths, the overall χ^2 statistics showed a better fit of the model, χ^2 (7) = 24.16, p = <.001, RMSEA = .077 and CFI = .98. Figure 1 presents findings from this modified model. The standardized path coefficients for the significant paths and the R^2 values for each endogenous variable (maternal health and child mental health variables) from the SEM are presented in the Figure.

After adjusting for demographic confounders, all 5 domains of ACEs were associated with some aspects of maternal health, and all maternal mental health and physical health were significantly associated development of child mental health problems. Specifically, we found expected mediation links that higher ACEs (i.e., neglect, psychological distress of family members, violence at home, violence in community) were associated with higher adulthood mental disorders, which further associated with higher offspring's internalizing problem. In addition, exposure to violence at home and sexual abuse during childhood were associated with poor adulthood physical health, which further associated with more offspring internalizing and externalizing problems. Furthermore, higher level of neglect during childhood was associated with increase likely to have underage pregnancy, which further associated with higher offspring's internalizing problem.

There were also two unexpected findings that we found childhood sexual abuse experience was associated with lower adulthood mental disorder, and experience with psychological distress of family members was associated with fewer offspring's internalizing problem.

Discussion

Our findings have several implications for maternal and child mental health. Our maternal caregivers had experienced adversities covering on an average five ACEs risk areas (out of 13 risk areas). Violence experienced at home was the most prevalent ACE followed by experience of psychological distress associated with family or caregivers. Both these domains imply a high level of interpersonal violence and traumatization experience that can lead to mental health problems in adulthood. Given that 50 % of our sample had experienced early motherhood and got pregnant as adolescents, we can see that their developmental trajectory was impacted in significant ways. Early pregnancy and motherhood in the Kenyan context are often associated with dysfunctional families, high poverty and violence exposure [26–29]. The odds for poor maternal health increase as number of ACEs increase was another critical finding of our work implying that the ACEs have a bearing on the current functioning of adult caregivers. A number of other studies have found that childhood adversity links to a wide range of health problems in adulthood [30]. Early pregnancy and motherhood are known adverse experiences for women that was later added in the expanded ACE questionnaire by WHO.

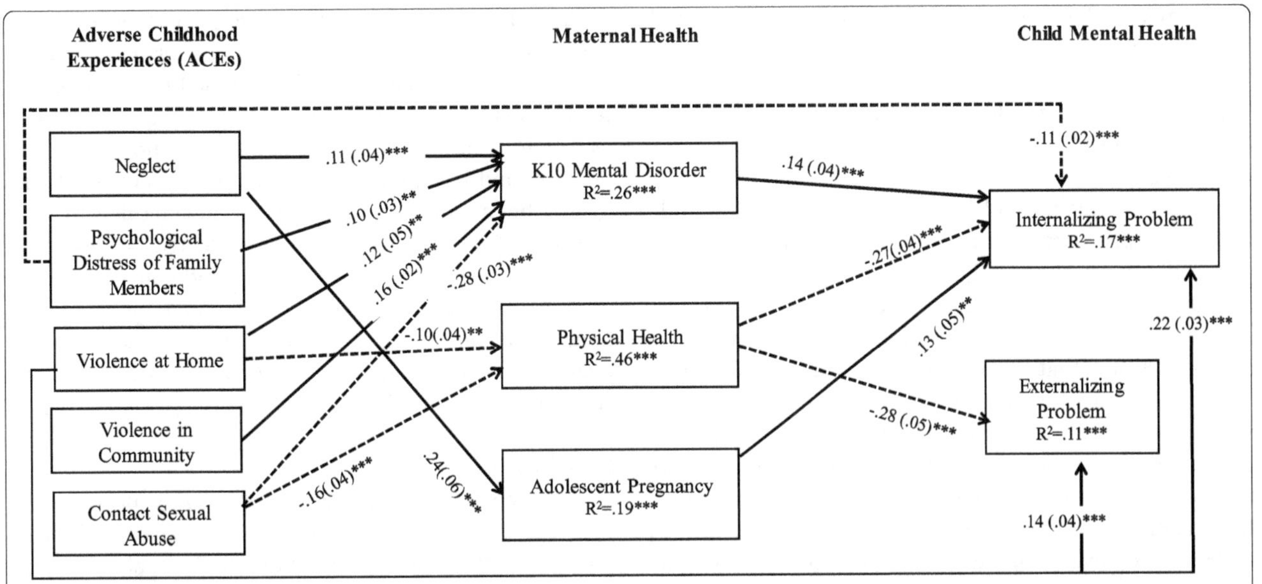

Fig. 1 Structural Equation Modeling for Association among ACEs, Maternal Health, and Child Mental Health. *Note.* Maternal mental and physical health and child mental health variables were continuous variables. Adolescent pregnancy was a dichotomized variable (1=underage pregnancy). Model controlled for maternal age, education status, marital status, and employed status. Standardized path coefficients and standard errors (in parentheses) are presented. A dash path indicates a negative association. Paths that did not reach significance are not shown in this figure. * $p < .05$ ** $p < .01$ *** $p < .001$. Inter-correlations (r) among ACE variables ranged from .07 to .26, among maternal health variables ranged from .09-.31, and between child outcomes was .61

Importance of ACEs in understanding adult well-being and child development

A number of ACE factors such as physical and emotional abuse and neglect, sexual abuse and parental separation or divorce or orphan-hood have been associated with pregnancy and motherhood experience in adolescence. These factors have been well-articulated in the literature on risk factors leading towards adolescent motherhood [31]. In our study we also found that in addition to ACEs predicting poor maternal mental health, other experiences such as physical neglect, emotional abuse and bullying were contributory factors. A number of studies have shown that children exposed to maternal depression are at risk for a wide range of negative cognitive, emotional and behavioral outcomes [32, 33]. Internalizing and externalizing problems are both implicated when caregivers have been through adversities and currently experience mental health problems. Overall all four ACE domains were significantly implicated with development of problem behaviors in the children as found in our analyses. While by and large a number of overlapping ACE domains were common to development of internalizing and externalizing problems, studies have shown that the level of caregiver depressive symptoms may also change over time and result in different trajectories of parenting behaviors [32, 34]. We did not assess changes longitudinally but perhaps a future study would take this into account. This may explain that some may lead to internalizing and others to externalizing problems. We also found that current mental health problems mediated the relationship between maternal ACEs and development of child mental health problems.

Exposure to violence at home and community has implications for development of depression in maternal caregivers

Exposure to violence and interpersonal trauma in childhood is a precursor for depression and mental health problems in adulthood [35]. Given that our female participants experienced variable and protracted adversities, such as high stress, anxiety and food insecurity, the K10 scores indicate that there may be other comorbidities impacting their functioning. In another study where such relationship was explored the chronic life events course, implies more severe depression symptoms, and that would mean less recovery as compared to when there is depression only [36].

There are several limitations of the study. The ACE data were collected using retrospective data collection method, we relied on caregivers' memory, which may not fully exclude recall bias. In addition, the assessment for maternal health and child mental health were concurrent assessments. Future research needs to include longitudinal data to better understand the causal mechanisms. This study was also limited to a maternal sample. Future studies should include fathers to better understand overall familial adversity experience on family functioning and offspring's health and development. In such studies, ways of engaging fathers would need to be identified as caregiving is largely left to mothers in the Kenyan context. Finally, our sample was drawn from a peri-urban informal settlement and there may be variable patterns in rural poor or more geographically diverse pockets in Kenya. To have broader generalizability, further studies would need to include diverse populations.

Clinical implications

Our study findings have several implications for clinical service development and intervention adaptation or engagement strategies development for women in Kenya. *Women with high adversities and stress need greater support to prevent intergenerational transmission of mental illness.* The adversity and stress experience of Kenyan women living in informal settlements has been well-documented. Interventions such as Problem Management Plus have been developed and championed by WHO to address adversity experiences and to bolster social support and treat depression in vulnerable women [37]. Low dose interventions delivered by community health workers or trained parent peer who may be able to factor in experience of adversities and ongoing depression and psychosocial functioning would be promising for women represented in our sample.

Similarly, a number of interventions focusing on maternal functioning have found positive impact on offspring well-being in recent times [38]. Parent peers can be a potential resource to deliver evidence-based psychosocial interventions [39]. Recent literature shows that ACEs could feed into more trauma-and-stress-mitigation informed practices and when this is combined with intergenerational approaches a number of interventions in clinical, early care, educational, and community contexts could be developed [40]. The especial focus on resilience and coping has been championed with ACE framework [41]. Parenting interventions targeting prosocial parenting and behavior development in families living in resource constraint and multiple adversity context would be helpful [42].

Conclusion

Adverse childhood experiences are highly prevalent in the lived experience of adult caregivers based in Kenyan informal settlements. Our study findings also support the integrated ACE and Family Stress model that maternal ACEs being a strong predictor for poor maternal health and child mental health. Preventive interventions for child mental health would benefit if consideration was given to understanding more deeply entrenched maternal trauma and adversities so that their impact on parenting and child health outcomes could be addressed. Interventions targeting poor health or mental health of women living in low resource settings need to target adverse childhood experiences of adult women in addition to their ongoing stress to provide the right psychosocial and mental health support. To have more generalizable causal influence, future studies need to utilize longitudinal design, and include mothers and fathers from diverse regions. Future studies need to also include other mental disorders (e.g., trauma, conduct disorders) in addition to anxiety and depression disorders to better understand impacts of ACEs on adulthood mental health.

Abbreviations

ACE: Adverse Childhood Experiences; ACE-IQ: Adverse Childhood Experiences International Questionnaire; CBCL: Child Behavior Checklist; K10: Kessler Psychological Distress Scale Overall Health and Quality of Life items; KVACS: Kenya Violence against Children Survey; MCH: Maternal and Child Health; SEM: Structural Equational Modeling; SSA: Sub-Saharan Africa; WHO: World Health Organization

Acknowledgements

We would like to acknowledge and appreciate the assistance our research assistants and volunteer community health workers at the Kangemi and Kariobangi North health centers. We thank the caregivers for participating in the study.

Funding

No external funding.

Authors' contributions

The proposal was jointly written by BM, APW, MK and HKY and reviewed by DB, BA, FW. The data was collected by BM, APW, JO, GNW, and MK. Data was analyzed by MK and HKY and written by MK and HKY and all authors read, reviewed and approved the paper.

Consent for publication

Not applicable.

Competing interests

The authors declare that they have no competing interests.

Author details

[1]Department of Psychiatry, University of Nairobi, Nairobi, Kenya. [2]Research Department of Clinical Health and Educational Psychology, University College London, London, UK. [3]Department of Pharmacy, University of Nairobi, Nairobi, Kenya. [4]Department of Food and Nutrition Sciences, University of Nairobi, Nairobi, Kenya. [5]Department of Clinical, Neuro- & Developmental Psychology, Vrije University of Amsterdam, Amsterdam, Netherlands. [6]Head VCT and HIV Care, Kenyatta National Hospital, Nairobi, Kenya. [7]College of Health Sciences, University of Nairobi, Nairobi, Kenya. [8]Department of Population Health, New York University School of Medicine, New York, USA.

References

1. Amendah DD, Buigut S, Mohamed S. Coping Strategies among Urban Poor: Evidence from Nairobi, Kenya. PLoS ONE. 2014;9(1):e83428 https://doi.org/10.1371/journal.pone.0083428.Accessed on 3 Nov 2018.
2. United Nations Children's Fund [UNICEF]. UNICEF Annual Report 2017. *https://www.unicef.org/about/annualreport/files/Kenya__2017_COAR*.pdf. Accessed 9 Aug 2018.
3. United Nations Children's Fund [UNICEF]. State of the world's Children 2016. https://www.unicef.org/publications/files/UNICEF SOWC_2016.pdf, Accessed 9 Aug 2018.
4. Mberu B, Ciera J, Elungata P, Ezeh A. Patterns and determinants of poverty transitions among poor urban households in Nairobi, Kenya. Afr Dev Rev. 2011;26:172–85. https://doi.org/10.1111/1467-8268.12073.
5. UNHABITAT. The *State of African Cities 2008 - A framework for addressing urban challenges in Africa. Nairobi* https://unhabitat.org/books/the-state-of-the-african-cities-report-2008/ Accessed 3 Nov 2018.
6. Shinsugi C, Matsumura M, Karama M, Tanaka J, Changoma M, Kaneko S. Factors associated with stunting among children according to the level of food insecurity in the household: a cross-sectional study in a rural community of southeastern Kenya. BMC Public Health. 2015;15:441 https://doi.org/10.1186/s12889-015-1802-6.
7. The Kenya Violence against Children Study : *Violence against Children in Kenya Findings from a 2010 National Survey.* https://www.unicef.org/esaro/VAC_in_Kenya.pdf. Accessed on 3 Nov 2018.
8. Mbagaya C, Oburu PO, Bakermans-Kranenburg MJ. Child physical abuse and neglect in Kenya, Zambia and the Netherlands: A cross-cultural comparison of prevalence psychopathological sequalae and mediation by PTSS. Int J Psychol. 2013;48(2):95–107.
9. Conger RD, Conger KJ, Martin MJ. Socioeconomic Status, Family Processes, and Individual Development. J Marriage Fam. 2010;72(3):685–704. https://doi.org/10.1111/j.1741-3737.2010.00725.x.
10. Conger RD, Wallace LE, Sun Y, Simons RL, VC ML, Brody GH. Economic pressure in African American families: a replication and extension of the family stress model. Dev Psychol. 2002;38:179–93 McLoyd VC. The impact of economic hardship on black families and children: psychological distress, parenting, and socioemotional development. Child Development, 1990: 61, 311–346.
11. McLoyd VC, Vonnie C. Socioeconomic disadvantage and child development. Am Psychol. 1998;53:185–204.
12. Butchart A.:- *Addressing adverse childhood experiences to improve public health*: Expert consultation, 4–5 May 2009: Meeting report. WHO; http://www.who.int/violence_injury_prevention/violence/activities/adverse_childhood_experiences/global_research_network_may_2009.pdf?ua=1. Accessed on 8 Aug 2018.
13. WHO (2017):- *Adverse Childhood Experiences International Questionnaire (ACE-IQ).* Retrieved from http://www.who.int/violence_injury_prevention/violence/activities/adverse_childhood_experiences/en/.
14. Conger RD, Elder GH. Families in troubled times: adapting to change in rural America. New York: Aldine; 1994.
15. Nurius PS, Logan-Greene P, Green S. ACEs within a social disadvantage framework: distinguishing unique, cumulative, and moderated contributions to adult mental health. J Prev Interv Community. 2012;40(4):278–90 https://doi.org/10.1080/10852352.2012.707443.
16. Shonkoff JP, Boyce WT, BS ME. Neuroscience, molecular biology, and the childhood roots of health disparities: Building a new framework for health promotion and disease prevention. J Am Med Assoc. 2009;301:2252–9.
17. Slopen N, Williams DR, Seedat S, Moomal H, Herman A, Stein DJ. Adversities in Childhood and Adult Psychopathology in the South Africa Stress and Health Study: Associations with First-Onset DSM-IV Disorders. Soc Sci Med. 2010;71(10):1847–54 https://doi.org/10.1016/j.socscimed.2010.08.015.
18. Alegria M, Vila D, Woo M, Canino G, Takeuchi D, Vera M, et al. Cultural relevance and equivalence in the NLAAS instrument: integrating etic and emic in the development of cross-cultural measures for a psychiatric epidemiology and services study of Latinos. Int J Methods Psychiatr Res. 2004;13(4):270–88.
19. Wolf EJ, Harrington KM, Clark SL, Miller MW. Sample size requirements for structural equation models: an evaluation of power, bias, and solution propriety. Educ Psychol Meas. 2013;76:913–34.
20. Kiburi SK, Molebatsi K, et al. Adverse childhood experiences among patients with substance use disorders at a referral psychiatric hospital in Kenya. BMC Psychiatry. 2018;18:197 https://www.ncbi.nlm.nih.gov/pmc/articles/PMC6007077/ Accessed on 3 Nov 2018.
21. Vissoci JRN, et al. Cross-cultural adaptation and psychometric properties of the Kessler Scale of Psychological Distress to a traumatic brain injury

population in Swahili and the Tanzanian Setting. Health Qual Life Outcomes. 2018;16:147 https://www.ncbi.nlm.nih.gov/pmc/articles/PMC6062865/ Accessed on 3 Nov 2018.

22. Kessler RC, Andrews G, Colpe LJ, Hiripl E, Mroczek DK, Normand SL, Zaslavsky AM. Short screening scales to monitor population prevalences and trends in non-specific psychological distress. Psychol Med. 2002;32:959–76.
23. Huang KY, Abura G, Theise R, Nakigudde J. Parental depression and associations with parenting and children's physical and mental health in a sub-Saharan African setting. Child Psychiatry Hum Dev. 2017;48:517–27.
24. Achenbach TM. Manual for Child Behavior Checklist/ 2-3 and 1992 Profile. Burlington, VT: University of Vermont, Dept. of psychiatry; 1992.
25. Ballard T, Coates J, Swindale A, & Deitchler M . *Household Hunger Scale: Indicator definition and measurement guide. in FANTA III Food and Nutrition Technical Assistance*, ed USAID (USAID & Fhi360, Washington DC).
26. United Nation Population Fund [UNFPA] *Motherhood in Childhood; Facing the challenge of Adolescent Pregnancy.* https://www.unfpa.org/publications/state-world-population-2013. Accessed 4 Aug 2018.
27. Kumar M, Huang K-Y, Othieno C, Wamalwa D, Madeghe B, Osok J, et al. Adolescent Pregnancy and Challenges in Kenyan Context: Perspectives from Multiple Community Stakeholders. Glob Soc Welf : Research, Policy & Practice. 2018;5(1):11–27 http://doi.org/10.1007/s40609-017-0102-8.
28. Osok J, Kigamwa P, Stoep AV, Huang K-Y, Kumar M. Depression and its psychosocial risk factors in pregnant Kenyan adolescents: a cross-sectional study in a community health Centre of Nairobi. BMC Psychiatry. 2018;18:136 http://doi.org/10.1186/s12888-018-1706-y.
29. Hunt TKA, Berger LM, Slack KS. Adverse Childhood Experiences and Behavioral Problems in Middle Childhood. Child Abuse Negl. 2017;67:391–402 https://doi.org/10.1016/j.chiabu.2016.11.005.
30. Mumah J, Kabiru CW, Mukiira C, Brinton J, Mutua M, Izugbara C, Birungi H, Askew I. Unintended Pregnancies in Kenya: A Country Profile, STEP UP Research Report. Nairobi: African Population and Health Research Center; 2014. http://www.popcouncil.org/uploads/pdfs/2014STEPUP_KenyaCountryProfile.pdf Accessed on 4 Aug 2018
31. Azak S, Raeder S. Trajectories of parenting behavior and maternal depression. Infant Behav Dev. 2013;36(3):391–402. https://doi.org/10.1016/j.infbeh.2013.03.004 Epub 2013 Apr 17.
32. Elgar FJ, McGrath PJ, Waschbusch DA, Stewart SH, Curtis LJ. Mutual influences on maternal depression and child adjustment problems. Clin Psychol Rev. 2004;24:441–59.
33. NICHD Early Child Care Research Network (2009). Chronicity of maternal depressive symptoms, maternal sensitivity, and child functioning at 36 months. Dev Psychol. 1999;35:1297–310.
34. Ellsberg M, Jansen HA, Heise L, Watts CH, Garcia-Moreno C, et al. Intimate partner violence and women's physical and mental health in the WHO multi-country study on women's health and domestic violence: an observational study. Lancet. 2008;371(9619):1165–72. https://doi.org/10.1016/S0140-6736(08)60522-X.
35. Pollack MH. Comorbid anxiety and depression. J Clin Psychiatry. 2005; 66(Suppl. 8):22–9.
36. Sijbrandij M, Bryant RA, Schafer A, Dawson KS, Anjuri D, Ndogoni L, et al. Problem Management Plus (PM+) in the treatment of common mental disorders in women affected by gender-based violence and urban adversity in Kenya; study protocol for a randomized controlled trial. Int J Mental Health Sys. 2016;10:44 http://doi.org/10.1186/s13033-016-0075-5. Accessed on 3 Nov 2018.
37. Rahman A, Fisher J, Bower P, Luchters S, Tran T, Yasamy MT, et al. Interventions for common perinatal mental disorders in women in low- and middle-income countries: a systematic review and meta-analysis. Bull World Health Organ. 2013;91(8):593–601I https://doi.org/10.2471/BLT.12.109819.
38. Atif N, Krishna RN, Sikander S, Lazarus A, Nisar A, Ahmad I, et al. Mother-to-mother therapy in India and Pakistan: adaptation and feasibility evaluation of the peer-delivered thinking healthy Programme. BMC Psychiatry. 2017;17:79 https://doi.org/10.1186/s12888-017-1244-z.
39. Bethel C, Gombojav N, Solloway M, Wissow L. Adverse childhood experiences, resilience and mindfulness-based approaches: common denominator issues for children with emotional, mental, or behavioral problems. Child Adolesc Psychiatr Clin N Am. 2016;25(2):139–56 https://doi.org/10.1016/j.chc.2015.12.001.
40. Garner AS, Forkey H, Szilagyi M. Translating developmental science to address childhood adversity. Acad Pediatr. 2015;15(5):493–502.
41. Pastorelli C, Lansford JE, Luengo Kanacri BP, Malone PS, Di Giunta L, Bacchini D, et al. Positive parenting and Children's prosocial behavior in eight countries. J Child Psychol and Psychiatry, and Allied Disciplines. 2016; 57(7):824–34 http://doi.org/10.1111/jcpp.12477.
42. Kumar M, Madeghe B, Osok J, Wambua GN, Amugune B. Shifting parental roles, caregiving practices and child development in low resource informal settlements of Nairobi: experiences of community health workers and school teachers. 2018. BMC Annals of General Psychiatry. https://doi.org/10.1186/s12991-018-0219-x.

9

The impact of immigration detention on mental health

M. von Werthern[1], K. Robjant[1], Z. Chui[1], R. Schon[1], L. Ottisova[2], C. Mason[1] and C. Katona[1,3*]

Abstract

Background: The number of asylum seekers, refugees and internally displaced people worldwide has increased dramatically over the past 5 years. Many countries are continuing to resort to detaining asylum seekers and other migrants, despite concerns that this may be harmful. In light of the considerable body of recent research, this review aims to update and expand on a 2009 systematic review on the mental health consequences of detention on adult, adolescent and child immigration detainees, which found (on the basis on 9 studies) that there was consistent evidence that immigration detention had adverse effects on mental health.

Methods: Three databases were searched using key terms relating to immigration detention and mental health. Electronic searches were supplemented by reference screening. Studies were included if they were quantitative, included individuals detained for immigration purposes, reported on mental health problems and were published in peer-reviewed journals. Two reviewers independently screened papers for eligibility, and a further two reviewers completed quality appraisals for included studies.

Results: Twenty- six studies (21 of which were not included in the 2009 review) reporting on a total of 2099 participants were included in the review. Overall, these studies indicated that adults, adolescents and children experienced high levels of mental health problems. Anxiety, depression and post-traumatic stress disorder were most commonly reported both during and following detention. Higher symptom scores were found in detained compared to non-detained refugees. In addition (and more clearly than was evident in 2009), detention duration was positively associated with severity of mental symptoms. Greater trauma exposure prior to detention was also associated with symptom severity.

Conclusions: The literature base reviewed in this paper consistently demonstrated severe mental health consequences amongst detainees across a wide range of settings and jurisdictions. There is a pressing need for the proper consideration of mental health and consequent risk of detention-related harm in decisions surrounding detention as well as for improved care for individuals within detention facilities. Recommendations based on these findings are presented, including increased focus on the identification of vulnerability and on minimising the duration of detention.

Keywords: Mental health, Vulnerability, Immigration detention, Asylum seekers, Refugees

Background

The number of people forcibly displaced worldwide as a result of persecution, conflict, generalized violence or human rights violations has increased dramatically in the last 5 years. The UNHCR estimates that there are currently (July 2018) 68.5 million forced migrants around the world [1].

Many countries detain asylum seekers in immigration detention centres whilst their applications are processed or following a decision to refuse them protection. At present the total number of third-country nationals held in immigration detention in the European Union is estimated to be 158,792 [2]. In the UK alone, this figure is 32526 people, representing 20% of total EU detainees, despite a much smaller percentage of asylum applications.

There is robust and consistent evidence that refugees are more vulnerable to mental illness, particularly depression and PTSD, as compared to the general

* Correspondence: cornelius@helenbamber.org
[1]Helen Bamber Foundation, Bruges Place, 15-20 Baynes Street, London NW1 0TF, UK
[3]Division of Psychiatry, University College London, London, UK
Full list of author information is available at the end of the article

population [3, 4]. Recent evidence indicates that vulnerability to non-affective psychoses is also increased in refugees compared to other migrants, reflecting their severe and often repeated exposure to adversity [5]. In addition to pre-migration factors such as exposure to torture or human trafficking, post-migration factors, including prolonged asylum procedures, prohibition from working, poverty and poor housing are significantly associated with poor mental health [6–9]. Research from the UK also indicates that post-migration and asylum-related stressors are associated with PTSD symptoms and emotional distress in asylum seekers and refugees [10].

Time spent in immigration detention in the host country is a particular post-migration stressor that entails loss of liberty and the threat of forced return to the country of origin. For many asylum seekers with a history of major trauma, it is reminiscent of contexts in their country of origin where they had been deprived of their liberty and human rights [11]. Immigration detention also exposes asylum seekers to possible abuse from staff and violence from fellow detainees, social isolation, and forceful removal. In the UK, the Medical Justice charity has documented these problems in a series of reports [12].

The practice of detaining asylum seekers, a group with a pre-existing vulnerability to mental health problems due to higher exposure to trauma pre- and peri-migration, [4] risks further exacerbating their mental health difficulties. The experience of detention may act as a new stressor, which adds to the cumulative effect of exposure to trauma, leading to an increased likelihood of developing mental health difficulties such as PTSD as a result of the 'building block effect' [13]. Indeed, a 2009 systematic review reporting on the effects of immigration detention on mental health found detainees to have high levels of anxiety, depression and post-traumatic stress disorder [14]. Suicidal ideation and deliberate self-harm were also common. Severity of distress was significantly greater in those who had been detained for relatively long periods [14]. The studies reviewed outlined the extent and severity of the mental health problems observed in detained people. The authors noted this research area was still in its infancy and highlighted the urgent need for further research on both the acute and longer-term impact of immigration detention on mental health, as well as its independence or otherwise from other risk factors.

Since 2009, a number of new studies have been published in the context of rising levels of forced migration globally and the frequent use of immigration detention to manage the increasing numbers of asylum seekers.

These findings have led to increasing concern that immigration detention may constitute a significant component of the post-migration adversity experienced by some asylum seekers. Such concerns over the treatment, support and management of both children and adults within detention facilities have been continuously expressed by numerous institutions across several countries, with many calling for legislative amendments to end immigration detention, particularly of children [15–17]. More recently, the UNHCR has also voiced concern over the physical and psychological effects of possible mandatory detention of all asylum seekers in Hungary [18]. The European Commission have reviewed the (very variable) use of alternatives to detention across the European Community. [19]

There has also been very extensive recent concern at the potential adverse consequences and human rights implications of the separation of migrant children from their parents by the USA authorities [20]. This led to this practice being discontinued [21].

In 2002, Australia was unique in its policy of indefinite, non-reviewable, mandatory detention of asylum seekers without valid entry documents arriving by boat. Clinical observation raised initial concerns, followed by the publication of research demonstrating the high prevalence of mental disorder in detention [22, 23]. Whereas the Australian authorities have since made changes to the law [24] that could be considered progress, the British government have sought to expand the capacity of immigration detention centres [25].

Although concerns have been raised over the mental health implications of immigration detention globally [26], we have taken the UK as a more in-depth example due to our familiarity with it and to the relatively large number of people detained there, incongruent with the comparatively small total number of asylum applications.

In 2015 a cross-party inquiry found that the UK detains too many people and for too long, and is more costly and less efficient than alternative systems operating in countries such as Australia and Sweden that have introduced community-based programmes to monitor asylum seekers and irregular migrants [27]. UK policy developments, therefore, provide an indicative illustration of these developing concerns.

In 2013, the Royal College of Psychiatrists issued a position statement on the detention of people with mental disorders in Immigration Removal Centres, which concluded that 'detention centres are likely to precipitate a significant deterioration of mental health in the majority of cases, greatly increasing both the suffering of the individual and the risk of suicide and self-harm' and therefore that 'people with mental disorder should only be subjected to immigration detention in very exceptional circumstances' [28].

In 2016, a government-commissioned review on the welfare of immigration detainees [29] highlighted the 'evident ethical, policy and practical implications' of medical research showing that immigration detention itself can seriously damage the mental health of detainees. A narrative review included within the report highlighted the particular vulnerability of people with a history of trauma and those with pre-existing mental or physical health problems to the adverse mental health effects of detention [30].

The UK Home Office published a Policy Guidance document on adults at risk in immigration detention [31]. which identified several 'conditions or experiences which will indicate that a person may be particularly vulnerable to harm in detention'. 'Immigration factors' enabled decisions to detain to be made and maintained despite substantial vulnerability factors being present. The Royal College of Psychiatrists issued a Position Statement expressing concern that the definition of torture within the new Adults at Risk policy added 'unnecessary and inappropriate complexity that does not assist in identifying those who are particularly vulnerable to the adverse effects of detention' [32]. In response to legal challenge, The UK Home Office has since changed this definition [33].

This review was conducted to provide a fuller and more up-to-date synthesis of the evidence. Its specific aims were to document (a) the prevalence and types of mental health problems among child and adult immigration detainees and (b) risk factors associated with mental health problems among immigration detainees. We looked particularly for evidence about the possible effects of pre-existing trauma and/or mental health problems and of duration of detention. Since detention systems vary between countries and nomenclature surrounding detainees vary across studies, the review takes a broad and inclusive stance and includes material on people detained within an immigration context (spanning asylum seekers, refugees and other migrants).

Methods

A systematic literature review following a modified version of the PRISMA guidelines [34] was conducted between October 2015 and May 2018 (PROSPERO Registration No: CRD42017056444).

Inclusion and exclusion criteria

Studies were included if they (a) included male or female adults or children detained for immigration purposes; (b) reported the prevalence of mental health problems; and (c) presented results of published peer-reviewed research based on one or more of the following study designs: cross-sectional survey; case–control study; cohort study; case series analysis; experimental study with baseline measures for the outcomes of interest; or secondary analysis of organisational records (Table 1). No restrictions were placed on country setting, country of origin of the immigration detainees, or method of measuring mental health outcomes. Since research in this area remains scarce, studies were not excluded on the grounds of their quality (though this is reported in Table 2). Qualitative studies will be presented in a subsequent paper.

Studies that did not report specifically on people held in immigration detention or removal centres (i.e. facilities detaining foreign national citizens for administrative purposes under immigration powers) were excluded. Studies that did not examine the impact of detention on mental health specifically were also excluded. Therefore any studies examining multi-morbidity involving both mental health disorders and physical disorders (e.g. infectious diseases) were excluded, as were studies focused on the attitudes and experiences of health professionals working within immigration detention. Reviews, grey literature, commentaries, conference abstracts, letters, editorials, books and short surveys were also excluded. We have however referred to relevant grey literature in the introduction and discussion sections.

Studies concerning child and adult detainees have been presented separately for the sake of clarity.

Search strategy

Relevant studies were identified through electronic searches of Embase (1980 to 2018 week 22), Ovid MEDLINE (1946 to May week 3 2018) and PsycINFO (1806 to May week 3 2018). Searches were limited to English language only. No other restrictions were applied to the searches. All search terms related to the following two main areas: mental health and immigration detention. The full electronic search strategy is presented in Additional file 1.

Electronic searches were supplemented by screening of reference lists of all included primary studies. In addition, the following journals published between 2013 and 2018 were hand searched: Forced Migrant Review, International Migration Review, International Migration, Journal of Refugee Studies, Journal of Traumatic Stress, Refuge, and Torture. Six International experts working in the field of forced migration and health (i.e. psychiatry, psychology and criminology) were contacted to nominate further papers eligible for inclusion. One response was received.

Data extraction and quality appraisal

Three reviewers (CM, RS, ZC) were involved in the process of independently screening titles and available abstracts of identified articles. If it was unclear whether a reference was relevant for the review, texts were retrieved in full. The same team of reviewers (CM, RS, ZC) independently assessed full texts to verify eligibility based on the above selection criteria. Disagreement was resolved either by discussion or with assistance of a third

Table 1 Mental Health Problems in Immigration Detainees: Characteristics of 26 quantitative studies

Author and year	Study Design	Sample	Country of Origin	Country of Study	Outcomes of interest	Method of assessing outcome
Brabeck & Xu [59]	Cross sectional survey	$N = 132$ immigrant parents who accessed immigrant community organisations Detention Duration: unknown	Various Latin American countries	United States	Impact of detention / deportation on Latino immigrant families	Self-report survey informed by Brabeck et al. [59] Translated and back translated
Cleveland & Rousseau [38]	Cross-sectional, comparison survey	$N = 122$ detained adult asylum seekers, $N = 66$ non-detained adult asylum seekers Detention Duration: mean 31.2 days, median 17.5 days	Unknown	Canada	Anxiety, depression & PTSD	HTQ, HSCL-25, modified DEC
Coffey et al. [40]	Cross-sectional semi-structured interview and survey	$N = 17$ refugees Detention Duration: mean 3 years 2 months, range 1.6 – 4.5 years	Afghanistan, Iraq, Iran and neighbouring countries	Australia	Experience of detention PTSD, depression, anxiety, quality of life	Semi-structured interviews; HSCL-25, HTQ, WHOQOL-Brief
Cohen [50]	Data comparison	$N = 231$ self-harm incident reports $N = 12$ suicide incident reports from IRCs $N = 38$ suicides from coroners and ombudsman reports	Unknown	UK	Rates of self-harm and suicide	Analysis of records, coroner's files and ombudsman's reports
Cwikel et al. [37]	Cross-sectional, comparison survey	$N = 47$ female brothel workers in detention, $N = 55$ female brothel workers Detention Duration: unknown	Former Soviet Union	Israel	PTSD, depression, somatic symptoms, suicidality	PCL, CES-D, constructed scale of physical symptoms, constructed scale of both past trauma and work trauma Russian speaking psychiatrist
Graf et al. [47]	Cross-sectional survey	$N = 80$ males detained for violation of the Swiss Aliens Act Detention Duration: 4 days	31 different countries	Switzerland	Prevalence rates of mental health disorders	BJMHS, CIDI (clinical psychologist), SCL-90R, subjective mental health questionnaire within 4 days of detention, SCL-90R and self-report again 6 months later where possible Material professionally translated into several languages
Green & Eager [36]	Cross-sectional analysis of health records	$N = 720$ Detention Duration: range 3 – 24 months	58 different countries	Australia	Estimated incidence rates of new health conditions, new mental health conditions and new injuries for each cohort	Health records coded by clinical coder
Hedrick [49]	Analysis of incident reports	Unknown	Unknown	Australia	Self-harm	Self-harm incident reports
Ichikawa et al. [41]	Cross-sectional, comparison survey	$N = 18$ former detained asylum seekers, $N = 37$ non-detained asylum seekers Accessible through a group of voluntary lawyers representing them and two NGO's Detention Duration: median 7 months, range 4 – 10 months	Afghanistan	Japan	Anxiety, depression, PTSD	HSCL-25, HTQ Translated into Dari and read out to participants by NGO caseworkers

Table 1 Mental Health Problems in Immigration Detainees: Characteristics of 26 quantitative studies *(Continued)*

Author and year	Study Design	Sample	Country of Origin	Country of Study	Outcomes of interest	Method of assessing outcome
Keller, Rosenfeld et al. [44]	Cross-sectional survey	*N* = 70 detained asylum seekers Detention Duration: median 7 months, range 2 – 42 months	Multiple countries	USA	Anxiety, depression, PTSD	HSCL-25, HTQ (+ two month follow up) Scales translated by interpreter, interviewed by experienced physician
Lorek et al. [52]	Cross-sectional survey	*N* = 11 detained children, *N* = 9 parents who responded to free legal assistance Detention Duration: range 11 – 115 days	Multiple	Britain	Mental and physical health of children held within immigration detention centre	Clinical diagnostic interviews, SCAS, DSRS, R-IES-13, SDQ, CORE, observations Psychologist and paediatricians had all been trained in carrying out cross-cultural assessments and worked regularly with asylum seeking children and families
Mares [54]	Secondary analysis of Australian Human Rights Commissions Data Set	*N* = 131 adults and *N* = 35 completed K10 N = 70 completed SDQ Detention Duration: mean 8 months, range 90-390 days	Unknown	Australia	Psychological distress, behavioural difficulties	K10, SDQ
Mares & Jureidini [53]	Assessment of referrals into CAMHS	*N* = 16 adults, 20 children, 10 families Detention Duration: mean 1 year 3 months, range 12 – 18 months	Iran, Iraq, Afghanistan, Palestine	Australia	Clinical assessment	Clinical instrument unknown
Momartin et al. [51]	Cross-sectional survey	*N* = 49 former immigration detainees on temporary protection visas and *N* = 67 granted permanent protection visas Detention duration: mean 12 months	Unknown	Australia	PTSD, anxiety, depression, general health, living difficulties and experiences of detention	HTQ, HSCL-25, GHQ-30, MOSSF-12, PMDC, DEC
Puthoopparambil et al. [46]	Cross-sectional survey	*N* = 127 immigration detainees Detention Duration: mean 37.8 days	46 different countries	Sweden	Quality of life	WHOQOL-BREF – incl. Six psychological questions Authorised telephone interpreters (used by 77 participants)
Robjant et al. [11]	Cross-sectional, comparison survey	N = 67 detained asylum seekers, *N* = 30 detained former prisoners, N = 49 asylum seekers living in the community Detention Duration: unknown	Unknown	UK	PTSD, depression, anxiety	HADS, IES-R, PDS English
Rojas-Flores [57]	Cross sectional comparison survey	*N* = 39 children of detained or deported parents *N* = 42 unauthorised no history of detention or deportation N = 16 Legal permanent resident Detention Duration: unknown	Mexico or Central America	US	PTSD, depression, behavioural difficulties, daily functioning	UCLA PTSD-RI, CES-DSC, BASC-2 PRS-C, TSCYC-SP, BASC-2 TRS-C, CAFAS
Rothe et al. (2002a)	Cross sectional survey	*N* = 74 adolescents Detention Duration: 4-6 months	Cuba	US	PTSD, psychological distress	PTSDRI, checklist of PTSD symptoms
Rothe et al. (2002b)	Cross sectional survey	*N* = 87 adolescents Detention Duration:	Cuba	US	PTSD, behavioural difficulties	PTSDRI, CBCL-TRF

Table 1 Mental Health Problems in Immigration Detainees: Characteristics of 26 quantitative studies *(Continued)*

Author and year	Study Design	Sample	Country of Origin	Country of Study	Outcomes of interest	Method of assessing outcome
		mean 6-8 months				
Sen et al. [45]	Observational, Cross-sectional	*N* = 101 male detained in immigration removal centre Detention Duration: unknown	27 different countries	UK	Neurodevelopmental	MINI v6, SAPAS, AQ-10, ASRS, LDSQ, CANFOR No interpreters
Sobhanian et al. [42]	Cross-sectional survery	*N* = 150 former refugee detainees Detention Duration: mean 11.3 months, range 2 – 21 months	Iran, Afghanistan	Australia	Psychological status and quality of life	T-FAST, QOLI, POMS, SIS Translated and back translated into Farsi, self report administered under supervision of clinical psychologist
Steel et al. [23]	Cross-sectional	N = 10 families (14 adults, 20 children) held for in immigration detention for more than two years Detention Duration: mean 2 years 4 months, range 2 years 2 months – 2 years 8 months	Unknown	Australia	Psychiatric Status	DEC, DSC, K-SADS-PL, SCID-IV, Parenting Questionnaire, Over the telephone by same language-speaking psychologists with prior professional experience working with refugees
Steel et al. [43]	Cross-sectional, comparison survey	*N* = 241 Arabic-speaking Mandaean refugees Detention Duration: median 6 months	Mainly Iran and Iraq	Australia	Anxiety, depression & PTSD	HTQ, HSCL-25, MOSSF-12, PMLD, DEC, DSC Translated and back translated by certified Arabic-speaking healthcare interpreter
Steel et al. [39]	Longitudinal survey	N = 47 former immigration detainees on temporary protection visas and *N* = 57 granted permanent protection visas attending a state-wide early intervention program in New South Wales Detention Duration: meadian 8 months, range 1 – 30 months	Iran, Afghanistan	Australia	Anxiety, depression and PTSD	HTQ, HSCL-25, GHQ-30, PSWQ, PMLD Baseline and 2-year follow up Measures translated by experienced clinical psychologist fluent in both dialects, and back translated. Interviews undertaken by Fasi / Dari speaking psychologists
Young & Gordon [48]	Secondary analysis of Australian Human Rights Commissions Data Set	*N* = 1354 detained refugees, asylum seekers and 'others'	Unknown	Australia	PTSD, mental health	K10, HTQ, HoNOS, HoNOSCA
Zwi et al. [58]	Cross sectional survey	*N* = 48 detained children N = 38 child asylum seekers in community	Eastern Mediterranean, South East Asia, Pacific, Africa, Stateless origin	Australia	Behavioural difficulties	SDQ

ASRS Adult ADHD Self-Report Scales, *AQ-10* Autism-Spectrum Quotient 10, *BASC-2 PRS-C* Behaviour Assessment System for Children-2nd Edition, Parent Rating Scales-Child, *BASC-2 TRS-C* Behaviour Assessment System for Children-2nd Edition, Teacher Rating Scales-Child, *BJMHS* Brief Jail Mental Health Screen, *CAFAS* Child and Adolescent Functional Assessment Scale, *CAMHS* Child and Adolescent Mental Health Services, *CANFOR* Camberwell Assessment of Needs – Forensic Version, *CBCL-TRF* Child Behavioral Check List – Teachers Report Form, *CES-D* Center for Epidemiologic Studies Depression, *CES-DSC* Centre for Epidemiologic Studies Depression Scale for Children, *CIDI* Composite International Diagnostic Interview, *CORE* Clinical Outcomes in Routine Evaluation, *DEC* Detention Experience Checklist, *DSC* Detention Symptom Checklist, *DSRS* Birleson Depression Self-Rating Scale, *GHQ-30* General Health Questionnaire 30, *HADS* Hospital Anxiety Depression Scale, *HSCL-25* Hopkins Symptoms Checklist 25, *HoNOS* Health of Nation Outcomes Scale, *HoNOSCA* Health of Nation Outcomes Scale for Children and Adolescents, *HTQ* Harvard Trauma Questionnaire, *IES-R* Impact of Events Scale Revised, *K10* Kessler 10, *K-SADS-PL* Schedule for Affective Disorders and Schizophrenia for School-Aged Children-Present and Life Time Version, *LDSQ* Learning Disability Screening Questionnaire, *MOSSF-12*Medical Outcomes Study – Short Form, *MINI v6* Mini International Neuropsychiatric Interview v6.0, *NGO* Non-governmental Organisation, *PCL* PTSD checklist, *PDS* Posttraumatic diagnostic scale, *PMDC* Post Migration Difficulties Checklist, PMLD – Post-migration living difficulties and detention experiences checklist, *POMS* Profile of Mood States, *PSWQ* Penn State Worry Questionnaire, *PTSDRI* Posttraumatic Stress Disorder Reaction Index, *QOLI* Quality of Life Inventory, *R-IES-13* Revised Impact of Events Scale-13, *SAPAS* Standardized Assessment of Personality Abbreviated Scale, *SCAS* Spence Children's Anxiety Scale, *SCID-IV* Structured Clinical Interview for DSM-IV Axis I Disorders, *SCL-90-R* Symptoms Checklist-90-R, *SDQ* Strengths and Difficulties Questionnaire, *SIS* Suicide Ideation Scale, *T-FAST* Truncated Firestone Assessment of Self destructive Thoughts, *TSCYC-SP* Trauma Symptom Checklist for Young Children – Spanish Version, *UCLA PTSD-RI* UCLA Posttraumatic Stress Disorder Reaction Index, *WHOQOL-Brief* World Health Organisation Quality of Life Short Version

reviewer (CK, KR or MW). Data from all included studies was double extracted by a team of four reviewers (CM, MW, RS, ZC) into a standardised electronic spreadsheet. The following information was extracted from each study: first author, year of publication, population sampled, country where study was carried out, study design, measures used to assess mental health or psychological domains of quality of life, outcomes and length of immigration detention. The quality of studies which met the inclusion criteria was appraised independently by two from a team of three reviewers (CK, CM, MW) using a modified version of the qualitative Critical Appraisal Skills Programme Checklist [35].

Each item was rated as high (2), intermediate (1) or low (0) quality, resulting in a maximum potential total score of 26 (see Table 2 for breakdown of scores). Discrepancies in scores between reviewers were resolved by discussion.

Results

The study selection process is outlined in Fig. 1. Twenty-six relevant studies reporting on a total of 2099 participants were included in the review. Of these, 16 studies reported on adults, 9 studies on children and families and one reported on both. Studies were conducted in Australia, Canada, Israel, Japan, Sweden, Switzerland, the UK and the US. Not all studies listed individual countries of origin, yet as many as 58 countries were represented within a single study [36]. Key characteristics of all included studies can be found in Table 2.

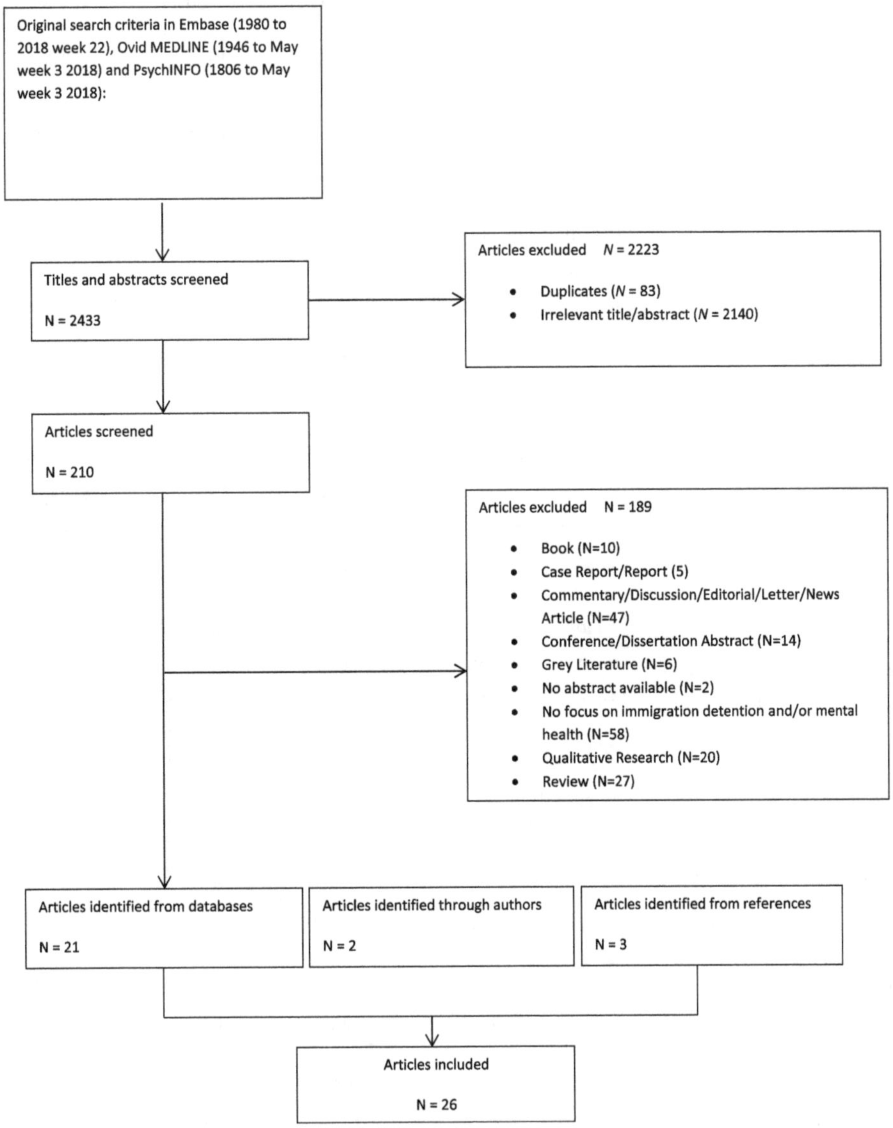

Fig. 1 Study flow chart

Table 2 Quality Review of 26 studies

Quality Question 1-7

Study	Clear focus on question	Appropriate design	Appropriate sampling method	Appropriate sample	Tolerable level of non-participation	Exposure (detention) appropriately addressed	Outcomes (mental health symptoms and disorders) appropriately addressed
Brabeck & Xu [59]	High	High	High	Intermediate	Intermediate	Intermediate	Low
Cleveland & Rousseau [38]	High	High	Intermediate	High	Intermediate	High	High
Coffey et al. [40]	High	High	Intermediate	Intermediate	Intermediate	High	High
Cohen [50]	Intermediate	Low	Low	Low	Low	Intermediate	Intermediate
Cwikel et al. [37]	High	High	Low	Intermediate	Low	High	High
Graf et al. [47]	High	High	High	Intermediate	Low	High	High
Green & Eagar [36]	High	Intermediate	High	Intermediate	High	High	Intermediate
Hedrick [49]	High	High	High	Intermediate	High	Intermediate	Intermediate
Ichikawa et al. [41]	High	High	High	High	High	High	High
Keller et al. [44]	Intermediate	High	Intermediate	High	High	High	High
Lorek et al. [52]	High	High	Intermediate	Intermediate	Low	High	Intermediate
Mares [54]	High	Intermediate	Intermediate	Intermediate	Low	High	High
Mares & Jureidini [53]	High	High	Intermediate	Intermediate	Intermediate	High	Intermediate
Momartin et al. [51]	High	High	Intermediate	Intermediate	High	High	High
Puthoopparambil et al. (2009)	High	High	High	Intermediate	Intermediate	High	High
Robjant et al. [11]	High	High	Intermediate	High	High	High	High
Rojas-Flores, L. [57]	High	High	Intermediate	Intermediate	Low	Intermediate	High
Rothe et al. [55]	Intermediate	High	Intermediate	Low	Low	High	Intermediate
Rothe et al. [56]	High	High	Low	Low	Low	High	High
Sen et al. [45]	High	High	Intermediate	Intermediate	Intermediate	High	High
Sobhanian et al. [42]	High	Intermediate	Low	Intermediate	Low	High	High
Steel et al. [23]	High	High	High	Intermediate	High	High	Intermediate
Steel et al. [43]	High	High	High	Intermediate	High	High	High
Steel et al. (2011)	High	High	High	High	High	High	High
Young & Gordon [48]	High	High	High	Intermediate	Intermediate	Intermediate	High
Zwi et al. [58]	High	High	Intermediate	High	Intermediate	High	High

Quality Question 8-13

Study	Consideration of cofounders	Appropriate conduction of statistical analyses	Reporting of confidence intervals	Consideration of ethical issues	Adequate support for conclusions	Generalisability of findings	Total Score
Brabeck & Xu [59]	High	High	High	Intermediate	High	Intermediate	19/26
Cleveland & Rousseau [38]	High	High	High	High	High	High	24/26
Coffey et al. [40]	Low	High	High	High	High	Intermediate	20/26
Cohen [50]	Low	Low	Low	Intermediate	High	Intermediate	7/26
Cwikel et al. [37]	High	High	Intermediate	Intermediate	High	Intermediate	18/26

Table 2 Quality Review of 26 studies *(Continued)*

Graf et al. [47]	Low	High	Low	High	High	High	19/26
Green & Eagar [36]	High	High	High	Intermediate	High	High	22/26
Hedrick [49]	Intermediate	High	Low	Intermediate	High	High	19/26
Ichikawa et al. [41]	High	High	High	High	High	Intermediate	25/26
Keller et al. [44]	High	High	High	High	High	High	23/26
Lorek et al. [52]	Intermediate	Low	Low	Intermediate	High	Intermediate	14/26
Mares [54]	Low	High	Low	High	High	Intermediate	16/26
Mares & Jureidini [53]	Low	Intermediate	Low	Low	High	Intermediate	14/26
Momartin et al. [51]	High	High	High	Intermediate	High	Intermediate	22/26
Puthoopparambil et al. [46]	High	High	High	High	High	High	24/26
Robjant et al. [11]	High	High	High	High	High	High	25/26
Rojas-Flores, L. [57]	High	High	Intermediate	Intermediate	High	Intermediate	18/26
Rothe et al. (2002a)	Low	Low	Low	Low	High	Low	9/26
Rothe et al. (2002b)	High	High	Low	Intermediate	High	Low	15/26
Sen et al. [45]	Intermediate	High	Low	High	High	High	19/26
Sobhanian et al. [42]	High	High	Low	Intermediate	High	High	15/26
Steel et al. [23]	Intermediate	Intermediate	Low	High	High	Intermediate	19/26
Steel et al. [43]	High	High	Intermediate	High	High	Intermediate	23/26
Steel et al. [39]	Intermediate	Intermediate	High	High	High	Intermediate	24/26
Young & Gordon [48]	Low	High	Low	Intermediate	High	Intermediate	17/26
Zwi et al. [58]	Intermediate	High	High	Intermediate	High	High	22/26

Adults

A total of 17 studies reported data on the mental health consequences of immigration detention in adults. These studies involved a total of 1168 participants (Note: this number only includes studies in which primary data was collected). Three studies on parental health are discussed separately in the 'Child and Families' subsection below. Six studies were conducted as comparison studies, with a total of 331 non-detained controls. Ten studies were conducted during detention, six were conducted following detention, and one included both current and past detainees. Reasons given for detention varied widely and were not consistently reported. Many were asylum seekers and some studies also included foreign national prisoners or ex-prisoners awaiting deportation, illegal workers and undocumented entrants. Participant ages ranged from 15 to 80 years of age. Approximately two thirds of all participants were male. One study focused exclusively on females, who were illegal sex workers detained in Israel and awaiting deportation [37]. Studies differed widely in the participants' duration of detention. Some studies reported average duration in terms of the mean, others reported median durations. For those reporting mean durations, these ranged between 4 days to 3.2 years. Reported median durations ranged between 6 to 8 months. Reported ranges fell between 2- to 4 months. Various pre-migratory traumatic events were reported, including but not limited to torture. Where reported, subjection to torture ranged from 12.2–100%.

Overall, 11 studies employed self-report measures, one used self-report measures along with clinical assessment, one used clinical assessments only and four analysed health records. These studies are reviewed below in terms of method of measuring mental health outcomes (self-report and clinical assessments), use of a control design, detention duration and release, and gender.

Self-report (see Table 3)

Self-report data (predominantly using clinically validated rating scales) relating to detention experiences

Table 3 Assessment and Prevalence Rates of Mental Health Difficulties in currently detained and formerly detained Adults

Mental Health Difficulty	Cleveland & Rousseau [38]	Coffey et al. [40]	Cwikel et al. [37]	Ichikawa et al. [41]	Keller et al. [44]	Robjant et al. [11]	Sen et al. [45]	Steel et al. [43]	Steel et al. [39]
Depression	√	88%	79%	√	86%	√	52.5%	√	√
Anxiety	√	–	–	√	77%	72%	12%	√	√
PTSD	√	70%	17%	√	50%	76%	20.8%	√	√
Specific Phobia	–	–	–	–	–				–
Psychotic or Depressive Affective Disorder	–	–	–	–	–	–	10%	–	–
Personality Disorder	–	–	–	–	–	–	34.7%	–	–
Suicidal Ideation	–	–	47%	–	26%	–	–	–	–
Suicide Attempt	–	–	19%	–	3%	–	–	–	–
Somatisation	–	–	40-60%	–	–	–	–	–	–
Autism	–	–	–	–	–	–	15%	–	–
ADHD	–	–	–	–	–	–	14%	–	–
OCD	–	–	–	–	–	–	9%	–	–

consistently identify severe levels of mental health problems amongst detainees. Most studies ($N = 9$) reported on symptoms of anxiety, depression and PTSD, which appear to be the most common forms of mental health difficulties experienced by detainees both during [36–39] and following detention (see below; [40–43]. Whilst not differentiating between types of traumatic experiences, greater trauma exposure prior to detention was significantly associated with higher rates of such symptoms [37, 38, 41]. Gaining temporary protection rather than permanent protection was an independent contributor to the risk of on-going depression and PTSD [43]. Isolation from family members and living alone were also associated with higher rates of such symptoms [41, 43].

Somatization, suicidal ideation, substance use, personality disorder and neurodevelopment disorders were also reported in some studies [37, 44, 45].

Three studies measured the quality of life of detainees and uniformly reported low quality of life ratings, particularly across psychological domains [40, 42, 46]. One of these studies found that levels of quality of life were mediated by the level of perceived support and satisfaction with the care received from detention staff [46].

Clinical assessments

Two of the identified studies involved diagnostic clinical assessments. Both of these were restricted to male detainees. Graf and colleagues [47], using the WHO Composite International Diagnostic Interview (CIDI), found a 76% point prevalence of mental health disorders in detainees, with 26.2% meeting criteria for serious mental illness within 4 days of admission. The most common disorders were found to be affective disorders (36%), anxiety disorders (34%) and PTSD (23%). Similar prevalence rates were found in a study by Sen et al. [45], which combined self-report measures with clinical assessments. They found the prevalence of any mental health, developmental or personality disorder to be 74.3%, with over half of the sample screened positive for more than one disorder. Seventy-three percent of the sample reported unmet psychological needs.

Secondary health data

Four studies analysed pre-existing health data obtained from detention centres. Data recording was poor across most studies, with authors facing flawed and unsystematic documentation. One study drew on data obtained from health records within detention centres [36]. Despite the reported lack of available records spanning the entire detention period of many detainees, the findings suggest that mental health issues were identified in 6% of detainees. The reason for being detained was also found to contribute to new mental health problems, with unauthorised boat arrivals displaying the highest rates of psychiatric morbidity (27%). Asylum seekers had more health problems including mental health problems than other detainees. Only 7% of all recorded detention centre interventions included formal mental state examinations. A further study reported much higher numbers, with approximately half the detainees suffering from PTSD symptoms [48]. Two studies looked at rates of suicide and/or self-harm using data extracted from incident reports within detention centres in Australia [49] and the UK [50]. Self-harm was estimated to occur in 22% (including attempted hanging) and 12.8% respectively. Where provided, precipitating factors to self-harm revolved around detention conditions and procedural related factors (such as duration of claims) and negative decisions [49]. Suicides in immigration detention were estimated at 222 per 100,000 between 2002 and 2004, with the majority of deaths being caused by hanging [50]. Of the deaths in detainees reported in coroner's reports and Prisoner's Ombudsman's reports, the majority had a history of mental health difficulties including depression, psychosis and PTSD. Overall however, these figures are likely to reflect only the most severe cases in which the mental health difficulties were sufficiently prominent to be identified and recorded by detention staff. Moreover, they are likely to represent the perspective of detention staff rather than of asylum seekers themselves.

Comparison studies

Six studies compared the self-reported levels of PTSD, depression and anxiety of detainees to those in a comparison group of non-detained refugees or migrants from a similar background. All six studies showed higher symptom scores and rates of meeting clinical threshold for mental health disorders in the detained groups. This held true when comparing detained asylum seekers with non-detained asylum seekers [38, 41] detained asylum seekers and detained former prisoners with non-detained asylum seekers [11], detained sex workers with non-detained sex workers [37] and detained temporary protection visa holders with non-detained permanent protection visa holders [39, 43, 51]. All but one study [11] found no significant difference in levels of pre-migration trauma exposure between the groups, suggesting that detention contributed independently to PTSD over and above the impact of past traumatic experiences. However, whilst the number of traumatic events may not have differed across groups, the frequency, severity and context of those events were often not assessed.

Whilst no direct comparison between detainees and prison populations have been conducted to date, one study compared findings obtained from one immigration removal centre in the UK against results from prison-based studies utilising the same screening tools [45]. Despite methodological shortcomings and difficulties in making direct comparisons, prevalence rates of depression and PTSD were higher among immigration detainees than in prison populations. Levels of suicidal ideation were high in both groups.

Detention duration and release

Eight studies reported on the relationship between length of detention or release from detention and mental health and/or quality of life. Four studies conducted in Australia and the USA found a significant positive correlation between detention duration and symptomatology [36, 43, 44, 48], suggesting that psychological functioning deteriorates with prolonged detention. A UK study found an interaction effect between exposure to interpersonal trauma and length of detention, suggesting that experience of interpersonal trauma and prolonged time in detention resulted in higher anxiety and depression scores [11] . The authors suggest that the interaction they found may also reflect the complex relationship between stage of claim and detention duration within the UK. However, even brief detention (median 17.5 days) has been found to have negative mental health consequences [38].

In contrast, two studies did not find a statistically significant correlation between detention duration and quality of life [42, 46], although a decreasing trend was found in one of these studies [46]. Here, the small sample size as well as the use of quality of life scales rather than mental symptom measures may have resulted in reduced sensitivity to the effects of detention. Furthermore, one of the two 'negative' studies indicated a significant increase of suicidal ideation with detention duration [42].

One study employed a longitudinal design with a two-month follow up, indicating not only that detention exacerbates psychological symptoms over time, but also that these symptoms were markedly reduced in those participants who had been released prior to the follow-up rating [44]. However, another longitudinal study suggests that symptomatology and social isolation remained higher in former detainees following release when compared to their non-detained counterparts [39].

Three studies conducting single assessments following release from detention suggest that symptoms of depression, anxiety and PTSD endure beyond the detention period, and persist at 10 months [41], 3 years [43] or almost 4 years [40] after release. In the two latter studies, numerous anxiety-related symptoms, such as avoidance of related triggers, nightmares and flashbacks were linked directly to the detention experience. The severity of such long-term impacts, along with continuing sadness, hopelessness, and anger were again found to correlate with detention duration [43].

Despite this, an improvement in quality of life following release was found when asking former detainees to give retrospective ratings of their quality of life during detention and current ratings following release from detention [42]. After release, participants exhibited more satisfaction, improved mood and a decline in suicidal ideation.

Gender

To date, an overwhelming proportion of research focuses on males in detention. In those studies in which female detainees were also included, analysis by gender was usually not conducted. In one study, females were deliberately excluded from the sample due to differing experiences in comparison to men [41].

Only two studies specifically examined gender differences, with one finding no significant differences between genders [38] and the other reporting higher rates of trauma/PTSD in females [48]. Female detainees were also found to be more vulnerable to the effects of more prolonged detention when compared to males.

One study concentrated exclusively on female sex workers in detention, finding high rates of substance abuse, depression, somatic symptoms and PTSD amongst the women [37]. However, this sample of Russian sex workers in Israel differs substantially from other groups of detainees, complicating the generalizability and comparability of these findings. The mental health consequences of detention for female detainees specifically therefore remain unknown based on the studies reviewed.

Children and families

Ten studies reported data on the mental health of children and/or families within the context of detention. This review reports on 629 children and young people (across 9 studies) and 302 parents (across 5 studies).

Table 4 Prevalence Rates of Mental Health Difficulties in Children and Families

	Steel et al. [23] *Diagnostic Interview*		Mares & Jureidini [53] *Diagnostic Interview*		Lorek et al. [52] *Diagnostic Interviews, Parent-report, Self-report*	
	Prevalence Rates in Children (*N* = 20)	Prevalence Rates in Parents (*N* = 14)	Prevalence Rates in Children (N = 20)	Prevalence Rates in Parents (N = 16)	Prevalence Rates in Children (N = 11)	Prevalence Rates in Parents (N = 9)
Mental Health Difficulty						
Major Depressive Disorder	95%	100%	100%	87%	100%	100%
Post-traumatic Stress Disorder	50%	86%	100%	56%	17%	55%
Anxiety Disorder	50% (separation anxiety)	100%	70%	–	36-100%	100%
Sleep Related Difficulties	65%	–	100%	–	91%	–
Eating Related Difficulties	–	–	–	–	100%	–
Oppositional Defiant Disorder / Conduct Problems	45%	–	30%	–	55%	–
Psychotic Symptoms	–	14%	–	25%	–	–
Suicidal Ideation	+ 50%	93%	–	–	–	100%
Self-harm	25%	36%	80%	31%	–	–
Somatic Complaints	–	–	50%	–	91%	–
Hyperactive Behaviour	–	–	–	–	27%	–
Peer Relationship Problems	–	–	–	–	64%	–
Developmental Concerns						
Enuresis	50% of children in middle childhood	n.a.	30% of children aged 6-17	–	13% of children aged 1-4	n.a.
Encopresis	–	n.a.	–	–	13% of children aged 1-4	n.a.
Food Refusal	–	n.a.	–	–	38% of children aged 1-4	n.a.
Return to Nappies	–	n.a	–	–	38% of children aged 1-4	n.a.
Language Regression	–	n.a.	50% of children aged under 5	–	50% of children aged 1-4	n.a.
Attachment Problems	–	n.a.	30% of children aged under 5	n.a.	–	n.a.

Two studies were conducted as comparison studies, with a total of 96 controls. Seven studies were conducted while participants were held in detention, and three were conducted following detention. Again, detention duration was differentially reported. Where reported, the means fell between 6 months and 2 years and 4 months and the ranges spanned from 11 days to 2 years and 8 months across studies. The ages of children spanned from childhood to adolescence, ranging from 11 months – 19 years. Both male and female children were represented, yet gender distributions were largely unreported.

Overall, 5 studies used either self-report or parent/teacher report measures Two studies combined clinical assessment with self-report measures to evaluate psychiatric vulnerability [23, 52]. This allowed not only for an estimation of prevalence rates of psychiatric disorders, but also for retrospective accounts of mental health difficulties preceding detention. One study reported clinical outcomes of referrals into Child and Adolescent Mental Health Services (CAMHS) from a detention centre [53]. Two further studies reported on data collected as part of an Australian Human Rights Commission Data Set [48, 54].

A wide range of psychological disturbances mirroring and extending those of adults was found across all three studies which also all included clinical assessments (see Table 4). All children evidenced at least one psychiatric disorder, most frequently depression, anxiety, PTSD and somatization, depending on the diagnostic categories used. The overwhelming majority also struggled with sleeping (65–100%) and eating problems (100%), suicidal ideation (50%), and self-harm (25–80%). Drawing on data from telephone-administered psychiatric interviews and self-report measures from a near-complete sample of detained families of unspecified ethnicity, Steel et al. [23] found psychiatric disorders to be ten times more likely to occur subsequent to detention when compared to prior to detention. Although based on retrospective reports, such difficulties appeared to be specifically linked to detention experiences. Combining clinical assessments with parent-report and, where possible, triangulating these with self-report measures of mental health in a small sample of child and adolescent detainees, Lorek et al. [52] further identified age-related differences in mental health difficulties. Specifically, whilst elevated levels of emotional and behavioural problems and somatic complaints were common across all age groups, developmental delay and regression were more apparent in younger detainees (aged 3–6). These included frequent crying and withdrawal (100%), disturbed sleep routines (100%), language delays (50%,), loss of previously acquired cognitive skills (33%) return to nappies (38%), enuresis (13%) and encopresis (13%). Amongst older children (aged 7–11), self-report questionnaires suggested high levels of depression (100% not within normal range, 50% above the cut off for clinical depression), anxiety (66% above cut off for clinical anxiety) and PTSD symptomatology (17% approaching clinical cut off) [52]. Though this study did not have a control group, the reported lack of pre-existing mental health problems again suggests that sudden mental health deterioration may be attributable to detention experiences.

Similar developmental differences in psychiatric morbidity were also found in the study of CAMHS assessments of 10 detained families [53]. Developmental concerns such as language regression (50%), attachment problems (30%) and enuresis (30%) were reported in children under 5 years of age, whereas symptoms of PTSD (100% above clinical cut off), depression with suicidal ideation (100% above clinical cut-off), self-harm (80%) anxiety (70%), and somatic symptoms (50%) were more common in older children (aged 6–17).

Regressive behaviours such as enuresis (45% boys, 48% girls) and encopresis (8% boys, 11% girls) were also self-reported by a group of adolescents referred into an infirmary during their time in detention in one study, alongside the more common symptoms of severe to very severe PTSD (very severe 94% boys, 96% girls; severe 6% boys, 4% girls; Rothe et al., 2002a). Following release from detention, 57% of adolescents within the same detention facility were considered to continue to meet a diagnosis of PTSD [56].

A secondary analysis of an Australian Human Rights Commission data set indicated very high rates of severe psychological distress amongst adolescents, evidenced by severe disorders for 85.7% of adolescents [54]. All met criteria for mixed anxiety and depression. Additionally, parent reports suggested a high probability of psychiatric disorder in 75% of their children, and significant emotional symptoms int 78.6%. Drawing on a different subset of the collected data, it was estimated that a third of detained children had sufficient clinical symptoms to necessitate tertiary outpatient assessments [48].

Comparison studies

Two studies compared the mental health of children within the detention context against those outside it; both found elevated psychological symptoms within the detained groups [57, 58]. When comparing children of detained or deported parents with peers whose parents were either legal permanent residents or undocumented yet without prior contact with immigration enforcement, parent reports indicated higher levels of PTSD symptoms and trauma in children of detained or deported parents than the other two groups [57]. Parents and clinicians also rated detained children as scoring more highly on internalising problems and negative moods. However, the grouping of detention with deportation in this study makes it difficult to tease out the specific effects of the experience of detention as against those of removal or deportation. The authors concluded that forced separation from parents due to immigration enforcement may be particularly adverse to child mental health.

Similarly, a study comparing detained children to child asylum seekers in the community found detained children to have significantly impaired social-emotional wellbeing as measured by conduct disorder, emotional problems and hyperactivity than their non-detained counterparts [58]. Interestingly, detained children scored higher on peer relations and pro-social subscales, which may be essential skills for children living in challenging circumstances to have, particularly if their parents are unable to adequately meet their needs.

Parental mental health

Parents displayed high rates of psychopathology across the three studies (see Table 3). There was a substantial increase in reported suicidal ideation. Further, whilst in one study all parents reported the ability to care adequately for and support their children prior to detention, only one of 14 parents remained able to do so during detention [23].

One study reported on the effects of actual or threatened detention and deportation on family units using self-report measures [59]. Multiple regression analysis revealed that parents' legal vulnerability has an impact on the family environment including the quality of the parent-child relationship (27.1% of variance), as well as on overall child well-being (30.6% of variance). In other words, the greater the parents' legal vulnerability, the greater the reported consequences of detention and deportation. However, the interchangeable use of the terms 'detention' and 'deportation' again make it difficult to discern the specific effect of detention.

In keeping with reports on children and adolescents, the secondary analyses revealed 83% of parents to have severe disorders [54]. Again, all participants met criteria for mixed anxiety and depression. When asked about concerns surrounding their child's emotional wellbeing, mental health and development, 67% identified concerns around emotional and mental health (e.g. nightmares, worry, sadness) and 23% identified concerns around development (e.g. poor eating and low weight).

Detention duration and release

Four studies investigated the relationship between detention duration and mental health difficulties. One study found that at 12-month follow up, the mental health of families who remained in detention further deteriorated during incarceration [53]. The three remaining studies did not find a significant correlation between length of detention and mental health problems [54, 56, 58]. However, the authors concluded that this might be due to small sample sizes, the lack of available data on detention duration as well as the possibility of a ceiling effect demonstrating extensive mental health difficulties.

Discussion

Key findings of this review

Adverse mental health consequences of immigration detention are consistently recognised across the literature. Such findings prevail even in countries where detention standards are regarded as relatively benign [46, 52]. Much of the clinical literature reports high levels of anxiety, depression and PTSD and poor quality of life. Whilst such mental health difficulties cannot be viewed in isolation from past histories and pre-detention traumas, which are not consistently measured across studies, controlled studies with non-detained controls uniformly suggest greater symptoms and 'caseness' (i.e. meeting diagnostic criteria for a specific mental health condition) in detained samples. This indicates that detention plays an independent role in contributing to poor mental health outcomes amongst asylum seekers. Nonetheless, being an asylum seeker or having greater trauma exposure of any kind (whether torture or other exposure) prior to detention seems to be associated with higher rates of anxiety, depression and PTSD in the context of such detention (e.g. [41]). Similarly, greater isolation from families and living alone has been found to increase such symptoms in immigration detainees (e.g. [43]).

All adult studies examining the association between detention duration and mental health severity ($N = 5$) demonstrate a significant relationship between detention duration and mental health deterioration. No such correlation was found for length of detention and quality of life ($N = 2$), although a negative trend was found in one of these studies [46]. Additionally, perceived support from detention staff was found to impact positively on quality of life, highlighting the importance of staff behaviour on the wellbeing of detainees but not necessarily having any effect on their mental health problems. Symptom severity has been found to decrease and quality of life to increase following release, but mental health difficulties persist well beyond release. Despite the prominence of mental health disorders amongst detainees, significant barriers to the identification and treatment of those needs remain [47].

The comparatively smaller body of research on detained children and families ($N = 10$ and a total of 629 children studied) echoes the findings in adults summarised above. It should be noted however that the detention of children is fairly uncommon across several countries including the UK, yet remains relatively widely practiced in some European countries [60] and, as recently widely publicised, in the USA. Across those settings and jurisdictions where it remains permitted, profound and far-reaching mental health difficulties are found amongst detained children and young people. Only one in four studies found the severity of mental health difficulties to increase with time the children spent in detention [53]. The other three studies found no correlation between detention duration and mental health. While this has not been researched, this may be explained by the possibility that even small durations of detention are traumatic and harmful to children. The nature of the mental health difficulties found differs across age groups; whereas younger children display developmental regression and primarily externalising behaviours, symptoms of depression, anxiety and PTSD are prominent in older children. Psychosomatic symptoms or somatization appear to be common across developmental stages. This may reflect the difference in experiencing and communicating psychological difficulties in children and young people [61, 62], but may also be understood as a reflection of the somatic component within the symptom pattern of complex PTSD [63]. Whilst detention itself may compromise child development and psychosocial health, as well as aggravating existing trauma, it may also lead to a breakdown of family units. The detention environment may therefore undermine adequate parenting abilities and leave parents feeling disempowered, as they struggle with their own mental health difficulties. Taken together, this may prevent parents from being able to provide support necessary for healthy child development, leaving children at risk of adverse mental health outcomes [64]. It remains unclear however, whether detaining children together with their parents or forcibly separating children from their families is more harmful to the children's mental health. Further, it is currently unknown how rates of parental mental health difficulties compare to those of single adults and those whose families are not detained. Finally, there is a dearth of quantitative research on the mental health of unaccompanied minors who are detained. With the current number of unaccompanied minors rising across the globe, research into the effects of immigration detention on this subgroup of children is of high importance, particularly with view to the possibility that some unaccompanied minors may be inappropriately treated as though they were adults, consequently increasing their risk of exploitation and harm [65].

Overall, the findings suggest that detention exacerbates the mental health burden of asylum seekers and refugees and that such detention should be viewed as a traumatic experience in and of itself. This may be particularly true for those detainees who are particularly vulnerable prior to detention. Individuals with pre-existing mental health difficulties may also be less effective self-advocates and therefore more likely to be detained [11], despite recommendations and policies to the contrary [31].

Key strengths and limitations of this review

A comprehensive search strategy, as well as independent screening, data extraction and quality appraisals were applied to ensure a systematic approach to synthesising the literature on the mental health consequences of immigration detention. Adherence to the PRISMA guidelines further increased the methodological rigour and clarity of the review. We sought to ensure that all research that met out criteria was identified through additional contact with expert researchers in the field. Finally, the exclusion of grey literature, as well as confining the search to papers written in English, inevitably resulted in the exclusion of some papers which may have limited the overall understanding of detainee mental health.

What this review adds to existing reviews

To the best of our knowledge, the current review is the first systematic review on the mental health of immigration detainees since our previous review published in 2009 [14]. Although excluding grey literature, it includes a larger number of clinical studies than previous reviews [30] and is not limited to detainees with a recorded history of torture [66]. The current review supports findings from the 2009 review and additionally highlights the importance of considering the impact of immigration detention on the mental health of families. It also includes multiple comparison studies which highlight the independent effect of such detention on mental health over and above that of uncertain immigration status. However, it also highlights the dearth (and consequent future importance) of further high quality research directly investigating vulnerability within the immigration detention context.

Key limitations of the available evidence and their implications for future research

Numerous methodological problems exist at primary study level, which may restrict the conclusions that can be drawn in this review but also indicate where further research is needed. The evidence to date remains sparse due to the multiple obstacles hindering such research. These include restricted access opportunities into detention facilities as well as the prohibiting of random sampling (e.g. [38, 44]). This may have led to an increased reliance on qualitative rather than quantitative methods, particularly in the study of detained children. Such studies have not been included in this review. With regards to studies conducted within detention centres, participants are often recruited through community areas within the detention centres (e.g. [11]), possibly introducing a bias towards those detainees who are most healthy. Recruitment of participants in studies conducted following release from detention, often occurs through lawyers, community organisations or other support services (e.g. [41]). Most studies did not describe the detention regime in sufficient detail to allow for this to be considered as a potential influencing factor. This, together with clearer differentiation between the traumatic effects of detention itself from those of the detention environment) is an important focus for future research. It also carries the implication that future studies should provide as much information as possible about the detention environment in order to facilitate judgment as to the generalisability of the findings. Participation rates are often unknown. It is therefore possible that the recruited samples differed systematically from detainees who did not access community facilities or come into contact with support services. Samples may therefore represent only the most vulnerable individuals in need of support, or conversely, the most highly functioning who are able to access appropriate services. Further research in more representative populations is needed to allow more confident generalisation of the findings to the detainee population as a whole. Additionally, the probability of being detained depends to some extent to sex and nationality, resulting in predominantly male populations of certain national origins [38]. Whilst a broad range of nationalities is represented across studies, a paucity of research focusing on women is evident. Differing nationalities contribute to the vast heterogeneity of samples, along with varying past experiences and traumatic histories, migration statuses, and detention systems and immigration policies within host countries. Correspondingly, language may be an important complicating factor, acting both as a prominent exclusion criterion or a possible cause of misinterpretation or inability to express mental health difficulties clearly [47]. Communicating mental health problems may additionally be compounded by differing expressions of distress and trauma, alongside differing attitudes and experiences of mental health within countries of origin [67]. However, participants from a wide range of cultural backgrounds seem to endure similar psychological ill-health when subjected to detention.

Multiple designs as well as a diversity of methodology and instruments used are evident across studies. Whilst these may differentially contribute to the overall understanding of mental health problems amongst detainees, they also limit comparability. The majority of research is conducted as cross-sectional studies, which warrant caution in the drawing of casual inferences. The suggested causal link between detention and worsening of mental health is however consistent with a limited number of longitudinal studies and comparison studies, implying that detention not only exacerbates existing mental health disorders, but also contributes independently to the onset of new ones. Nonetheless, isolating the effects of detention alone remains a complex task and additional longitudinal research is needed in order to establish the mental health trajectories of detainees, from the very early days of being arrested and detained. This may also include investigating the adverse effects of being detained multiple separate times at different lengths, as well as the effects that experiences in detention may have on people's ability to navigate and integrate into new societies. Finally, the frequent reliance on a range of self-report questionnaires, which have often not been validated specifically for the use with detainee populations, may be problematic though it is in our view unlikely that this significantly affects the overall validity of the findings. Moreover, measures often focus solely on symptoms of PTSD, depression and anxiety, which may fail to investigate other disorders such as schizophrenia and other non-affective disorders as may be the case in refugees as a whole [5]. Whilst self-report questionnaires are undoubtedly useful for the purpose of screening for mental health problems, outcomes of such self-report measures should not be equated with formal psychiatric diagnoses, which require clinician-administered interviews. To date, there is a limited use of diagnostic clinical assessments to complement self-report measures, and where these are conducted, the samples are restricted to adult male detainees only.

Conclusions and practical recommendations

Taken as a whole, the body of research reviewed in this paper consistently illustrates severe mental health consequences amongst detainees across a wide range of settings and jurisdictions. In view of this, in terms of provision of care, consideration of mental health disorders and their sequelae should become routine in making the decision whether or not to detain, and in monitoring the welfare of those already in detention. Comprehensive sociocultural assessments should be carried out by care providers with transcultural knowledge, skills and practices [68]. These assessments should lead to adequate treatment for individuals in detention who suffer from mental health difficulties. Additionally, there is a need to identify and address vulnerability within an overall asylum policy and more specifically a detention policy that avoids or minimises further harm being done to vulnerable people. For this, it is important to take into account multiple varying expressions of distress and vulnerability, which should not be reduced to Western conceptualisations. Moreover, a broad concept of past trauma is needed which is not restricted to the definition of torture according to Article 1 of the Convention Against Torture [69], but rather focuses on the severity of harm to which the individual has been subjected [70]. Further, there should be a greater focus on minimizing length of detention. Our findings add weight to the call in the UK and other countries to introduce a statutory limit of duration of detention, such as exists in all other EU countries [71]. The increasing evidence for the negative impact of immigration detention on vulnerable populations is particularly policy-relevant. Similarly, there is insufficient attention paid to child protection and safety, or to adequate education and health protection in countries where children continue to be detained, despite the recognised vulnerability and risk of children and young people and their protection under the UN Convention on the Rights of the Child [72].

Abbreviations

CAMHS: Child and Adolescent Mental Health Service; EU: European Union; PTSD: Post-traumatic stress disorder; UK: United Kingdon; UNHCR: United Nations High Commissioner for Refugees; USA: United States of America; WHO: World Health Organization

Acknowledgements

We are grateful to Erin Dexter and Dafni Katsampa for their help in preparing this paper for final submission.

Funding

This study was supported by a research grant to the Helen Bamber Foundation from the Oak Foundation (Grant number: OCAY-15-286).

Authors' contributions

MvW, KR, ZC, RS, LO, CM and CK contributed to the conception and design of the review. ZC,RS and CM undertook the systematic search, screening and selecting articles. MvW, CM and CK assessed study quality. MvW interpreted the data and drafted and revised all versions of the manuscript. KR, ZC, RS, CM and CK critically reviewed the manuscript. LO independently reviewed the drafts. All authors have read and approved the final manuscript.

Authors' information

The Helen Bamber Foundation (HBF), based in London, supports people who have experienced extreme human cruelty, such as torture or human trafficking, who are refugees and asylum seekers. We are a human rights charity with clinical and legal expertise and we deliver a specialist Model of Integrated Care (MoIC) to meet the complex needs of some of the most vulnerable people in the world. HBF's experts deliver this MoIC tailored to each client which includes:

- Clinical: specialist psychological care; medical advisory services and physical rehabilitation therapies
- Legal protection and medico-legal assessment and documentation
- Safeguarding and prevention of social deprivation
- Community integration through life, employment and creative skills

We support the most marginalised people in our society to secure their needs and rebuild their lives. We amplify the impact of our work to benefit survivors more widely through advocating for policy change, research, and dissemination of best practice.

Consent for publication

Not applicable.

Competing interests

The authors declare that they have no competing interests.

Author details

[1]Helen Bamber Foundation, Bruges Place, 15-20 Baynes Street, London NW1 0TF, UK. [2]Health Services and Population Research Department, Kings College London, London, UK. [3]Division of Psychiatry, University College London, London, UK.

References

1. The United Nations High Commissioner For Refugees. Figures at a glance. 2017. http://www.unhcr.org/uk/figures-at-a-glance.html. Accessed 17 Sept 2017.
2. Global Detention Project. https://www.globaldetentionproject.org/organisations-alliances/european-union-eu. Accessed 17 Sept 2017.
3. Fazel M, Wheeler J, Danesh J. Prevalence of serious mental disorder in 7000 refugees resettled in western countries: a systematic review. Lancet. 2005; 365:1309–14.
4. Priebe S, Giacco D, El-Nagib R. Health evidence network synthesis report 47. Public health aspects of mental health among migrants and refugees: A review of the evidence on mental health care for refugees, asylum seekers and irregular migrants in the WHO European Region. Geneva: World Health Organization; 2016.
5. Hollander AC, Dal H, Lewis G, Magnusson C, Kirkbride JB, Dalman C. Refugee migration and risk of schizophrenia and other non-affective psychoses: Cohort study of 1.3 million people in Sweden. BMJ. 2016;352:i1030.
6. Song SJ, Kaplan C, Tol WA, Subica A, de Jong J. Psychological distress in torture survivors: pre-and post-migration risk factors in a US sample. Soc Psych Psych Epid. 2015;50:549–60.
7. Schick M, Zumwald A, Knöpfli B, Nickerson A, Byrant RA, Schnyder U, et al. Challenging future, challenging past: the relationship of social integration and psychological impairment in traumatized refugees. Eur J Psychotraumatol. 2016;7:28057.
8. Laban CJ, Gernaat HB, Komproe IH, van der Tweel I, de Jong JT. Postmigration living problems and common psychiatric disorders in Iraqi asylum seekers in the Netherlands. J Nerv Ment Dis. 2005;193:825–32.
9. Warfa N, Curtis S, Watters C, Carswell K, Ingleby D, Bhui K. Migration experiences, employment status and psychological distress among Somali immigrants: A mixed-method international study. BMC Public Health. 2012;12:749.
10. Carswell K, Blackburn P, Barker C. The relationship between trauma, post-migration problems and the psychological well-being of refugees and asylum seekers. Int J Soc Psychiatr. 2011;57:107–19.
11. Robjant K, Robbins I, Senior V. Psychological distress amongst immigration detainees: a cross-sectional questionnaire study. Br J Clin Psychol. 2009;48:275–86.
12. Medical Justice. http://www.medicaljustice.org.uk/about/what-we-do/research-and-campaigning/publications/. Accessed 17 Sept 2017.
13. Schauer M, Neuner F, Karunakara U, Klaschik C, Robert C, Elbert T. PTSD and the 'building block' effect of psychological trauma among West Nile Africans. Eur J Psychotraumatol. 2003;10:5–6.
14. Robjant K, Hassan R, Katona C. Mental health implications of detaining asylum seekers: a systematic review. Brit J Psychiat. 2009;194:306–12.
15. Australian Association of Social Workers. Position Statement: Children in immigration detention. 2015. https://www.aasw.asn.au/document/item/7264. Accessed 17 September 2017.
16. Canadian Council for Refugees. Ending immigration detention of children: Call for legislative amendment. 2016. http://ccrweb.ca/sites/ccrweb.ca/files/ending-detention-children-proposal.pdf. Accessed 17 Sept 2017.
17. American Orthopsychiatric Association. The impact of immigration enforcement on children and families. 2010. http://www.bhjustice.org/assets/docs/positionstatements/immigration%20enforcement.pdf. Accessed 17 Sept 2017.
18. The United Nations High Commissioner For Refugees. UNHCR deeply concerned by Hungary plans to detain all asylum seekers. 2017. http://www.unhcr.org/uk/news/briefing/2017/3/58be80454/unhcr-deeply-concerned-hungary-plans-detain-asylum-seekers.html. Accessed 17 September 2017.
19. European Commission. The use of detention and alternatives to detention in the context of immigration policies. Synthesis report for the EMN Focused Study 2014. https://ec.europa.eu/home-affairs/sites/homeaffairs/files/what-we-do/networks/european_migration_network/reports/docs/emn-studies/emn_study_detention_alternatives_to_detention_synthesis_report_en.pdf. Accessed 17 Sept 2017.
20. Immigration Detention. Human Rights First. 2018. https://www.humanrightsfirst.org/topics/immigration-detention. Assessed 22 Jul 2018.

21. USA Today. 2018. https://eu.usatoday.com/story/news/2018/06/27/immigrant-children-family-separation-border-timeline/734014002/. Accessed 27 June 2018.
22. Sultan A, O'Sullivan K. Psychological disturbances in asylum seekers held in long term detention: a participant-observer account. Med J Australia. 2001;175:593–6.
23. Steel Z, Momartin S, Bateman C, Hafshejani A, Silove DM, Everson N, et al. Psychiatric status of asylum seeker families held for a protracted period in a remote detention Centre in Australia. Aust NZ J Pub Heal. 2004;28:527–36.
24. Migration Amendment (Detention Arrangements) Act 2005. 2008. Legislation.gov.au https://www.legislation.gov.au/Details/C2005A00079. Accessed 22 Jul 2018.
25. Fazel M, Silove D. Detention of refugees. BMJ. 2006;332(7536):251–2.
26. Immigration Detention News, Research and Analysis - The Conversation. The Conversation. 2018. https://theconversation.com/topics/immigration-detention-12212. Accessed 22 Jul 2018.
27. All Party Parliamentary Group on Refugees & the All Party Parliamentary Group on Migration. The Report of the Inquiry into the Use of Immigration Detention in the United Kingdom. 2015. https://detentioninquiry.files.wordpress.com/2015/03/immigration-detention-inquiry-report.pdf. Accessed 23 Jul 2018.
28. The Royal College of Psychiatrists. Position Statement on detention of people with mental disorders in immigration removal centres. 2013. http://www.medicaljustice.org.uk/wp-content/uploads/2016/06/Appendix-A-The-Royal-College-of-Psychiatrists-Position-Statement-on-detention-of-people-with-mental-disorders-in-Immigration-Removal-Centres.pdf. Accessed 28 Nov 2018.
29. Shaw S. Review into the welfare in detention of vulnerable persons. 2016. https://www.gov.uk/government/uploads/system/uploads/attachment_data/file/490782/52532_Shaw_Review_Accessible.pdf. Accessed 17 Sept 2017.
30. Bosworth M. Mental health in immigration detention: a literature review. Review into the welfare in detention of vulnerable persons, cm 9186. London: HSMO; 2016.
31. Immigration Act 2016: Guidance on adults at risk in immigration detention. Home Office 2016. https://www.gov.uk/government/uploads/system/uploads/attachment_data/file/547519/Adults_at_Risk_August_2016.pdf. Accessed 17 Sept 2017.
32. Royal College of Psychiatrists. Definition of torture in the context of immigration detention policy. Position Statement 07. 2016. http://www.rcpsych.ac.uk/pdf/PS07_2016.pdf. Accessed 17 Sept 2017.
33. The Detention Centre (Amendment) Rules 2018. 2018. Legislation.gov.uk. http://www.legislation.gov.uk/uksi/2018/411/article/2/made. Accessed 22 Jul 2018.
34. Moher D, Liberati A, Tetzlaff J, Altman DG. Preferred reporting items for systematic reviews and mental-analyses: the PRISMA statement. PLoS Med. 2009;6:E1000097.
35. Critical Appraisal Skills Programme. http://www.casp-uk.net/casp-tools-checklists. Accessed 17 Sept 2017.
36. Green JP, Eagar K. The health of people in Australian immigration detention centres. Med J Australia. 2010;192:65–70.
37. Cwikel J, Chudakov B, Paikin M, Agmon K, Belmaker RH. Trafficked female sex workers awaiting deportation: comparison with brothel workers. Arch Womens Ment Health. 2004;7:243–9.
38. Cleveland J, Rousseau C. Psychiatric symptoms associated with brief detention of adult asylum seekers in Canada. Can J Psychiatr. 2013;58:409–16.
39. Steel Z, Momartin S, Silove D, Coello M, Aroche J, Tay KW. Two year psychosocial and mental health outcomes for refugees subjected to restrictive or supportive immigration policies. Soc Sci Med. 2011;72:1149–56.
40. Coffey GJ, Kaplan I, Sampson RC, Tucchi MM. The meaning and mental health consequences of long-term immigration detention for people seeking asylum. Soc Sci Med. 2010;70:2070–9.
41. Ichikawa M, Nakahara S, Wakai S. Effect of post-migration detention on mental health among afghan asylum seekers in Japan. Aust NZ J Psychiat. 2006;40:341–6.
42. Sobhanian F, Boyle GJ, Bahr M, Fallo T. Psychological status of former refugee detainees from the Woomera detention Centre now living in the Australian community. Psychiatr Psychol Law. 2006;13:151–9.
43. Steel Z, Silove D, Brooks R, Momartin S, Alzuhairi B, Susljik I. Impact of immigration detention and temporary protection on the mental health of refugees. Brit J Psychiat. 2006;188:58–64.
44. Keller AS, Rosenfeld B, Trinh-Shevrin C, Meserve C, Sachs E, Leviss JA, et al. Mental health of detained asylum seekers. Lancet. 2003;362:1721–3.
45. Sen P, Arungnanaseelan J, Connell E, Katona C, Khan A, Morna P, et al. Mental health morbidity amongst people subjected to immigration detention in the UK. Epidemiol Psychiatr Sci. 2017. https://doi.org/10.1017/S2045796017000269.
46. Puthoopparambil SJ, Bjerneld M, Kaellestal C. Quality of life among immigrants in Swedish immigration detention centres: a cross-sectional questionnaire study. Glob Health Action. 2015;8:28321.
47. Graf M, Wermuth P, Haefeli D, Weisert A, Reagu S, Pflueger M, et al. Prevalence of mental disorders among detained asylum seekers in deportation arrest in Switzerland and validation of the brief jail mental health screen BJMHS. Int J Law Psychiat. 2013;36:201–6.
48. Young P, Gordon M. Mental health screening in immigration detention: a fresh look at Australian government data. Aust Psychiatry. 2016;24(1):19–22.
49. Hedrick K. Getting out of (self-) harm's way: a study of factors associated with self-harm among asylum seekers in Australian immigration detention. J Forensic Legal Med. 2017;49:89–93.
50. Cohen J. Safe in our hands?: a study of suicide and self-harm in asylum seekers. J Forensic Legal Med. 2008;15(4):235–44.
51. Momartin S, Steel Z, Coello M, Aroche J, Silove DM, Brooks R. A comparison of the mental health of refugees with temporary versus permanent protection visas. MJA. 2006;185(7):357–61.
52. Lorek A, Ehntholt K, Nesbitt A, Wey E, Githinji C, Rossor E, et al. The mental and physical health difficulties of children held within a British immigration detention Centre: a pilot study. Child Abuse Negl. 2009;33:573–85.
53. Mares S, Jureidini J. Psychiatric assessment of children and families in immigration detention – Clinical, administrative and ethical issues. Aust NZ Pub Heal. 2004;28:520–6.
54. Mares S. The mental health of children and parents detained on Christmas Island: secondary analysis of an Australian human rights commission data set. Health Hum Rights. 2016;18(2):219–32.
55. Rothe EM, Castillo-Matos H, Busquets R. Post-traumatic stress symptoms in Cuban adolescent refugees during camp confinement. Adolescent Psychiatry. 2002a;26:97.
56. Rothe E, Lewis J, Castillo-Matos H, Martinez O, Busquets R, Martinez I. Posttraumatic stress disorder among Cuban children and adolescents after release from a refugee camp. Psychiatr Serv. 2002b;53(8):970–6.
57. Rojas-Flores L, Clements M, Hwang Koo J, London J. Trauma and psychological distress in Latino citizen children following parental detention and deportation. Psychol Trauma Theory Res Pract Policy. 2017;9(3):352–61.
58. Zwi K, Mares S, Nathanson D, Tay A, Silove D. The impact of detention on the social–emotional wellbeing of children seeking asylum: a comparison with community-based children. Eur Child Adolesc Psychiatry. 2017;27(4):411–22.
59. Brabeck KM, Xu Q. The impact of detention and deportation on Latino immigrant children and families: a quantitative exploration. Hispanic J Behav Sci. 2010;32:341–61.
60. End Immigration detention of children. https://www.hrw.org/world-report/2016/children-behind-bars. Accessed 17 Sept 2017.
61. Campo VJ. Annual research review: functional somatic symptoms and associated anxiety and depression – developmental psychopathology in pediatric practice. J Child Psychol Psyc. 2012;53:575–93.
62. Van der Kolk BA. The body keep the score: memory and the evolving psychobiology of posttraumatic stress. Harvard Rev Psychiat. 1994;1:253–65.
63. Cloitre M, Courtois CA, Ford JD, Green BL, Alexander P, Briere J, et al. The ISTSS Expert Consensus Treatment Guidelines for Complex PTSD in Adults. 2012. http://www.istss.org/ISTSS_Main/media/Documents/ISTSS-Expert-Concesnsus-Guidelines-for-Complex-PTSD-Updated-060315.pdf. Accessed 17 Sept 2017.
64. International Detention Coalition. Captured Childhood. 2012. https://idcoalition.org/wp-content/uploads/2012/03/Captured-Childhood-FINAL-June-2012.pdf. Accessed 17 Sept 2017.
65. Zwi K, Mares S. Stories from unaccompanied children in immigration detention: a composite account. J Paediatr Child H. 2015;51:658–62.

66. Storm T, Engberg M. The impact of immigration detention on the mental health of torture survivors is poorly documents – a systematic review. Dan Med J. 2013;60:A4728.
67. Summerfield D. The invention of post-traumatic stress disorder and the social usefulness of a psychiatric category. BMJ. 2001;322:95–8.
68. Wylie L, Van Meyel R, Harder H, Sukhera J, Luc C, Ganjavi H, Elfakhani M, Wardrop N. Assessing trauma in a transcultural context: challenges in mental health care with immigrants and refugees. Public Health Rev. 2018;39(1):22.
69. United Nations Human Rights Office of the High Commisioner. Convention against torture and other cruel, inhumane or degrading treatment or punishment. 1987. http://www.ohchr.org/EN/ProfessionalInterest/Pages/CAT.aspx. Accessed 17 Sept 2017.
70. The Royal College of Psychiatrists. Position Statement 07. Definition of torture in the context of immigration detention policy. 2016. http://www.rcpsych.ac.uk/pdf/PS07_2016.pdf. Accessed 17 Sept 2017.
71. All Party Parliamentary Group. Refugees welcome? The experience of new refugees in the UK. 2017. https://www.refugeecouncil.org.uk/assets/0004/0316/APPG_on_Refugees_-_Refugees_Welcome_report.pdf. Accessed 17 Sept 2017.
72. United Nations Human Rights Office of the High Commissioner. Convention on the Rights of the Child. 1989. http://www.ohchr.org/en/professionalinterest/pages/crc.aspx. Accessed 17 Sept 2017.

10

"Happy feet": evaluating the benefits of a 100-day 10,000 step challenge on mental health and wellbeing

K. T. Hallam[1,2], S. Bilsborough[3] and M. de Courten[1*]

Abstract

Background: An increased awareness of the health benefits of walking has emerged with the development and refinement of accelerometer equipment. Evidence is beginning to highlight the value of promoting walking, particularly focusing on the Japanese mark of obtaining 10,000 steps per day. Workplace based step challenges have become popular to engage large cohorts in increasing their daily physical activity in a sustainable and enjoyable way. Findings are now highlighting the positive health effects of these medium-term programs (typically conducted over a few months) in terms of cardiovascular health, reducing diabetes risk and improving lifestyle factors such as weight and blood pressure. As yet, research has not focused on whether similar improvements in psychological health and wellbeing are present.

Methods: This study investigated the impact of a 100-day, 10,000 step program on signs of depression, anxiety and stress as well as general wellbeing using standardised psychological scales.

Results: The results indicated a small but consistent effect on all of these measures of mental health over the term of the program. This effect appeared irrespective of whether a person reached the 10,000 step mark.

Conclusions: These results highlight improved mental health and wellbeing in people undertaking this 100-day 10,000 step program and indicates the efficacy and potential of these programs for a modest, yet important improvement in mental health. Notably, targets reached may be less important than participation itself.

Keywords: Depression, Stress, Anxiety, Wellbeing, Physical activity, Health promotion

Background

By 2030, mental illness is projected to cost the global community over US$ 6 T [1]. This places mental illnesses impacts above cardiovascular disease, chronic respiratory disease, cancer and diabetes [1]. People experiencing mental illness are also known to be at a much higher risk for morbidity and early mortality from physical health issues than the general population [2]. This risk may be further exacerbated by the medications utilised in the treatment of these illnesses [2, 3]. Associated with this high treatment cost is the emerging equity and access issue in low income countries associated with psychiatric disability or sub syndromal functional decline. In these contexts, 75%–85% of people with mental health issues are untreated [4]. Paired with a shortfall of mental health specialists in low and middle income countries [5], these data point to the importance of primary prevention and population level interventions to improve mental health and wellbeing. Physical activity (PA) has become an increasingly important focus in the prevention of non-communicable diseases, yet these strategies are often underutilised in the mental illness (and mental health) domain [6–8]. Epidemiological studies demonstrate that adequate PA is associated with fewer depressive symptoms [9], and conversely, the development of depressive symptoms many result from insufficient PA [10]. Four Cochrane Database Systematic reviews, titled "Exercise and Depression", have been undertaken in the past 10 years. The most recent of these meta-analyses showed that in clinically depressed individuals, exercise has a

* Correspondence: maximilian.decourten@vu.edu.au
[1]Centre for Chronic Disease, College of Health and Biomedicine, Victoria University, Melbourne, Australia
Full list of author information is available at the end of the article

moderate effect on symptoms of depression, highlighting its place as an adjunct treatment option [11].

Physical activity likely exerts its impact on mood via reducing the activity of the sympathetic nervous system and associated hypothalamic-pituitary-adrenal axis reactivity in the brain [12]. In terms of monoaminergic activity, animal models highlight the role of exercise in increasing both serotonin and noradrenalin levels in the brain in a similar fashion to antidepressant medications [13]. On a clinical level, this serotonergic activity may explain why exercise is as effective as serotonergic focused antidepressant medications for mild to moderate symptoms [14]. Evidence also indicates increased brain derived neurotrophic factor (BDNF) levels associated with single sessions of exercise that improve further with regular exercise. This increased BDNF level is associated with both cognitive and mood improvements in the brain and behaviour [15]. Smits and colleagues (2008) have demonstrated that with as little as six, 20 min sessions of treadmill exercise (at 70% maximum health rate) over two weeks has a positive impact on mood factors such as anxiety [16]. It is clear that promoting PA for both clinical and sub-clinical mood disturbance is a valuable goal.

Stress is a precipitating factor in susceptibility and exacerbation of mental health issues. Stress is more commonly experienced than depression and anxiety and is associated both with poorer mental health and wellbeing, an important linkage as wellbeing itself is associated with better physical and psychological health over the lifespan [17]. Notably, stress is very responsive to PA [18] and regularly engaging in PA has been recommended by many government and health authorities for improving mental and physical health and wellbeing [19, 20].

The World Health Organisation [21] has identified a valuable role for workplace based interventions in improving the health of the whole workforce. Pedometer based programs can significantly improve physical activity and physical health including reducing sitting time, reducing weight, improving blood lipid levels and reduced diabetes risk indicators [22–24]. Glance and colleagues [24] have also indicated an improvement in wellbeing, implying an impact on stress levels in participants. Within step challenge programs, the 10,000 step goal roughly equate to 8 km of walking per day (around 1.5 to 2 h of walking). This level of activity well exceeds the WHO Global Strategy on Physical Health, Diet and Activity recommendations of 150 min of moderate physical activity per week [25]. Despite clear physical improvements associated with 10,000 step programs, to date no research has investigated possible important impacts of these workplace programs or the 10,000 daily step benchmark on the psychological factors of wellbeing, stress, anxiety and depression. Whether 10,000 steps are sufficient to elicit changes in these (perhaps more complex) psychological domains remains unknown at this time [26].

The aim of this investigation was to assess the impact of a 100-day workplace based 10,000 step challenge on mental health and wellbeing in an international workplace community sample. Based on evidence indicating positive physical health effects from 10,000 step programs four hypotheses were developed. Firstly, it was hypothesised that participants involved in a 10,000 step program for 100 days would see benefits in their levels of depression, anxiety and stress and consequent improvements in wellbeing scores. Further, it was hypothesised that increasing amounts of exercise in these programs would lead to improved outcomes on these. Thirdly it was hypothesised that those who on average completed more than 10,000 steps per day throughout (the recommended level for these programs) would perform better in terms of mental health and wellbeing than those who did not reach this threshold. Finally, it was hypothesised that when controlling for demographic factors of age and gender, this improved outcome in people who engaged in more stepping exercise would be maintained.

Methods

Participants

Of the 2379 respondents who consented to participate in this research, 1963 participants made up the final sample size. This number accounted for 416 who either did not complete 70% of the 100-day challenge or those who did not complete the demographic or mental health survey.

Materials

Stepathlon is a company headquartered in Mumbai, India running globally organized team-based walking programs at participating workplaces. Stepathlon has also offices in Australia where the workplace health and wellbeing policies are developed. Hence, the study sample are predominantly from these two countries.

Through the Stepathlon corporate challenge (http://www.stepathlon.com), routine data are obtained relating to age, gender, location and daily step counts as recorded by participants on a password protected website based on readings from pedometer (clip-on) or other fitness monitors (e.g. wrist accelerometer). On completion of the 100-day step challenge in 2015 and 2016, digital assets management staff of Stepathlon extracted de-identified data from their server and provided this de-identified database to Victoria University as per research agreement.

Symptoms of depression, anxiety and stress were assessed using the short form of the Depression, Anxiety Stress Scales (DASS [27]). The short form DASS is a 21-item, self-report, symptom-oriented measure consisting of three sub scales: Depression, Anxiety and Stress.

Participants rated their experience of each indicator across a four-point frequency (from 0 [did not apply to me at all] to 3 [applies very much to me or most of the time]). The DASS has strong construct validity [28], adequate discriminant and convergent validity [27] and internal consistency (Cronbach's α of 0.96, 0.89, 0.93 for the depression, anxiety and stress subscales respectively [29]). It has strong factor structure in both non-clinical [27] and clinical samples [29].

The Warwick-Edinburgh Mental Wellbeing Scale (WEMWBS) is a 14-item measure rated on a 1–5 scale (from 'none of the time' to 'all of the time'). The scale focuses on positive elements of wellbeing and is positively worded throughout. The scale provides a one factor model for measuring wellbeing [30, 31]. The WEMWBS shows strong criterion validity with the WHO Wellbeing Index-5, Positive and Negative Affect Schedule and is negatively correlated with the General Health Questionnaire-12 measure of mental ill health [30]. Finally, internal consistency (Cronbach's $\alpha = 0.91$) and one-week test-retest reliability (0.83) of the scale were strong [30].

Procedure

Participants were recruited from the established international Stepathlon program. This workplace activity challenge was promoted at participating sites via posters, e-flyers, and through engagement of senior management through visits to sites by health & wellbeing managers.

Participants of this workplace activity challenge were provided with a participant information and consent forms inviting them to this research charting the impacts of the 10,000 step challenge on their mental health and wellbeing. The project was approved by the Victoria University Human Research Ethics Committee (HRE15–168). All participants completed the standard demographics questionnaire and logged their daily step count for as many of 100 days during the challenge. Participants could use their own pedometer, or activity monitoring device throughout the challenge and recorded their daily totals via the Stepathlon user portal. Through this portal they received regular newsletters, updates and motivational articles for the duration of the challenge. In addition to the standard step challenge package, consenting participants completed a pre-and post 100-day challenge questionnaire regarding their mental health using the DASS-21 and WEMWBS questionnaires in English.

Design

The results of the study were analysed using a number of repeated measures ANOVAs. Firstly, the data were assessed to see if there were overall changes in mood and wellbeing from pre to post testing over the activity challenge. Following this, a repeated measures ANOVA focusing on the 10,000 step threshold (between subjects factor) and change over time (within subjects factor) was used to evaluate the 10,000 step criterion. Further, a series of Pearson product moment correlation coefficients were utilised to assess overall relationships between number of steps completed on average by participants and changes in mental health and wellbeing scores. Finally, a repeated measures ANCOVA was utilised to assess the factors in the 10,000 steps over time but covarying for age and gender. All analysis was conducted in SPSS version 21.

Results

The final sample of 1963 participants was screened for univariate outliers via box plot analysis on the outcome scales. Data inspection indicated no outliers (+ 2 SD) in the sample, presumably due to the large sample size. Data were assessed for the assumptions of normality and skewness. The data did not violate the assumptions of asymmetry and kurtosis of ±2 using threshold defined by Field [32]. Tests of within subject violations of the assumption of sphericity indicated no violations of this measure, hence parametric analysis was appropriate for the within subjects analysis. Finally, violation of the assumption of homogeneity was assessed using Levene's equality of error variance estimates. Due to the large sample size in the study, the Levene's significant level was adjusted to 0.001 as per the recommendations of Warner [33]. The results after correction showed no violations of homogeneity of variance, hence parametric analysis was used for all statistical analysis.

Demographics

The final sample represented 1458 males and 505 females who ranged in age from 16 to 74 years (M = 36.6, SD = 8.9). Participants represented numerous countries of origin with the majority being from India ($n = 1610$) and Australia ($n = 227$) along with 21 other countries.

Change in mental health and wellbeing over 100 day challenge

A repeated measures ANOVA demonstrated improvements on all measures of the DASS over the 100-day challenge period. This included a significant 7.6% improvement in levels of depressive symptoms based on a reduction from an average of 4.59 (S.D. = 3.52) to 4.24 (S.D. = 3.44), $F(1, 1962) = 67.385$, $p < .001$, $\eta^2 = .033$, *power* = 1.0. In relation to anxious symptoms, the data showed a 5.04% improvement after the 100 day challenge, reducing from an average of 4.56 (S.D. = 3.13) to 4.33 (S.D. = 3.08), $F(1, 1962) = 34.416$, $p < .001$, $\eta^2 = .0017$, *power* = 1.0. Stress symptoms were the most responsive to the 100-day challenge with the data showing an 8.96% improvement in stress levels on the DSS following the program. This equated to a reduction from an average of 5.47 (S.D. = 3.19) to 4.98 (S.D. = 3.05), $F(1, 1962) = 117.593$, $p < .001$, $\eta^2 = .057$, *power* = 1.0. Finally, there was a 2.13% improvement in overall wellbeing on the WEMWBS, associated with an increase in average wellbeing scores from 50.01 (S.D. = 10.29) to 51.08 (S.D. = 10.45), $F(1, 1962) = 103.555$, $p < .001$, $\eta^2 = .050$, *power* = 1.0.

Relationship between mental health and wellbeing score changes and average amount of walking

To investigate if these clear mental health improvements over the challenge were associated with increasing levels of walking exercise a series of correlation analyses were conducted contrasting change scores on each of these measures from pre to post testing versus the average number of steps taken per day. The results indicated no significant overall correlations between average steps and depression ($r^2 = -0.026$, $p = .254$), anxiety ($r^2 = -.029$, $p = .205$), stress ($r^2 = -.026$, $p = .247$) and WEMWBS ($r^2 = .026$, $p = .256$). While all measures trend in the direction of improvement with increasing steps, it is notable that the range (2775 average steps to 112,831 average steps) of steps taken on average varied markedly, impacting clear correlations.

Do people who walk over 10,000 steps on average have greater improvements in mental health and wellbeing?

It is contended in 10,000 step programs that reaching 10,000 steps has a certain significance for participants. This "stepping goal" was assessed to elucidate any meaningful differences between those who reached less than or greater than this goal on average across the program. This research question was assessed with a repeated measures ANOVA that compared the between subject factor of number of steps (less than 10,000 versus equal to or more than 10,000 steps). These results are depicted in Table 1.

The results highlighted an interaction effect between group (less than 10,000 steps versus 10,000 or more steps) and time (pre and post testing) for DASS stress (F [1, 1961] = 3.982, $p = .046$, $\eta 2 = .002$, *power* = .514) with the participants who completed equal to or more than 10,000 steps showing a 10.13% improvement in stress levels whilst the individuals who completed less than 10,000 steps daily only achieved a 5.36% improvement.

Likewise, the interaction effect around anxiety showed that those who completed equal to or more than 10,000 steps daily had a significantly better improvement in anxiety over the challenge, improving their anxiety levels by 5.89% versus only 1.34% for those who completed less than 10,000 steps. (F [1, 1961] = 5.421, $p < .001$, $\eta 2 = .003$, *power* = .643). Interaction effects for depression and overall wellbeing scores were not evident in the analysis. Finally, between subjects differences profiling overall levels of psychological distress and wellbeing in those who did less than 10,000 steps on average versus those who did more showed that the participants in the greater than 10,000 steps group had better scores on wellbeing, $F(1, 1961) = 4.017$, $p = .045$, $\eta 2 = .002$, *power* = .517, and stress levels, $F(1, 1961) = 21.795$, $p < .001$, $\eta 2 = .011$, *power* = .997. There were no overall differences in anxiety, $F(1, 1961) = .001$, $p = .975$, $\eta 2 = .000$, *power* = .050 and depression scores, F (1, 1961) = 1.876, $p = .171$, $\eta 2 = .001$, *power* = .278.

Do 10,000 step differences remain when age and gender are accounted for?

A final analysis was conducted to see if adding demographic factors other than the 10,000 steps model impacted the importance of meeting this threshold in relation to mental health and wellbeing. Gender was divided into male and female participants whilst age was categorised as 18–30 years ($n = 519$), 31–45 years (1096), 46–60 years ($n = 292$) and 60 plus ($n = 24$ years). This analysis continued to use pre and post-depression/anxiety/stress and WEMWBS levels as the within subjects factors and now included threshold (i.e. more or less than 10,000 steps achieved on average) as the between subjects factor as above. Gender and age were covariates in the model.

The ANCOVA analysis of depression continued to reflect no significant change in depression levels over time (within subjects factor) whilst gender and age category were both significant between subjects predictors of depression scores overall, F (1, 1927) =13.402, $p < .001$, $eta^2 = .007$, *power* .955 and F (1, 1927) =22.725, $p < .001$, $eta^2 = .012$, *power* = .997 respectively. Whether people had reached 10,000 steps daily on average had no added significant effects. Finally, there were no interaction effects with the between subjects covariates and the

Table 1 Change in mental state and wellbeing scores across 100-day challenge based on participant's average 10,000 step goal

	Depression		Anxiety		Stress		WEMWBS	
	Pre	Post	Pre	Post	Pre	Post	Pre	Post
< 10,000 steps ($n = 435$)	4.72(0.17)	4.49(0.16)	4.47(0.15)	4.41(0.15)	5.97(0.16)	5.65(0.15)	49.30(0.47)	50.08(0.47)
≥ 10,000 steps ($n = 1528$)	4.55(0.10)	4.17(0.09)	4.58(0.08)	4.31(0.08)	5.33(0.08)	4.79(0.08)	50.22(0.27)	51.37(0.27)
Change over time	$F(1, 1961) = 62.462$, $p < .001$, $\eta^2 = 0.031$		$F(1, 1961) = 12.831$, $p < .001$, $\eta^2 = 0.007$		$F(1, 1961) = 62.462$, $p < .001$, $\eta^2 = 0.031$		$F(1, 1961) = 58.47$, $p < .001$, $\eta^2 = 0.029$	

10,000 step threshold factor and change in depression levels over time.

The ANCOVA analysis of anxiety again revealed the overall decrease in anxiety over the challenge but no significant interactions between age, gender or the 10,000 step threshold in the changes observed in the within subjects analysis. In terms of between subjects effects of the threshold measure and the covariates of age and gender, the results highlight an overall impact of the age covariate, $F(1,1927) = 52.363$, $p < .001$, $eta^2 = .026$, $power = 1$ but no significant impacts from whether people achieve the 10,000 step threshold or their gender.

The ANCOVA related to stress highlighted that with the fuller model, the former significant change over time was no longer observable. Further, there were no significant interaction effects in relation to stress changes for whether people reached the 10,000 step threshold or related to the covariates age and gender. The between subjects analysis highlighted that age and whether people walked over 10,000 had significant impacts on stress levels. in terms of overall stress levels, both age and gender impacted, $F(1,1927) = 13.707$, $p < .001$, $eta^2 .007$, $power = .959$ and $F(1,1927) = 23.616$, $p < .001$, $eta^2 = .012$, $power = .998$. Notably, the participants who were in the group that had averaged over 10,000 steps were those with lower stress levels overall.

Finally, wellbeing scores were assessed. The data from the WEMWBS indicated that the wellbeing scores were unchanged by participation in the program overall and there were no significant interactions between other factors and the results on this scale. Both covariates showed impacts on the between subjects results of the WEMWBS including those for gender, $F(1,1927) = 56.608)$, $p < .001$, $eta^2 = .004$, $power = 1.0$ and age $F(1,1927)7.315$, $p = .007$, $eta^2 = .004$, $power = .771$. Notably, being in the above the 10,000 step threshold group did not infer any differences.

Discussion

The results of this study highlight some psychological and wellbeing benefits of being engaged in work based 10,000 step programs. This effect appeared irrespective of the average number of steps achieved by the person over the program period. Mental health is related to a range of biopsychosocial factors and as a result a range of interventions and approaches may make up sustaining good mental health. This study demonstrated that engaging in a workplace based step program improved stress levels by 8.9%, signs of depression by 7.6%, anxiety by 5.0% and wellbeing by 2.1% from baseline. This reinforces the benefits of this type of exercise regimen as playing a small yet significant role in improving mental as well as physical health. It is notable that when considering the role of the 10,000 step threshold as a significant number to improve people on these psychological factors, there is little evidence from this study that this number holds any significant value. Further, evidence indicates that even the most basic demographic variables such as gender and age can impact the outcomes of this number of steps, again reinforcing the complex biopsychosocial milieu that makes up mental health and wellbeing.

The lack of a dose response highlights there may be multiple factors that lead to improvements associated with these programs outside activity level per se. This may include the enjoyment and connection obtained from meaningful group participation, teamwork, improved friendship, interpersonal support and networking that has been shown to significantly improve mental health and wellbeing [34]. Further, health promoting activities often lead to other behavioural change (e.g. improved diet) to potentially further improve outcomes. The goal of these public health campaign approaches is exactly this, the creation of a gestalt (i.e. the end result being more than just the parts, e.g. doing 10,000 steps specifically) of external and internal change to improve both individual and collective group health. Further research into this cohort needs to explore which combination of internal and external factors most predict successful behavioural change in work based programs. A limitation of this study is the lack of follow-up after the program has ceased to see if mental health gains and behavioural change have been maintained or if they only exist within the workplace challenge. Put plainly, 10,000 steps is not a magic number for the gains in mental health and wellbeing we observed but being part of a health program is clearly positive for mental health and wellbeing by the end of a program.

This workplace health challenge highlights the mental health benefits in a similar way to physical health benefits of these programs. This shows a greater impact than previously demonstrated. Mental health and wellbeing issues play a significant part in absenteeism, reduced productivity and overall decreased quality of life for many individuals. Cost savings for workplaces in terms of mental health are evident with these programs. In combination with other workplace mental health initiatives, these may contribute to the suite of different resources and approaches that improve mental health for those with sub threshold concerns and potentially some benefit for those with more serious mental health issues. This spectrum also requires further investigation.

Evidence indicates that workplace based health promotion programs reduce absenteeism and organisational health care expenditure as described in a systematic review of interventions in large US based firms with an average program duration of 3 years: there the average employee health care costs fell by US$ 3.3 for every 1$ spent on employee wellness programs [35]. However, the real value of workplace wellness programs should include outcomes beyond financial or economic factors, such as physical and mental health, quality of life and other, non-health related factors that improve employee wellbeing, satisfaction and reduce turnover [36].

Our research benefited from a large sample size of participants across a number of countries to fully assess the hypotheses. In terms of limitations, this study did not record diagnoses of mental health issues (including depression and anxiety) which would further elucidate the impact of the program on clinical levels of distress. Secondly, the research did not report on the individual's overall level of activity. This may have been an important consideration as there are clearly individuals who were more active before commencing the program. Ideally this would be co-varied in future studies. Further, all activity levels are self-report and, as participants were involved in the challenge as teams, the data may reflect social desirability biases. Finally, longitudinal follow up of whether people continue to exercise and experience mental health benefits after participating in a workplace based activity challenge needs to be explored to ascertain the sustainability and return of investments of such workplace wellbeing programs. An eight-months follow-up evaluation after a comparable 4-months pedometer-based workplace health program has demonstrated sustained improvement in chronic disease risk factors indicating that such programs can have a long-term benefit [37].

Conclusions

The increasing prevalence of non-communicable diseases such as mental ill health has heightened the need to change lifestyle behaviours and increase physical activity. With most adults spending at least half of their life working, the workplace is an important setting for promoting mental health and wellbeing change [38]. The results of this research indicate that 10,000 step challenges may significantly and meaningfully improve mental health and wellbeing through simple and inexpensive workplace based interventions.

Abbreviations

ANCOVA: Analysis of covariance; BDNF: Brain derived neurotrophic factor; DASS: Depression, Anxiety and Stress Scales; PA: Physical Activity; WEMWBS: Warwick-Edinburgh Mental Wellbeing Scale; WHO: World Health Organization

Acknowledgements

We thank all study participants for their willingness to provide data for this research project and we are indebted to all co-workers for their enthusiastic support.

Funding

The analyses were funded by an unrestricted grant from Stepathlon Ltd. to Victoria University.

Authors' contributions

Conceptualization was carried out by MdC and KH. MdC, KH and SB were responsible for the methodology. Statistical analyses were carried out by KH, SB and MdC. Drafting of the manuscript was done by KH, SB and MdC. Manuscript was revised and finalized by MdC. All authors read and approved the final manuscript.

Consent for publication

Not applicable

Competing interests

Shane Bilsborough is employed by Stepathlon Ltd. Karen Hallam and Maximilian de Courten were benefactors from the unrestricted grant of Stepathlon to Victoria University.

Author details

[1]Centre for Chronic Disease, College of Health and Biomedicine, Victoria University, Melbourne, Australia. [2]Outlook Matters, Pty Ltd, Melbourne, Australia. [3]Stepathlon Private Limited, No. 2B 25E, Lorette Ville, Ground Floor, Village Bandra, Santacruz West, Main Avenue, Mumbai, India.

References

1. Bloom D, Cafiero E, Jané-Llopis E, Abrahams-Gessel S, Bloom L, Fathima S, et al. The global economic burden of noncommunicable diseases. Geneva: World Economic Forum; 2011.
2. De Hert M, Correll CU, Bobes J, Cetkovich-Bakmas M, Cohen D, Asai I, et al. Physical illness in patients with severe mental disorders. I. Prevalence, impact of medications and disparities in health care. World Psychiatry. 2011;10:52–77.
3. Correll CU, Detraux J, De Lepeleire J, De Hert M. Effects of antipsychotics, antidepressants and mood stabilizers on risk for physical diseases in people with schizophrenia, depression and bipolar disorder. World Psychiatry. 2015;14:119–36.
4. Funk M, Drew N, Knapp M. Mental health, poverty and development. J Public Mental Health. 2012;11:166–85.
5. Kakuma R, Minas H, van Ginneken N, Dal Poz MR, Desiraju K, Morris JE, et al. Human resources for mental health care: current situation and strategies for action. Lancet. 2011;378:1654–63.
6. Booth FW, Chakravarthy MV, Gordon SE, Spangenburg EE. Waging war on physical inactivity: using modern molecular ammunition against an ancient enemy. J Appl Physiol. 2002;93:3–30.
7. Callaghan P. Exercise: a neglected intervention in mental health care? J Psychiatr Ment Health Nurs. 2004;11:476–83.
8. Stanton S, Rosenbaum S, Kalucy M, Reaburn P, Happell B. A call to action: exercise as treatment for patients with mental illness. Aust J Prim Health. 2015;21:120–5.
9. Lucas M, Mekary R, Pan A, Mirzaei F, O'Reilly EJ, Willett WC, et al. Relation between clinical depression risk and physical activity and time spent watching television in older women: a 10-year prospective follow-up study. Am J Epidemiol. 2011;174:1017–27.
10. Hiles SA, Lamers F, Milaneschi Y, Penninx BWJH. Sit, step, sweat: longitudinal associations between physical activity patterns, anxiety and depression. Psychol Med. 2017;9:1–12.
11. Cooney GM, Dwan K, Greig CA, Lawlor DA, Rimer J, Waugh FR, et al. Exercise for depression. In: Mead GE, editor. Cochrane database Syst rev, vol. 62. Chichester: John Wiley & Sons, Ltd; 2013. p. CD004366.
12. Rimmele U, Zellweger BC, Marti B, Seiler R, Mohiyeddini C, Ehlert U, et al. Trained men show lower cortisol, heart rate and psychological responses to psychosocial stress compared with untrained men. Psychoneuroendocrinology. 2007;32:627–35.
13. Meeusen R, De Meirleir K. Exercise and brain neurotransmission. Sports Med. 1995;20:160–88.
14. Kvam S, Kleppe CL, Nordhus IH, Hovland A. Exercise as a treatment for depression_ a meta-analysis. J Affect Disord. 2016;202:67–86.
15. Szuhany KL, Bugatti M, Otto MW. A meta-analytic review of the effects of exercise on brain-derived neurotrophic factor. J Psychiatr Res. 2015;60:56–64.
16. Smits JAJ, Berry AC, Rosenfield D, Powers MB, Behar E, Otto MW. Reducing anxiety sensitivity with exercise. Depress Anxiety. 2008;25:689–99.
17. Steptoe A, Deaton A, Stone AA. Subjective wellbeing, health, and ageing. Lancet. 2015;385:640–8.

18. Salmon P. Effects of physical exercise on anxiety, depression, and sensitivity to stress: a unifying theory. Clin Psychol Rev. 2001;21:33–61.
19. Brown WJ, Bauman AE, Bull FC, Burton NW. Development of evidence-based physical activity recommendations for adults (18–64 years): report prepared for the Australian Government Department of Health, august 2012. Canberra: Commonwealth of Australia; 2013.
20. Fletcher GF, Balady G, Blair SN, Blumenthal J, Caspersen C, Chaitman B, et al. Statement on exercise: benefits and recommendations for physical activity programs for all Americans. A statement for health professionals by the committee on exercise and cardiac rehabilitation of the council on clinical cardiology, American Heart Association. Circulation. 1996;94:857–62.
21. Proper K, van Mechelen W. Effectiveness and economic impact of worksite interventions to promote physical activity and healthy diet. Geneva: World Health Organization; 2008.
22. Faghri PD, Omokaro C, Parker C, Nichols E, Gustavesen S, Blozie E. E-technology and pedometer walking program to increase physical activity at work. J Prim Prev. 2008;29:73–91.
23. Ganesan AN, Louise J, Horsfall M, Bilsborough SA, Hendriks J, McGavigan AD, et al. International mobile-health intervention on physical activity, sitting, and weight. J Am Coll Cardiol. 2016;67:2453–63.
24. Glance DG, Ooi E, Berman Y, Glance CF, Barrett HR. Impact of a digital activity tracker-based workplace activity program on health and wellbeing. DH '16. New York: ACM Press; 2016. p. 37–41.
25. Alwan A. Global status report on noncommunicable diseases 2010. Geneva: World Health Organization; 2011.
26. Otto MW, Church TS, Craft LL, Greer TL, Smits JAJ, Trivedi MH. Exercise for mood and anxiety disorders. Prim Care Companion J Clin Psychiatry. 2007;9:287–94.
27. Lovibond SH, Lovibond PF. Manual for the depression anxiety stress scales. Sydney: The Psychology Foundation of Australia; 1995.
28. Crawford JR, Henry JD. The depression anxiety stress scales (DASS): normative data and latent structure in a large non-clinical sample. Br J Clin Psychol. 2003;42:111–31.
29. Brown TA, Chorpita BF, Korotitsch W, Barlow DH. Psychometric properties of the depression anxiety stress scales (DASS) in clinical samples. Behav Res Ther. 1997;35:79–89.
30. Tennant R, Hiller L, Fishwick R, Platt S, Joseph S, Weich S, et al. The Warwick-Edinburgh mental well-being scale (WEMWBS): development and UK validation. Health Qual Life Outcomes. 2007;5:63.
31. Bass M, Dawkin M, Muncer S, Vigurs S, Bostock J. Validation of Warwick-Edinburgh mental well-being scale (WEMWBS) in a population of people using secondary care mental health services. J Ment Health. 2016;25:323–9.
32. Field A. In: Carmichael M, editor. Discovering statistics using IBM SPSS statistics. 4th ed. London: SAGE Publications. London; 2013.
33. Warner RM. Applied statistics: from Bivariate through multivariate techniques. Thousand Oaks: SAGE; 2012.
34. LaMontagne AD, Martin A, Page KM, Reavley NJ, Noblet AJ, Milner AJ, et al. Workplace mental health: developing an integrated intervention approach. BMC Psychiatry. 2014;14:131.
35. Baicker K, Cutler D, Song Z. Workplace wellness programs can generate savings. Health Aff. 2010;29:304–11.
36. Pronk NP. Placing workplace wellness in proper context: value beyond money. Prev Chronic Dis. 2014;11:E119.
37. Freak-Poli R, Wolfe R, Brand M, de Courten M, Peeters A. Eight-month postprogram completion: change in risk factors for chronic disease amongst participants in a 4-month pedometer-based workplace health program. Obesity (Silver Spring). 2013;21:E360–8.
38. Conn VS, Hafdahl AR, Cooper PS, Brown LM, Lusk SL. Meta-analysis of workplace physical activity interventions. Am J Prev Med. 2009;37:330–9.

11

Maternal mental health priorities, help-seeking behaviors, and resources in post-conflict settings

Wietse A. Tol[1,2*], BreeOna Ebrecht[1], Rebecca Aiyo[1], Sarah M. Murray[2], Amanda J. Nguyen[3], Brandon A. Kohrt[4], Sheila Ndyanabangi[5], Stephen Alderman[6], Seggane Musisi[1,7] and Juliet Nakku[1,8]

Abstract

Background: Limited knowledge exists to inform the selection and introduction of locally relevant, feasible, and effective mental health interventions in diverse socio-cultural contexts and health systems. We examined stakeholders' perspectives on mental health-related priorities, help-seeking behaviors, and existing resources to guide the development of a maternal mental health component for integration into non-specialized care in Soroti, eastern Uganda.

Methods: We employed rapid ethnographic methods (free listing and ranking; semi-structured interviews; key informant interviews and pile sorting) with community health workers ($n = 24$), primary health workers ($n = 26$), perinatal women ($n = 24$), traditional and religious healers ($n = 10$), and mental health specialists ($n = 9$). Interviews were conducted by trained Ateso-speaking interviewers. Two independent teams conducted analyses of interview transcripts following an inductive and thematic approach. Smith's Salience Index was used for analysis of free listing data.

Results: When asked about common reasons for visiting health clinics, the most salient responses were malaria, general postnatal care, and husbands being absent. Amongst the free listed items that were identified as mental health problems, the three highest ranked concerns were *adeka na aomisio* (sickness of thoughts); *ipum* (epilepsy), and *emalaria* (malaria). The terms epilepsy and malaria were used in ways that reflected both biomedical and cultural concepts of distress. Sickness of thoughts appeared to overlap substantially with major depression as described in international classification, and was perceived to be caused by unsupportive husbands, intimate partner violence, chronic poverty, and physical illnesses. Reported help-seeking for sickness of thoughts included turning to family and community members for support and consultation, followed by traditional or religious healers and health centers if the problem persisted.

Conclusion: Our findings add to existing literature that describes 'thinking too much' idioms as cultural concepts of distress with roots in social adversity. In addition to making feasible and effective treatment available, our findings indicate the importance of prevention strategies that address the social determinants of psychological distress for perinatal women in post-conflict low-resource contexts.

* Correspondence: wtol@pcaf.org
[1]Peter C. Alderman Foundation, plot 855, Mawanda Road, PO Box 20129, Nakawa, Kampala, Uganda
[2]Department of Mental Health, Johns Hopkins Bloomberg School of Public Health, 624 N Broadway, Baltimore, MD 21205, USA
Full list of author information is available at the end of the article

Background

Mental disorders are a leading contributor to ill health in women of reproductive age [1]. The burden of mental ill health in this population is likely higher in low- and middle income countries (LMIC). A recent systematic review and meta-analysis of studies in LMIC found a pooled prevalence of 25.3% for prenatal depression (51 studies from 20 LMIC, $n = 48{,}904$), and 19.0% for postnatal depression (53 studies from 23 LMIC, $n = 38{,}142$) [2]. Armed conflicts, which predominantly affect LMIC, are associated with an increased burden of mental ill health. In these settings, women have been found to have higher odds of poor outcomes than men [3].

There is a sizeable body of research on the mental health of populations in both ongoing and post-conflict LMIC settings, but very little of this research focuses specifically on maternal mental health, i.e. the mental health of women during pregnancy or the first post-partum year [4]. Poor maternal mental health, a crucial health concern in its own right, is associated with multiple poor child outcomes including: preterm birth and low birth weight [5]; suboptimal breastfeeding and immunization coverage [6]; being underweight or stunted [7]; higher rates of diarrhea and febrile illness [6, 8]; and, negative impacts on child development [6].

Effective prevention and treatment interventions exist to reduce the burden associated with maternal mental disorders [9, 10], but these are not available to the large majority of women at risk in LMIC. To increase access to care, global mental health researchers and practitioners have called for the integration of evidence-based mental health interventions into non-specialized health systems, such as primary care, maternal and child health care, and community care settings [11, 12]. Answering this call is fraught with multiple challenges. First, relatively little research is available to guide efforts to integrate evidence-based interventions into non-specialized care settings in LMIC. For example, although recent systematic reviews indicate that non-specialized health workers can effectively deliver maternal mental health interventions [13–15], the quality of the evidence is low overall and important gaps remain [15]. Specific gaps in knowledge relate to optimal care delivery models (e.g., collaborative vs. stepped care models), effective training and supervision models for health workers, and the cost-effectiveness of bringing different approaches to scale [15]. Most implementation science research in mental health has been conducted in high-income countries, where uptake of evidence-based interventions in routine clinical settings is also low and lessons learned might not be transferable to LMIC contexts [16, 17].

Second, and more fundamentally, considerable critique has been levied on the field of global mental health for a perceived lack of sensitivity to socio-cultural context. For example, critics have argued that phrasing mental health goals purely in terms of disorders described in psychiatric classification systems from industrialized countries fails to capture locally felt priorities and descriptions of mental health problems in socio-culturally diverse settings [18]. Similarly, viewing intervention options solely in terms of evidence-based mental health services that often originate from research conducted in high-income settings, may undermine existing ways of dealing with common mental disorders [18].

The overall objective of this paper is to describe formative qualitative research for a maternal mental health project in post-conflict Uganda that aimed to address some of these shortcomings in global mental health implementation research. Areas of northern and eastern Uganda experienced an insurgency by the Lord's Resistance Army between 1987 and 2006 that was associated with widespread human rights violations against the civilian population and the displacement of 1.9 million people at the height of the conflict [19]. The site of this study (the Teso sub-region) also suffered large-scale forced displacement during a 1987–1992 civil war between the Uganda People's Army and the then newly established government.

Studies in conflict-affected areas in Uganda seven to ten years after cessation of hostilities have found high prevalence of a range of mental health problems, including depression, anxiety, (complex) posttraumatic stress disorder, hazardous alcohol use, as well as suicide [20–22]. Previous qualitative research in Uganda has found that health workers perceive maternal mental health to be a priority, but that government mental health services are generally not available or accessible, prompting the recommendation to make maternal mental health services available at lower levels of the health system [23].

In response to this identified need, a partnership between the Peter C. Alderman Foundation (an international non-governmental organization focused on mental health of violence-affected populations in low-resource areas), the Ugandan Ministry of Health, and Johns Hopkins University was established to develop a mental health services component that can be integrated in the Ugandan maternal and child health care system. Despite challenges in reaching Millennium Development Goals specific to maternal and child health, 95% of pregnant women in Uganda attend at least one antenatal care visit, making antenatal screening an important access point for addressing maternal mental health [24]. Moreover, the government of Uganda is committed to further strengthening maternal and child health services through incorporating the Sustainable Development Goals in its Second National Development Plan [25]. The research described in this paper was implemented as an initial step in designing such a maternal mental health intervention. Our research was framed around two key objectives: (1) given the existence of limited resources and the potential for diverse maternal mental health needs in conflict-affected settings, we aimed to examine the perspectives of stakeholders regarding prioritization of maternal mental health problems; and (2) to build upon local resources and develop an acceptable intervention strategy, we sought to understand current help-seeking patterns for prioritized maternal mental health problems and perceptions of both available resources and gaps in support for women with these problems.

Methods

Setting and sampling

Research activities were conducted in Soroti district, a predominantly Ateso speaking area of the Teso sub-region of Uganda (Fig. 1, developed by BK) [26]. Uganda's health care system formally comprises seven levels, corresponding with government administrative divisions. At the village or Health Center I level (HC I), community health workers are organized into Village Health Teams. Village Health Teams are a voluntary health force that generally do not have a physical office and who mainly engage in community-based preventive, health awareness and basic curative activities. At the parish or HC II level, health centers are staffed by primary health care workers (e.g. general nurses or midwives), who deliver basic health services to catchment areas of approximately 5000 people. At the HC III (sub-county level), health centers have a clinical officer, a maternity unit, and unlike lower levels, separate wards for male and female patients (8 beds). Health centers at levels IV-VII have greater staff capacity and provide increasingly specialized care. In Soroti district, there are 14 HC IIs, 12 HC IIIs, two HC IVs, and one 195-bed regional referral hospital.

We estimated that including four of Soroti's ten sub-counties in our study would give us enough opportunity to identify commonalities and differences between sub-counties and reach data saturation among different participant groups of interest. As the majority of Uganda's population lives in rural areas where the gap between health needs and available services is greatest, we excluded all sub-counties that did not have a predominantly rural population ($n = 4$) [24]. For feasibility reasons, we then excluded one sub-county where the majority of residents did not speak Ateso. Of the five remaining sub-counties, we randomly selected four for inclusion. Together, these sub-counties represent a predominantly rural, Ateso-speaking population living at various distances from the regional hub in Soroti municipality.

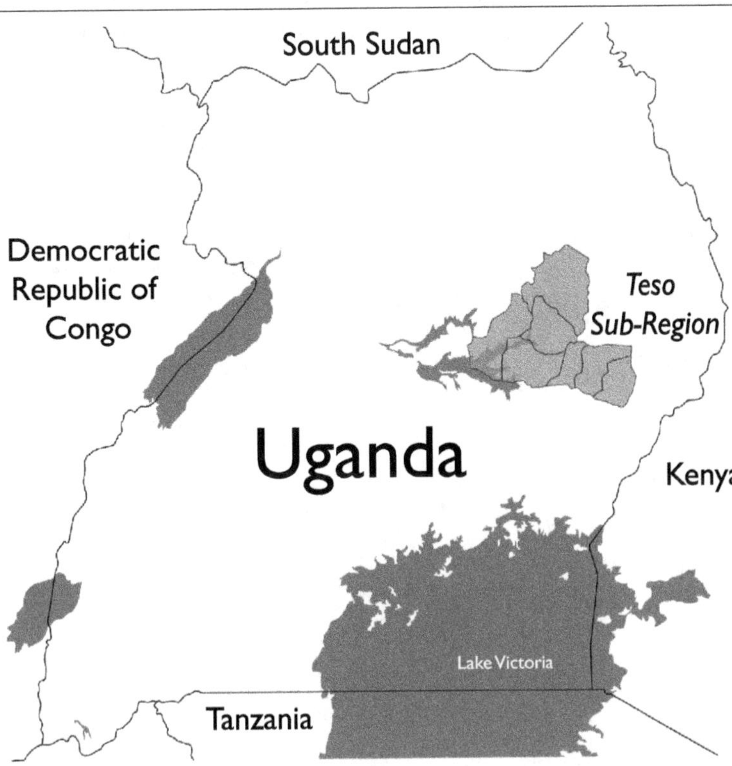

Fig. 1 The Teso sub-region study site in eastern Uganda

Within each sub-county, we conducted purposive and convenience sampling of stakeholders, including health workers, perinatal women seeking help at health centers, and religious and traditional healers. We aimed to include health workers from different healthcare system levels, with a focus on HCI to HCIII workers as rural women most commonly access antenatal care at these levels. HC IIIs were of particular interest, as these facilities have the highest rates of antenatal care visits. Among sub-counties with multiple HC IIs, HC IIs were randomly selected for study inclusion. In each sub-county, we started recruitment by visiting HC IIs and IIIs during working hours to introduce the study to the clinical officer in-charge of the facility. These clinical officers helped recruit other health workers from their facilities to be interviewed. Community health workers at the HC I level were recruited by liaising with the Village Health Team Sub-County Coordinator.

Free listing and ranking

An overview of participants and data collection activities can be found in Table 1. We first conducted free listing and ranking (cf. [27, 28]) embedded in semi-structured interviews with 22 primary and 22 community health care workers from HC Is, IIs, and IIIs in each sub-county. Free listing was conducted individually with the exception of one group exercise with community health care workers (Table 1). Specifically, we asked participants *"what are the most common problems for which pregnant women, or women who have just given birth, visit the health center?"* Participants were invited to provide as many answers as possible and were probed to include all of the (physical) health, mental health, social and spiritual or supernatural problems that may lead perinatal women to visit the health center. The interviewer wrote down answers verbatim. Among the problems that were listed, interviewers asked the participants which problems they considered to be related to thoughts, feelings or behaviors (i.e. mental health problems) and to rank the three mental health problems that they felt were most important. Participants were then asked about help-seeking and current health center resources for the three most highly prioritized maternal mental health problems.

Semi-structured interviews

We conducted individual semi-structured interviews with perinatal women to gather information on help-seeking behaviors and available services for maternal mental health problems. We aimed to recruit four perinatal women from each included sub-county as they were waiting to receive antenatal care at the HC III. In these interviews, we presented participants with a fictitious case vignette about a woman in Soroti district experiencing mental health problems. The vignette was developed based on descriptions of the most highly prioritized problems identified in the free list interviews with health workers. Participants were asked to describe (1) what the woman in the case vignette could herself do about her problems; (2) their thoughts about where the

Table 1 Overview of participants and methods

Research activities	Location	Participants
Free listing and key informant interviews with primary health care workers (AI 1)	Health Center III in SC1, SC2, SC3, SC4 Health Center II in SC1, SC2	$N = 22$ (13 female, 9 male)
Free listing and key informant interviews with community health care workers (AI 2)	Health Center I (Village Health Team) in SC1, SC2	$N = 22$ (7 female, 15 male) – 10 individual interviews and one group interview (12 participants – 8 male and 4 female)
Semi-structured interviews (case vignette) with perinatal women (AI 3)	Health Center III antenatal services in SC1, SC2, SC3, SC4	$N = 16$ perinatal women (4 from each sub-county)
Key informant interviews with primary health care workers (SI 4)	Health Center III in SC2 Health Center II in SC1, SC2	$N = 4$ (female)
Key informant interviews with community health care workers (AI 4)	Health Center I in SC3	$N = 2$ (male)
Key informant interviews with traditional and religious healers (round 1) (AI 5)	SC1, SC2, SC3, SC4	$N = 8$ (4 traditional healers, 4 religious healers; all male)
Key informant interviews with a subset of traditional and religious healers (round 2) (AI 4)	SC1, SC2	$N = 2$ (1 traditional healer, 1 religious healer; both male)
Key informant interviews with perinatal women (AI 6)	SC1, SC2, SC3, SC4	$N = 8$
Key informant interviews with mental health specialists (AI 7)	Health Center V (Soroti Regional Referral Hospital) Health Center VII (Butabika National Referral Hospital, Kampala)	$N = 9$ (3 female, 6 male)

AI Additional Information, *SC1* Sub-county 1, as a confidentiality safeguard, sub-counties are numbered

woman would likely seek help (first, second, third, and so on); (3) to provide details about what services could be obtained at each place where help might be sought; and, (4) what help the health center could offer for this woman and how the health center could improve its assistance.

Key informant interviews and pile sorting

We conducted key informant interviews with four groups of participants: traditional or religious healers, mental health specialists, community and primary health care workers, and perinatal women. Two traditional or religious healers were recruited through consultation with sub-county leaders and health center officials in each sub-county and nine mental health specialists were recruited from the regional and national referral hospitals. Specialists and healers participated in free listing and ranking exercises during their interviews that were similar in structure to the initial free listing interviews completed with primary and community healthcare workers. In this round of free listing interviews, greater focus was placed on eliciting symptoms of identified priority maternal mental health problems, what groups are particularly affected by these problems, and treatments provided for them.

We then conducted a second round of key informant interviews with a subset of the community and primary health workers who participated in the free listing interviews and traditional healers who participated in the initial key informant interviews. Health workers and healers were selected if they provided rich information about the mental health needs in their sub-counties. We also conducted key informant interviews with two older (more experienced) perinatal women from each sub-county. These women were recruited by health care workers and selected based on their ability to read and their experience with the antenatal care system, as determined by their age and number of previous births. Because free listing resulted in several terms that seemed closely related, we added a pile sorting activity to these key informant interviews. Pile sorting was intended to increase our understanding of how participants would classify various symptoms. Participants were provided with notecards with names of symptoms (in both Ateso and English) derived from descriptions of the three prioritized maternal mental health problems. Participants were asked to sort the cards into piles that made sense for them, in as many or few groups as they preferred, and to name to each pile. These key informant interviews subsequently focused on different idioms of distress used to describe the three prioritized maternal mental health problems; symptoms belonging to these problems; and groups of women particularly affected by them. Finally, participants were asked about the causes of the top three problems and possible solutions for each of the causes. Perinatal women were also probed about help-seeking behaviors for the prioritized problems.

Instruments, procedures, and ethics

Interviews were conducted using semi-structured interview guides (available as Additional files 1, 2, 3, 4, 5, 6, 7, 8) that contained interview questions, possible probes, and space for notes. They were conducted in Ateso or English, depending on the preferences of the participant. All interviews were audio recorded and transcribed verbatim. When using the guide, interviewers were instructed to still follow the narrative of the participants as much as possible. All interviews were conducted by locally recruited, Ateso-speaking interviewers who participated in a two-week training on research ethics and qualitative interviewing skills. The training provided ample opportunity for skill-based learning through feedback on role-plays, with a strong focus on asking open questions, probing, and giving non-judgmental responses.

All participants provided written informed consent before participating in interviews. Ethical approval for this study was granted by the Johns Hopkins Bloomberg School of Public Health Institutional Review Board, the Mildmay Uganda Research Ethics Committee, and the Uganda National Council for Science and Technology. In addition, we obtained approval from the District Health Officer before starting recruitment.

Analysis

To analyze free list data and rank priority maternal mental health problems, we used Smith's Salience Index (S), which ranks responses based on frequency of mention while also weighting items based on where it appeared on participants' lists. Under this method, frequently mentioned items among individuals are considered to indicate common knowledge or consensus, and items listed earlier are assumed to be more important to the participant. A higher S score is indicative of greater saliency [29]. Smith Salience index is calculated for each item as the total number of items in the list minus the rank order for item *A* divided by the total number of items in the list. Scores range from 0 to approximately 1, with scores closer to 1 indicating greater saliency.

Transcripts were analyzed using an emergent, inductive coding approach [30, 31]. This stage of the analysis was performed in parallel by two teams of analysts: one of postgraduate students based at the Johns Hopkins Bloomberg School of Public Health (JHBSPH) in the US; the other was comprised of one postgraduate student from JHBSPH and a Ugandan community psychology graduate based in Uganda. The US-based team began analysis by conducting an initial transcript review, in which they highlighted and summarized portions of text relevant to the research questions on a sub-set of interviews. Out of these summaries, they developed emergent codes and organized the codes into a framework or codebook. This codebook was utilized to code the interviews using Dedoose software [32]. The Ugandan team manually conducted line-by-line coding for the first three interviews and prepared a list of initial codes. These codes were combined and re-organized into focused codes and the revised code-book consisted of five topical and 41 response codes. New themes emerging from the data were discussed between the researchers and incorporated into the developing codebook as deemed appropriate (available as a Additional file 8). In the last step, the Uganda team coded all interviews using this final codebook, through the aid of the R package for Qualitative Data Analysis software [33].

Results

In total, 81 individual interviews and one 12-participant group interview were conducted. Participants included 51 women and 42 men with an average age of 38 years (Table 1). Of these interviews, 26 were conducted with primary health care workers, 24 with community health care workers, 24 with perinatal women, 10 with traditional healers, and nine with mental health specialists. An overview of the flow of data collection activities is provided in Fig. 2.

Maternal mental health priorities

The five most salient responses to free lists of common health problems for which women visit the health center were malaria (S = 0.51), general postnatal care (S = 0.32), husbands being absent (S = 0.32); general antenatal check-ups (S = 0.22); and, lower abdominal or stomach pain (S = 0.21). Saliency varied across the different types of participants. For example, "absent husbands" was not one of the five most salient problems listed by primary health care workers, but was the most salient problem for traditional healers. For community health care workers, bleeding and HIV were highly salient, but did not feature in the top five most salient problems for other types of participants.

Of the fifteen problems that were identified as being related to mental health and were listed by two or more respondents (of any type), *adeka na aomisio* (Ateso, literally sickness of thoughts) had the highest saliency (S = 0.28). About half of the participants (20 out of 41) listed *adeka na aomiso* as one of the top three most important mental health problems. The mental health problems with the next highest saliency scores were epilepsy *(ipum)* and malaria *(emalaria)* (Table 2). Although malaria had the highest saliency among the initial free list responses (focused on all health problems), participants ranked it the third most important problem when asked to rank the three most important mental health problems.

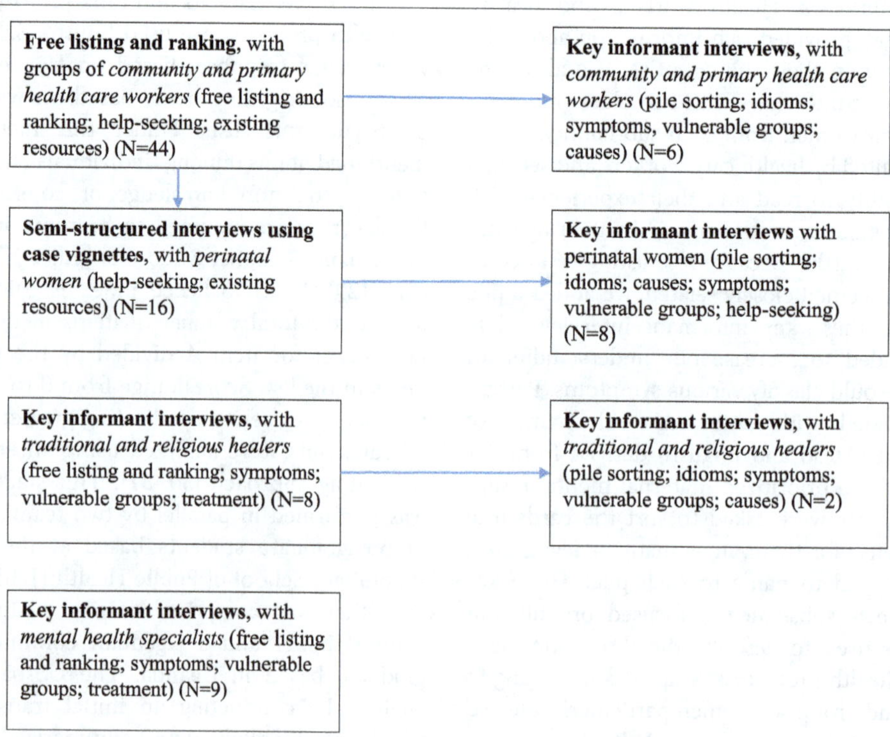

Fig. 2 Data collection flow

Table 2 Free listing saliency results for highest priority mental health conditions

Rank	All Respondents	Primary Health Care Workers	Community Health Care Workers	Mental Health Specialists	Traditional Healers
1	Sickness of thoughts (S = 0.28)	Sickness of thoughts (S = 0.38)	Epilepsy (S = 0.55)	Postpartum depression and (puerperal) psychosis (S = 0.59)	Absent husbands (S = 0.33)
2	Epilepsy (S = 0.25)	Malaria (S = 0.26)	Malaria (S = 0.37)	Stress (S = 0.26)	Gender based violence (S = 0.29)
3	Malaria (S = 0.20)	Absent husbands (S = 0.23)	Thinking too much and poverty (S = 0.17)	Epilepsy (S = 0.15)	Witchcraft/ spiritual problems (S = 0.29)

S=Smith Salience index

When free list responses from primary health care workers, community health care workers, traditional healers, and mental health specialists were analyzed separately, we found differences in which problems were most salient. Community health care workers listed epilepsy *(ipum)* (S = 0.55) as the most important mental health problem, followed by malaria (S = 0.37), and with *aomom na epol* (thinking too much) and poverty tied for third (S = 0.17). Primary health care workers believed the most important problem was sickness of thoughts (S = 0.38), the second most important was malaria (S = 0.26), and the third most important was absent husbands (S = 0.23). Mental health specialists said the most important problems were postpartum depression and (puerperal) psychosis (S = 0.58), followed by stress (S = 0.26), and epilepsy (S = 0.15). Traditional healers identified absent husbands as the most important mental health problem (S = 0.33), followed by gender-based violence (S = 0.29), and witchcraft or spiritual problems (S = 0.29).

Below we describe the three maternal mental health concerns most commonly prioritized by participants overall. For each concern, we describe participants' perspectives on common complaints accompanying the concern, causes of the concern, and ways of seeking assistance for managing the concern.

Sickness of thoughts

Sickness of thoughts *(adeka na aomiso)* was prioritized as the most important mental health problem among perinatal women. Reasons given for prioritizing sickness of thoughts were that it could lead to suicidal or homicidal tendencies and that its causes are highly prevalent in the community. The terms thinking too much *(aomom na epol)*, thinking *(aomom)*, over-thinking that leads to ulcers *(akwamakit aomom)* and depression appeared to be used interchangeably by most participants for sickness of thoughts. Perinatal women often referred to thoughts as a tangible force that could be taken away from a woman's life. They utilized phrases such as – "removing thoughts from the head", "reduce thinking in the mind", "remove thoughts from heart", "make your heart settled", or "remove burden from life". Mental health specialists did not utilize the phrase sickness of thoughts, but rather "maternity blues", which they referred to as distinctly different from postpartum depression.

Symptoms that were listed for sickness of thoughts by primary health care workers and maternity blues by mental health specialists included excessive sadness for longer than two weeks, crying more than usual, low moods, sleep disturbances, less interest in activities that a woman used to enjoy, feeling worthless, outbursts of anger, lack of appetite, weight loss, lack of energy, excessive worries, suicidal thoughts, social withdrawal, fearing life situations, and substance use. Other symptoms mentioned by only a few mental health specialists for maternity blues and only a few primary health care workers for sickness of thoughts were hallucinations, uncoordinated speech, and fever. In contrast, perinatal women and community health care workers were more likely to list behavioral symptoms of sickness of thoughts (sleeping less, crying, not eating and feeling weak) than emotional symptoms (sadness, feelings of worthlessness). One perinatal woman described the symptoms of sickness of thoughts as follows:

> The way I can tell that a woman's life is not okay, she's growing thin very slowly, she cries about the heart, feels pain in the heart, and also her eating reduces.
>
> Perinatal woman, Semi-Structured Interview

Primary health care providers were more likely to give detailed descriptions of symptoms that were consistent with Diagnostic and Statistical Manual fourth version (DSM-IV) criteria, such as stating that the symptoms must be consistently present for two or more weeks. Among both primary health workers and mental health specialists, infanticide (i.e., the drive of a woman to kill her newborn baby), was noted as a very severe symptom of sickness of thoughts or depression.

The most common cause of sickness of thoughts according to participants was absent or unsupportive partners. Perinatal women consistently reported that when husbands in the community provide no support, whether emotional, social or financial, sickness of thoughts was more likely. Because husbands are considered to be responsible for the financial welfare of families, but were perceived to provide very little to no money for the family, food was often reported to be scarce. Women were therefore unable to feed themselves and their growing fetus. One participant explained these burdens:

> Mostly here, you may find a mother is depressed... but I think that it's due to the way they are staying with their husbands in their families. One time a certain lady told me that my husband says I am rude to him, that I am carrying death.... They call pregnancy death... Most women here they get depressed because their husbands, there is a way people here behave. You can find a man and the woman is pregnant; the man goes to the lakeshores for fishing and stays there. You are remaining there, you are alone with the children, feeding becomes a problem, even when you are supposed to go to the hospital but there is nobody to take you, there is no money. Those are the problems they mostly get, you try to refer somebody from here, and she tells you now my husband is not at home and I have children, there is nobody to take care of the children.
>
> Enrolled Midwife, Female, Free listing and Ranking Interview

Other common causes given by participants were unwanted or unplanned pregnancies, experiencing domestic violence, being in a "quarreling" relationship, chronic sickness, and poverty.

Healthcare providers also described men refusing to escort their wives to antenatal care visits as a problem, particularly when the men refuse to be tested for HIV. Due to a governmental policy requiring men to be at antenatal care visits, women can be scolded or even turned away from antenatal care if their husbands are not present. Alternatively, if women push their husbands to attend antenatal care, they put themselves at risk for physical violence. Gender-based violence was listed as a very prevalent problem in the community, caused not only by women pushing their husbands to attend antenatal visits, but also by "drunkard" husbands. These men were described as spending most of the day out of the house drinking alcohol and acting violent upon returning home. Health care workers also explained that many women become depressed due to an accumulation of stress in their daily lives related to a combination of intimate partner violence, poverty, HIV, and other diseases that are common but often go untreated. Only mental health specialists mentioned biological causes of depression, such as hormonal imbalances. A Village Health Team member described a common combination of problems as follows:

> You find after the mother has got pregnant, you find that people argue, now the woman is pregnant and her mind is not stable. Maybe the husband says that 'I am not the one responsible for the pregnancy'. So you find her mind is disturbed. It disturbs her, maybe to predict the child, that me, I want a boy... so you find even that disturbs her, "what [gender] child will I produce?" I usually get such women worrying... And another is being attacked. Their husbands, when they come back from drinking they attack you when you are pregnant, you find that woman does not stay well, you find that her body is weak, maybe she is thinking outside that what am I going to do concerning this man's issues? Whenever he comes from drinking he attacks, whenever he comes you find that her mind is disturbed and not clear. And then after she has delivered, it will find that as he wanted the girl child, she has produced a boy. Then that starts torturing. You will find that such children remain when they have not been taken even for immunization because her mind has not settled to love this baby well.
>
> Community Health Care Worker, Male, Focus Group Discussion

Healthcare providers, mental health specialists, and traditional healers described young, single, unemployed, minimally educated women that lack social, financial and partner support as being at the highest risk of developing sickness of thoughts. A religious healer described the reason young women are more affected as:

> Most women which are affected, they are young women. These young ladies, you know for them they rush to marry not knowing the challenges which are going to face their families. So they enter in that marriage but the challenges come so they are not able to withstand all that... They are even two in this house here [pointing at a certain house in the neighborhood]. So the man brought one first, left and went and brought another one. This one is still young, one baby only and he has decided to go for another one. That one is also pregnant and the man just took off, he's not able to answer this problem. So the young ladies are there, they are both pregnant, one is about to give birth.
>
> Religious Healer, Male, Key Informant Interview

The most common, and usually first, suggestion made for women who have sickness of thoughts was to pray or talk with someone to "calm their disturbed heart." One perinatal woman had the following recommendations for a woman affected by sickness of thoughts:

> She should find strength. Sometimes she also must go aside and people will give her advice which will give her strength, because when she sits alone she cannot, she needs people to give her some advice which can make her also settle since she's pregnant. They can make her heart settled so she may stop over thinking. You know when you distance yourself from people you will have many thoughts as it is like that you are even pregnant, the man is treating you badly... now these people need to be near some people who can help you with ideas and others advise.
>
> Perinatal Woman, Semi-Structured Interview

Participants said that friends and family could provide encouragement and material or financial support to help a woman experiencing sickness of thoughts. After seeking help from her family and community, participants said the woman should seek out a traditional or spiritual healer. If this healer is unable to help, they should refer the woman to a community health care worker who could help them access the primary health care facility. A primary care nurse described these steps of care-seeking:

> What the women do, like some of them who are close to churches can go to churches, they can explain their problems to a pastor or to a spiritual leader who is around then they see how they can counsel her. At times they pray for them also. Then maybe when they see, the church members see that as if the situation is not coming down... They might see that maybe now it is a serious sickness, now, then they refer them to the hospital...then the hospital will now assess and see what the situation is. Like for us here when we assess and we see the situation is not to our handling, we now refer ahead so that that person can be helped.... Others can also walk to their friends. Some can explain to the friends and see how the friends can help them. With counseling maybe some of them can even just leave the home...aaah leave the home and go somewhere else because if the problem is within the home, that's why you see most women just end up maybe if you are married, somebody leaves that home and maybe goes back to their home where she thinks she can have what.... some peace.
>
> Enrolled Nurse, Female, Free Listing and Ranking Interview

Additional resources described at the community level for managing sickness of thoughts included group activities (e.g. village savings and loans or drama groups) and the government or non-governmental organizations that provide food, clothing, advice and protection.

The two health care services for sickness of thoughts described most often were counseling and medication, with medication being utilized most frequently. Primary health care workers described counseling as individual, couple, or family sessions utilized to talk to women about how to deal with their sickness of thoughts. Another reported strategy for managing sickness of thoughts was to treat the underlying diseases or causes of the depression, such as HIV or other chronic illnesses. Some primary health care workers talked about scheduling follow-up appointments or referring patients for care at a higher-level health center. The community health care workers' role for sickness of thoughts is to sensitize the community about going to the health facility.

Epilepsy

Epilepsy *(ipum)* was the second most salient mental health problem described by participants. The term epilepsy was used interchangeably with other terms, including falling sickness *(adeka na ebironor),* repeated fits or attacks *(adoenen aria ebironor na ebongonikini)* and fainting *(ailonor).* Though the majority of participants discussed epilepsy as a mental health problem in and of itself, some participants also described feelings of burden among caregivers of a family member or child living with epilepsy. One health care worker described severe consequences of epilepsy:

> You will find that people with epilepsy, most of them suffer a lot, most especially when they get the attack. You will find that they suffer a lot. You can find somebody maybe falling on the what? On the fire, some of them have even ended in... recently there is someone who died, he went to fetch water and he fell in a well, killing the person. That's why I say that number one [epilepsy] should also be dealt with.
>
> Enrolled Nurse, Male, Free Listing and Ranking Interview

Symptoms that participants commonly associated with epilepsy included convulsions, falling on the ground, headache, fever, and bruises all over the body. Less commonly, participants listed saliva coming out of the mouth and urinating as symptoms associated with epileptic episodes. Additionally, some perinatal women described that women with epilepsy would have visible wounds on the body due to multiple falls and would be more likely to isolate themselves due to fear of falling in public.

Common causes listed for epilepsy included physical trauma, conflict and war, alcoholism, stress, malaria, fevers, infections of the spinal cord, and family history.

One participant explained a perceived link between conflict exposure and the development of epilepsy:

> You find it's common here because the village was attacked by Kony so those bombs and the sound of those guns affected their brains, most of them... So it can be the cause because you will find that here children they have epilepsy but when you maybe ask their background, they cannot even explain it well, that's why am first querying maybe because the place was first attacked by those people, now that sound of those bombs it can affect their brains.
>
> Nursing Assistant, Female, Free Listing and Ranking Interview

Less commonly listed causes included flies, sleeping with someone who has epilepsy, a difficult delivery, and curses or other supernatural causes. Primary health care workers and mental health specialists generally attributed epilepsy to a biological or genetic cause, while community health care workers and perinatal women typically discussed epilepsy as attributable to spiritual or psychosocial factors.

Descriptions of care seeking behaviors for epilepsy were similar to those related to sickness of thoughts. Women were described as first seeking help from their family and friends, followed by a traditional or religious healer. In cases where healers are not able to help women, participants stated they would make health facility referrals. One traditional healer noted two possible treatments for epilepsy:

> The solution for the problem [Epilepsy]? As it is the devil, the first solution is to pray a deliverance prayer to the person who is sick or is affected. Another solution: that person can be taken to the hospital for a close checkup.
>
> Traditional Healer, Male, Key Informant Interview

Many respondents listed the importance of managing safety concerns for women with epilepsy. They talked of the importance of family and community support, both in reminding a woman to take her medication and in keeping her away from harm.

> For them, when somebody has realized they have epilepsy... they should not do risky work like cooking. Like when you are in the kitchen, you should not be alone, you have to be with somebody, when you're going to the well, make sure you move with somebody. Then there are signs, which happen when maybe if it wants to throw you down, so we always advise them that if you see that sign, you have to come to the hospital... [the families] always help them like fetching water. They always fetch for them water. Like the one I got here, even coming for antenatal they don't make her come alone. So that when they give them advice on how to feed, what and what, at least that person knows better. The community also always helps them like when a person of epilepsy gets an attack, or falls somewhere and the community is aware that that person has that problem, they will not leave that person. Like if she falls on the road, the community will at least pull that person away from that dangerous place. Because they are aware that she's having such and such a problem. Though some people have that fear, some of them have that misconception that when you step where that person has fallen you will also automatically get it.
>
> Enrolled Nurse, Female, Free Listing and Ranking Interview

Nearly all participants stated that epilepsy should be treated with medication, and that with medication, epilepsy is unlikely to be fatal. However, some health care workers mentioned not knowing the correct medication to give. Respondents also mentioned that risk factors for epilepsy are preventable. The role of health care workers was described as consisting of encouraging mothers with epilepsy to start antenatal care, telling them how to take their medication, and advising them on how to care for themselves. Health care workers also explained that mothers with epilepsy should give birth at facilities via cesarean section.

Malaria

Participants named both *Emalaria* and *eimiddi,* which translate to malaria, as problems of perinatal women. *Eimiddi* was less frequently listed than *emalaria*. Three women stated that the Ateso phrase *emusuja*, meaning fever, could also be used for malaria. Malaria was listed as a mental health problem by perinatal women, traditional healers, community and primary health care workers, but not by any mental health specialists. Health care workers described malaria as a mental health concern because, with delayed treatment, it was said to cause convulsions or "brain disturbances" and to "spoil the mind of that lady." Some primary health care workers and mental health specialists referred specifically to cerebral malaria, but most community health care workers and traditional healers referred to it as severe malaria. Aside from cerebral malaria, respondents described malaria as a mental health problem because it can cause stress in mothers.

> [In my view] malaria is the second most important problem because most of our mothers suffer from malaria because sometimes we lack drugs and somebody comes here, no treatment, no what, no money so that one also sometimes ends up with stress maybe can even end up with miscarriage.
>
> Enrolled Midwife, Female, Free Listing and Ranking Interview

Symptoms described as associated with malaria included: headache, general body weakness, fever, and loss of energy. When perinatal women were asked how they could recognize if someone had malaria, they asserted that infected women would feel warm and might prefer to sit in the sunshine. Participants also mentioned urine discoloration or blood in the urine, especially among pregnant women, and yellow or red discoloration of the eyes, as symptoms of malaria. Two women also reported seeing sores or wounds start to develop in the mouth of someone with malaria.

Nearly all participants reported malaria to be caused by mosquitoes. Less commonly listed causes of malaria were feeling cold, "bad air", or having the flu. These causes were more likely to be listed by perinatal women or community health care workers.

Health care workers stressed the importance of women coming to the health center when they have malaria. In contrast to sickness of thoughts or epilepsy, participants most commonly said that women with malaria should go directly to health facilities, rather than first going to a family member, friend, or traditional or religious healer. Nearly all participants described the importance of obtaining medication for malaria and taking it as directed by health care workers. The major role that families were seen as being able to take in supporting a woman was to prevent the spread of malaria by making changes to the environment, such as covering holes where standing water collects, shutting windows in the evening to keep mosquitoes out, and clearing bushes from near the house. One community health care worker stated:

> *The community needs each family, when the compound is clean, all those broken bottles to be removed from home. You slash the compound also and the home is clean...everyone needs to have a net they sleep under.*
>
> Community Health Care Worker, Male, Free Listing and Ranking Interview

Participants said that health facilities have a responsibility to conduct routine testing for malaria at a woman's first antenatal visit, provide mosquito nets, and give education on how to prevent malaria. Fansidar, coartem and quinine were the medicines reported to be given to mothers who test positive for malaria. Fansidar was mentioned most frequently as both a front-line treatment and prophylaxis for malaria among pregnant women. In complicated cases or in situations where medications are locally unavailable, participants said pregnant women might be referred to a higher level of care and/or a hospital. The role of community health care workers was described as handing out mosquito nets, providing malaria prevention education, and referring febrile women to health centers. Health workers noted that once women began treatment for malaria, clinics and health teams would provide case management and follow-up to ensure that they completed treatment.

Discussion

This qualitative study examined stakeholders' perspectives on maternal mental health priorities, as well as help-seeking and resources for these priorities, in a rural eastern Ugandan post-conflict setting.

Before discussing our findings, we note several study limitations. The study included more formal health actors than actors from outside the formal health system (e.g., traditional and religious healers). This may have led us to uncover biomedical explanatory models in lieu of other understandings of the cause of priority problems. Nonetheless, the main mental health concern we identified, sickness of thoughts, is not a recognized medical diagnosis. Further, malaria, which is not traditionally seen as a mental health concern by medical specialists, was highly prioritized. These findings suggest that we were successful in identifying concerns outside of biomedical perspectives. We did include perinatal women and a sizeable group of community health workers who have no training in mental health, and thus arguably are more likely to articulate lay perspectives than medical views on mental health problems. Second, perinatal women were recruited during antenatal visits and interviews were held at the health centers. This may have led to the inclusion of perinatal women with a more favorable opinion towards health centers or encouraged women to give responses perceived as desirable by health workers. Third, we employed a rapid ethnographic approach, involving locally trained interviewers from the same socio-cultural background as the participants. A hesitancy to explain concepts in detail to an interviewer who was perceived to share the same cultural knowledge may have limited our ability to understand complex social phenomena. Due to a lack of multiple follow-up interviews with participants, our process may also have produced a more superficial understanding of concepts than a longer-term ethnographic study. Further, only one Ugandan was involved in data analysis.

Our study does have several key strengths, including triangulation across different data collection techniques and types of participants, while also having sufficient breadth and depth of information to explore priorities and reach saturation in our analyses within each participant group. Analyses were conducted by two independent teams of analysts, strengthening the trustworthiness of the coding procedures.

Pertaining to our first research objective, we found *adeka na aomisio* (or sickness of thoughts) to be the most commonly prioritized maternal mental health concern. Although there was some variation across types of participants (e.g., traditional healers appeared to prioritize determinants of psychological distress rather than a specific psychological condition), there was broad consensus about the importance of sickness of thoughts. Sickness of thoughts was largely used interchangeably with thinking too much, an idiom of distress that has been identified in 138 studies across diverse socio-cultural contexts [34] and is listed as a cultural concept of distress in the DSM-5 [35]. In this study, psychological problems reported as associated with sickness of thoughts by non-health workers were primarily observable signs rather than symptoms of depression (e.g., eating less, crying, and sleep disturbance).

Social scientists have warned against conflating thinking too much idioms with psychiatric disorder categories, as idioms of distress can communicate important social dimensions of suffering and often do not exist as orderly syndromes [34]. Our findings indeed seem to indicate that the sickness of thoughts idiom conveys a constellation of social adversity experienced by pregnant and postpartum women in Soroti. This constellation includes high levels of intimate partner violence, unsupportive spouses (including for reproductive health) who potentially drink alcohol, financial stress, and physical illnesses (e.g. HIV/AIDS and malaria). Concerns on social origins of maternal distress expressed by traditional and religious healers overlapped with those expressed by health workers, specifically the perceived influence of unsupportive spouses and intimate partner violence. While epidemiological research in eastern Uganda has found that prior conflict experiences predicted higher levels of intimate partner violence [36], we note that this constellation of adversity for pregnant and postpartum women has been found to underlie maternal common mental disorders in low-resource settings more broadly [37–40]. More in-depth ethnographic and social epidemiological research would help elucidate the complex socio-cultural dynamics that underlie sickness of thoughts, including its etiology in the historical context of armed conflict and ongoing adversity.

Ipum (epilepsy), also referred to by participants as falling sickness (*adeka na ebironor*), repeated fits or attacks (*adoenen aria ebironor na ebongonikini*), and fainting (*ailonor*), was prioritized as the second most important perinatal mental health concern. Epilepsy is not a highly prevalent disorder in eastern Africa; a meta-analysis estimated its prevalence as 5.1 per 1000 people, though given the stigma associated with epilepsy, this may be an underestimation [41]. However, compared to other regions, epilepsy is about twice as common in sub-Saharan Africa [41], and an analysis of primary care health information system data found that it is the most common presenting mental, neurological, or substance use related complaint in refugee settings [42]. Given that participants in this study indicated that conflict, stress, and evil spirits may cause *ipum*, its high prioritization may be in part due to an overlap with non-epileptic fits in the context of spirit possession. Previous research in southern Uganda has found that dissociative complaints, which are linked to the experience of potentially traumatic events, may include fits [43, 44].

Similarly, the term malaria may be syncretic, reflecting both biomedical and cultural concepts of distress. In neighboring Kenya, Jenkins and colleagues have noted that common mental disorders are often misdiagnosed as malaria in primary care [45], and Ndetei and colleagues included reporting malaria in a screener for common mental disorders [46]. Likewise, Tesfaye and colleagues have hypothesized that malaria is often misdiagnosed in people with psychological symptoms visiting primary care facilities in Ethiopia [47].

Consistent with studies in other settings, we found that participants emphasized prayer and social support from family and community members (including emotional encouragement and financial support) to address *adeka na aomisio* [34]. Assistance from a traditional healer, religious healer, or community health worker was said to be sought in cases where sickness of thoughts persists. Descriptions of help-seeking pathways for epilepsy were similar, except that spiritual support was said to specifically address evil spirits as a cause of epilepsy, safety concerns were emphasized, and medication was a commonly discussed treatment option. For malaria, women were described as seeking help directly from health centers.

Based on these qualitative findings and international guidelines for managing perinatal depression, a treatment strategy can be developed that has local relevance (i.e., is focused on locally prioritized mental health concerns) and is feasible (i.e., considers existing help-seeking behaviors and resources). For example, the UK National Institute for Health and Clinical Excellence (NICE) guidelines for perinatal mental health emphasize a stepped care approach in which women, identified in primary care settings, receive progressively more specialized treatments depending on need [48]. In this context, identification of perinatal mental health problems in primary care should focus on sickness of thoughts. Because of the overlap of sickness of thoughts with perinatal depression, cultural adaptation of existing screening measures for major depressive episodes seems a feasible next step [49]. Identification of sickness of thoughts should take place in an accessible health care setting (e.g. routine antenatal care), given that help-seeking for sickness of thoughts only occurs at health centers at later stages.

In the process of intervention design, we feel it would be important to consult with local stakeholders to collaboratively design specific proposed intervention components. A promising public health strategy would be to address the identified constellation of social adversity as a determinant of sickness of thoughts through a preventive approach [50]. For example, research in urban Uganda found a community mobilization program effective in primary and secondary prevention of intimate partner violence [51]. A gender-informed psycho-educational intervention for both mothers and fathers focused on the spousal relationship and parenting in Australian primary care was found to have preventive benefits for perinatal mental health [52]. An important direction for future implementation science would be to assess whether socio-culturally adapted prevention interventions with demonstrated effectiveness in other settings [9, 53] can be successfully delivered in low-resource post-conflict contexts [17].

Conclusion

In conclusion, our qualitative study identified sickness of thoughts, epilepsy, and malaria to be the highest prioritized maternal mental health concerns in a post-conflict eastern Ugandan setting. Sickness of thoughts was perceived to result from a combination of social adversity including intimate partner violence, unsupportive spouses, alcohol misuse, poverty, and physical illnesses. In addition to integrating feasible and effective treatment strategies into existing maternal and child health care, a fruitful direction for mental health interventions concerns preventive interventions that address the social determinants of sickness of thoughts. Malaria and epilepsy deserve further study as syncretic idioms that incorporate both biomedical and cultural concepts of distress.

Additional files

Additional file 1: Key Informant Interviews. Primary Health Care Workers (HC-III).

Additional file 2: Group Interviews. Community Health Workers and Primary Health Care Workers.

Additional file 3: Semi-structured Interviews.

Additional file 4: Key Informant Interviews. Service Providers.

Additional file 5: Key Informant Interviews. Traditional and Religious Healers.

Additional file 6: Key Informant Interviews. Perinatal Women.

Additional file 7: Key Informant Interviews. Mental Health Specialists.

Additional file 8: CODEBOOK (Combined from Uganda and US-based teams).

Abbreviations

DSM-IV: Diagnostic and Statistical Manual of Mental Disorders - fourth version; HC: Health Center; JHBSPH: Johns Hopkins Bloomberg School of Public Health; LMIC: Low- and Middle- Income Countries; NICE: UK National Institute for Health and Clinical Excellence; S: Smith's Salience Index

Acknowledgements

We would like to thank Patricia Achan, Albert Erongu, and Joel Omoding for their assistance in data collection. We are grateful to the participants for taking part in the study.

Funding

This study was funded through a Faculty Innovation Fund award (WT) Johns Hopkins Bloomberg School of Public Health.

Authors' contributions

WT designed the study with inputs from BK, SN, SA, SM2, and JN. BE and RA supervised data collection. BE, RA, SM1, and AN conducted the qualitative data analysis. BE and WT wrote a first draft of the manuscript. RA, SM2, AN, BK, SN, SA, SM1, JN contributed substantially to manuscript drafting and revision. All authors read and approved the final manuscript.

Consent for publication

Not applicable

Competing interests

The authors declare that they have no competing interests

Author details

[1]Peter C. Alderman Foundation, plot 855, Mawanda Road, PO Box 20129, Nakawa, Kampala, Uganda. [2]Department of Mental Health, Johns Hopkins Bloomberg School of Public Health, 624 N Broadway, Baltimore, MD 21205, USA. [3]University of Virginia Curry School of Education, 405 Emmet St S, Charlottesville, VA 22904, USA. [4]Department of Psychiatry and Behavioral Sciences, George Washington University, 2120 L St NW Suite 600, Washington, DC 20037, USA. [5]Ministry of Health, Republic of Uganda, Plot 6, Lourdel Road, Nakasero, Kampala, Uganda. [6]Peter C. Alderman Foundation, New York, NY, USA. [7]Department of Psychiatry, Makerere University College of Health Sciences, P.O. Box 7072, Kampala, Uganda. [8]Butabika National Psychiatric Referral Hospital, Butabika Rd, PO Box 7017, Kampala, Uganda.

References

1. Whiteford HA, Degenhardt L, Rehm J, Baxter AJ, Ferrari AJ, Erskine HE, Charlson FJ, Norman RE, Flaxman AD, Johns N, et al. Global burden of disease attributable to mental and substance use disorders: findings from the global burden of disease study 2010. Lancet. 2013;382(9904):1575–86.
2. Gelaye B, Rondon MB, Araya R, Williams MA. Epidemiology of maternal depression, risk factors, and child outcomes in low-income and middle-income countries. Lancet Psychiatry. 2016;3(10):973–82.

3. Roberts B, Browne J. A systematic review of factors influencing the psychological health of conflict-affected populations in low- and middle-income countries. Glob Public Health. 2011;6(8):814–29.
4. Tol WA, Barbui C, Galappatti A, Silove D, Betancourt TS, Souza R, Golaz A, van Ommeren M. Mental health and psychosocial support in humanitarian settings: linking practice and research. Lancet. 2011;378(9802):1581–91.
5. Grote NK, Bridge JA, Gavin AR, Melville JL, Iyengar S, Katon WJ. A meta-analysis of depression during pregnancy and the risk of preterm birth, low birth weight, and intrauterine growth restriction. Arch Gen Psychiatry. 2010; 67(10):1012–24.
6. Parsons CE, Young KS, Rochat TJ, Kringelbach ML, Stein A. Postnatal depression and its effects on child development: a review of evidence from low- and middle-income countries. Br Med Bull. 2012;101:57–79.
7. Surkan PJ, Kennedy CE, Hurley KM, Black MM. Maternal depression and early childhood growth in developing countries: systematic review and meta-analysis. Bull World Health Organ. 2011;89(8):608–15.
8. Guo N, Bindt C, Te Bonle M, Appiah-Poku J, Hinz R, Barthel D, Koffi M, Posdzich S, Deymann S, Barkmann C, et al. Association of antepartum and postpartum depression in Ghanaian and Ivorian women with febrile illness in their offspring: a prospective birth cohort study. Am J Epidemiol. 2013; 178(9):1394–402.
9. Sockol LE. A systematic review of the efficacy of cognitive behavioral therapy for treating and preventing perinatal depression. J Affect Disord. 2015;177:7–21.
10. Barlow J, Smailagic N, Huband N, Roloff V, Bennett C. Group-based parent training programmes for improving parental psychosocial health. Cochrane Database Syst Rev. 2014;5:CD002020.
11. Rahman A, Surkan PJ, Cayetano CE, Rwagatare P, Dickson KE. Grand challenges: integrating maternal mental health into maternal and child health programmes. PLoS Med. 2013;10(5):e1001442.
12. Collins PY, Patel V, Joestl SS, March D, Insel TR, Daar AS, Anderson W, Dhansay MA, Phillips A, Shurin S, et al. Grand challenges in global mental health. Nature. 2011;475(7354):27–30.
13. Rahman A, Fisher J, Bower P, Luchters S, Tran T, Yasamy MT, Saxena S, Waheed W. Interventions for common perinatal mental disorders in women in low- and middle-income countries: a systematic review and meta-analysis. Bull World Health Organ. 2013;91(8):593–601I.
14. Clarke K, King M, Prost A. Psychosocial interventions for perinatal common mental disorders delivered by providers who are not mental health specialists in low- and middle-income countries: a systematic review and meta-analysis. PLoS Med. 2013;10(10):e1001541.
15. van Ginneken N, Tharyan P, Lewin S, Rao GN, Meera SM, Pian J, Chandashekar S, Patel V. Non-specialist health worker interventions for the care of mental, neurological and substance-abuse disorders in low and middle-income countries. Cochrane Database Syst Rev. 2013;11:CD009149.
16. Kane JC, Adaku A, Nakku J, Odokonyero R, Okello J, Musisi S, Augustinavicius J, Greene MC, Alderman S, Tol WA. Challenges for the implementation of World Health Organization guidelines for acute stress, PTSD, and bereavement: a qualitative study in Uganda. Implement Sci. 2016;11:36.
17. Murray LK, Tol WA, Jordans MJD, Sabir G, Amin AM, Bolton P, Bass JK, Bonilla-Escobar FJ, Thornicroft G. Dissemination and implementation of evidence based, mental health interventions in post conflict, low resource settings. Intervention: Journal of Mental Health and Psychosocial Support in Conflict Affected Areas. 2014;12(S1):94–112.
18. Kirmayer LJ, Pedersen D. Toward a new architecture for global mental health. Transcult Psychiatry. 2014;51(6):759–76.
19. Human Rights Watch. Uprooted and Forgotten: Impunity and Human Rights Abuses in Northern Uganda. New York: Human Rights Watch; 2005.
20. Mugisha J, Muyinda H, Malamba S, Kinyanda E. Major depressive disorder seven years after the conflict in northern Uganda: burden, risk factors and impact on outcomes (the Wayo-Nero study). BMC Psychiatry. 2015;15:48.
21. Mugisha J, Muyinda H, Wandiembe P, Kinyanda E. Prevalence and factors associated with posttraumatic stress disorder seven years after the conflict in three districts in northern Uganda (the Wayo-Nero study). BMC Psychiatry. 2015;15:170.
22. Murphy S, Elklit A, Dokkedahl S, Shevlin M. Testing the validity of the proposed ICD-11 PTSD and complex PTSD criteria using a sample from northern Uganda. Eur J Psychotraumatol. 2016;7:32678.
23. Nakku JE, Okello ES, Kizza D, Honikman S, Ssebunnya J, Ndyanabangi S, Hanlon C, Kigozi F. Perinatal mental health care in a rural African district, Uganda: a qualitative study of barriers, facilitators and needs. BMC Health Serv Res. 2016;16:295.
24. Uganda Bureau of Statistics, ICF International Inc. Uganda Demographic and Health Survey 2011. Kampala, Uganda/ Calverton. Maryland: UNBOS and ICF International Inc.; 2012.
25. Republic of Uganda: Second National Development Plan (NDPII). Kampala, Uganda: Republic of Uganda; 2015.
26. Mwakikagile G. Ethnicity and National Identity in Uganda: the land and its people. Dar Es Salaam, Tanzania: new Africa press; 2009.
27. WHO, UNHCR. Assessing mental health and psychosocial needs and resources: toolkit for humanitarian settings Geneva. Switzerland: WHO; 2012.
28. Adaku A, Okello J, Lowry B, Kane JC, Alderman S, Musisi S, Tol WA. Mental health and psychosocial support for south Sudanese refugees in northern Uganda: a needs and resource assessment. Confl Health. 2016;10(1):18.
29. Smith JJ. Using ANTHROPAC 3.5 and a spreadsheet to compute a free list salience index. Cultural Anthropology Methods. 1993;5(3):1–3.
30. Charmaz K. Constructing grounded theory. London, thousand oaks: New Delhi: Sage Publications; 2014.
31. Saldana J. The coding manual for qualitative researchers. Phoenix, AZ: Sage Pulbications Ltd.; 2013.
32. Dedoose Version 6.1.18, web application for managing, analyzing and presenting qualitative and mixed method research data. In. Los Angeles, CA: SocioCultural Research Consultants, LLC; 2015.
33. RQDA: R-based Qualitative DAta Analysis. R package version 0.2–7 [http://rqda.r-forge.r-project.org/]. Accessed 2 Feb 2018.
34. Kaiser BN, Haroz EE, Kohrt BA, Bolton PA, Bass JK, Hinton DE. "Thinking too much": a systematic review of a common idiom of distress. Soc Sci Med. 2015;147:170–83.
35. American Psychiatric Association. Diagnostic and Statistical Manual of Mental Disorders. 5th ed. Arlington, VA: American Psychiatric Publishing; 2013.
36. Kinyanda E, Weiss HA, Mungherera M, Onyango-Mangen P, Ngabirano E, Kajungu R, Kagugube J, Muhwezi W, Muron J, Patel V. Intimate partner violence as seen in post-conflict eastern Uganda: prevalence, risk factors and mental health consequences. BMC Int Health Hum Rights. 2016;16:5.
37. Silove DM, Rees SJ, Tam N, Mohsin M, Tay AK, Tol WA. Prevalence and correlates of explosive anger among pregnant and post-partum women in post-conflict Timor-Leste. BJPsych Open. 2015;1:34–41.
38. Silove DM, Rees SJ, Tay K, da Costa ZM, Soares C, Tol WA. Pathways to perinatal depressive symptoms in the medium-term following conflict in Timor-Leste: the roles of conflict-related trauma, intimate partner violence, current adversity, and PTSD symptoms. Lancet Psychiatry. 2015;2(2):161–7.
39. Davies T, Schneider M, Nyatsanza M, Lund C. "The sun has set even though it is morning": experiences and explanations of perinatal depression in an urban township, cape town. Transcult Psychiatry. 2016;53(3):286–312.
40. Kakyo TA, Muliira JK, Mbalinda SN, Kizza IB, Muliira RS. Factors associated with depressive symptoms among postpartum mothers in a rural district in Uganda. Midwifery. 2012;28(3):374–9.
41. Ba-Diop A, Marin B, Druet-Cabanac M, Ngoungou EB, Newton CR, Preux PM. Epidemiology, causes, and treatment of epilepsy in sub-Saharan Africa. Lancet Neurol. 2014;13(10):1029–44.
42. Kane JC, Ventevogel P, Spiegel P, Bass JK, van Ommeren M, Tol WA. Mental, neurological, and substance use problems among refugees in primary health care: analysis of the health information system in 90 refugee camps. BMC Med. 2014;12:228.
43. van Duijl M, Nijenhuis E, Komproe IH, Gernaat HB, de Jong JT. Dissociative symptoms and reported trauma among patients with spirit possession and matched healthy controls in Uganda. Cult Med Psychiatry. 2010; 34(2):380–400.
44. van Duijl M, Kleijn W, de Jong J. Unravelling the spirits' message: a study of help-seeking steps and explanatory models among patients suffering from spirit possession in Uganda. Int J Ment Health Syst. 2014;8:24.
45. Jenkins R, Kiima D, Okonji M, Njenga F, Kingora J, Lock S. Integration of mental health into primary care and community health working in Kenya: context, rationale, coverage and sustainability. Ment Health Fam Med. 2010;7(1):37–47.

46. Ndetei DM, Othieno CJ, Mutiso V, Ongecha FA, Kokonya DA, Omar A, Gakinya B, Mwangi J. Psychometric properties of an African symptoms check list scale: the Ndetei-Othieno-Kathuku scale. East Afr Med J. 2006; 83(5):280–7.
47. Tesfaye M, Hanlon C, Tessema F, Prince M, Alem A. Common mental disorder symptoms among patients with malaria attending primary care in Ethiopia: a cross-sectional survey. PLoS One. 2014;9(9):e108923.
48. NICE. Antenatal and postnatal mental health: clinical management and service guidance, vol. Last modified June 2015. National Institute for Health and Care Excellence; 2015. guidance.nice.org.uk/cg192. Accessed 2 Feb 2018.
49. Kohrt BA, Luitel NP, Acharya P, Jordans MJ. Detection of depression in low resource settings: validation of the patient health questionnaire (PHQ-9) and cultural concepts of distress in Nepal. BMC Psychiatry. 2016;16:58.
50. Tol WA. Stemming the tide: promoting mental health and preventing mental disorders in low- and middle-income countries. Global Mental Health. 2015;2:e11.
51. Abramsky T, Devries KM, Michau L, Nakuti J, Musuya T, Kyegombe N, Watts C. The impact of SASA!, a community mobilisation intervention, on women's experiences of intimate partner violence: secondary findings from a cluster randomised trial in Kampala, Uganda. J Epidemiol Community Health. 2016;70(8):818–25.
52. Fisher J, Rowe H, Wynter K, Tran T, Lorgelly P, Amir LH, Proimos J, Ranasinha S, Hiscock H, Bayer J, et al. Gender-informed, psychoeducational programme for couples to prevent postnatal common mental disorders among primiparous women: cluster randomised controlled trial. BMJ Open. 2016; 6(3):e009396.
53. Dennis CL, Dowswell T. Psychosocial and psychological interventions for preventing postpartum depression. Cochrane Database Syst Rev. 2013;2: CD001134.

12

Risk and protective factors associated with the mental health of young adults in Kabul, Afghanistan

Qais Alemi[1], Carl Stempel[2], Patrick Marius Koga[3*], Susanne Montgomery[1], Valerie Smith[4], Gagandeep Sandhu[1], Bianca Villegas[5] and Jessica Requejo[1]

Abstract

Background: We examined the mental health status and severity of psychological distress symptoms among young adults residing in Kabul, Afghanistan and determined how such outcomes might be influenced by an array of risk and protective factors.

Methods: A cross-sectional study design was adopted using convenience, snowball, and street-intercept recruitment techniques. Surveys were completed by 232 young adults between 18 and 35 years of age in September 2015. We used both etic (mental health component of the SF-8) and emic (Afghan Symptom Checklist) measures of mental health and psychological distress, respectively, and regressed these outcome measures against socio-demographic, physical health, and psychological variables (resilience, hope-optimism) using ordinary least squares (OLS) regression methods.

Results: We found that poor mental health is common in this sample, affecting 75% of participants; and, that distress symptoms (depressive, anxiety, and somatoform symptoms) occur often. Regression models were consistent in showing higher education as a risk-factor for both outcomes, whereas, age, ethnicity, and income significantly contributed only to the ASCL model as risk-factors. However, both outcomes were strongly influenced by protective factors such as good physical health status and higher perceived hope-optimism.

Conclusions: Our study provides further evidence of how current economic conditions in Kabul contribute to poor mental health and symptom severity, but also show how positive physical health and perceived hope-optimism can be protective. This study provides support for developing culturally-competent policies and interventions that build on protective factors.

Keywords: Afghanistan, Distress, Hope, Mental health, Resilience, Young adults

Background

War has a catastrophic effect on the health and well-being of nations by fragmenting communities and families, disrupting social and economic development, and by bringing long-term physical and psychological harm to children and adults [1]. This is epitomized in Afghanistan, a country ranking among the lowest (169 out of 188 countries) on the human development index [2] and where approximately 17% of the adult population suffers from mental health disorders [3].

Early household-based cross-sectional studies show that the prevalence of depression, anxiety, and post-traumatic stress disorder (PTSD) is high, with female gender and exposure to traumatic events being important risk-factors [4, 5]. More recent studies show that mental health problems for Afghans are not solely rooted in traumatic experiences. Rather, they are largely influenced by poor living conditions associated with a broken economy and poor governance [6]. Among their sample, Miller and Rasmussen [7] show that less than 15% of the variance in levels of PTSD symptoms are accounted for by war exposure, while

* Correspondence: pmkoga@ucdavis.edu
[3]Department of Public Health Sciences, UCD School of Medicine, University of California, One Shields Avenue, Med Sci 1-C, Davis, CA 95616, USA
Full list of author information is available at the end of the article

a significantly larger proportion is accounted for by ongoing daily stressors associated with unmet basic needs. Similar trends are observed among representative samples of children across various municipalities in Afghanistan, where a major risk-factor identified was residence in Kabul, described by the study's authors as a volatile setting where overcrowding, high living costs, and widening inequalities exacerbate war-related adversities [8].

Due to these conditions, many young people view Afghanistan's social atmosphere profoundly dispiriting and have become deeply cynical as a result [9], which explains the unprecedented exodus of young people seeking asylum in European nations [10]. Panter-Brick et al.'s [11] survey of young educated adults in Kabul shows that they are not only distressed, but disillusioned by conditions that prevent their social advancement. Surprisingly, however, Panter-Brick and colleagues find that the vast majority of young adults in their sample demonstrate a high degree of hope and fortitude about the future by endorsing the optimistic beliefs that socio-political conditions would improve (74.8%) and that they can be resilient (81.9%), despite adversity. The authors go on to describe young adults in Afghanistan as significant agents of change and economic power for the future of their country.

While these studies are informative, there is a paucity of research on the mental health of young adults in conflict-affected countries like Afghanistan. Patel et al. [12] indicate that a high global burden of mental health in young people is influenced by risk and protective factors within biological, psychological and social domains. The important public health implication of this, according to Patel et al. is that early interventions could reduce symptom severity and prevent comorbidity.

To this end, the present study examines the mental health of young adults between 18 and 35 years of age residing in Kabul, a setting that typifies Galea et al.'s [13] characterization of adverse urban environments known for concentrated disadvantage, crime, and a myriad of other factors that perpetuate chronic psychological and physiological stress. The aim of our work was to further current knowledge of the risk and protective factors affecting the mental health of young adults by exploring two distinct mental health outcome variables. The first is the mental health subscale from the *Short-Form/SF-8* [14], an etic scale which provides an overall assessment of mental health status; and, the other an emic scale of culturally-salient idioms and indicators of distress symptoms developed in Afghanistan, the *Afghan Symptom Checklist (ASCL)* [15]. Rasmussen et al. [16] recently examined the value of using this locally-developed emic measure versus an internationally-developed etic measure, the Self-Reporting Questionnaire-20 and found that the ASCL was a better measure of distress symptoms for women (given the ASCL's ability to tap into local conceptions of distress) while the two measures were similar for men. Here we intend to use etic and emic measures for providing a comprehensive account of mental health, which is conceptually in line with Kabul-based studies by Miller et al. [6] and Panter-Brick et al. [11].

Though compared to Panter-Brick et al.'s study, which focused solely on college educated young adults, our study sample varies by education, allowing us to test previous findings about educated young Afghans by comparing them to less educated Afghans. Our study also advances knowledge of protective factors for mental health, for example, how one's physical health, never-before-tested measures of individual resilience, as well as culturally-salient coping strategies such as hope and optimism operate in terms of mitigating mental health problems. As informed by previous studies conducted in Afghanistan, we theorize that poor outcomes on both measures will be determined by risk-factors such as female gender, not being married, higher education, unemployment, and unstable income; whereas, good physical health status, as well as psychological factors including measures of resilience and of hope and optimism will exert a protective effect on these outcomes. While these expected associations may be common in other regions, the significance of understanding them in this setting is highly pressing given that young adults are a burgeoning working-age population [17] who enter a job market that provides little hope for upward mobility amid a socio-political climate that does not ensure safety—consequently placing more and more people at risk of mental health problems. Young people are vital to Afghanistan's peace and prosperity, and unfortunately, current conditions are forcing many to seek asylum at unprecedented rates in western Europe [18], and among those who choose not to exit the country, growing numbers are joining the insurgency solely to earn an income, and engaging in other subversive behaviors such as drug trafficking [19]. Therefore, understanding mental health risk and protective factors in this setting is a starting point for mobilizing policy-makers and public health authorities alike to take action through promoting community-based programs that reduce symptoms, build on their resilience, and protective cultural assets.

Methods

Sample, setting, & procedures

In a cross-sectional design, participants were recruited in Kabul in September 2015 using a combination of convenience, snowball, and street-intercept techniques where two data collectors solicited participants with an information sheet providing details about the study, their rights, and the survey. Interestingly, an overwhelming number of individuals asked whether their participation would benefit them in any way with regard to their open immigration cases to the United States (U.S.), and in response we clearly explained that it would not. Upon gaining verbal consent, surveys were completed mainly through self-administration (wherever they were recruited, e.g. on the street, public venues, their places of employment), which took approximately 15 min for participants to complete, while some individuals with literacy challenges were interviewed, which usually lasted approximately 30 min. As a token of our appreciation for their time and in consideration of their real economic needs, participants were offered an equivalent of $10 for completing surveys.

Instrumentation

Dependent variables

Mental Health Status As mentioned, two distinct measures of mental health were used to test our hypotheses. One of these scales included the mental health component of the *SF-8* scale. This scale contains four items assessing: vitality (energy level), social functioning (ability to perform social activities with family or friends when facing physical health or emotional problems), role emotional (ability to perform work, school, or other daily activities when facing personal or emotional problems), and mental health (extent of emotional problems such as anxiety, depression, or irritability) [14]. Items are based on a four-week recall period asking participants to respond using a five or six-point ordinal set of response choices. A norm-based scoring procedure is used in order to generate Mental Component Summary (MCS) scores as indicated in the instrument's scoring guidelines [20]. Higher scores indicate better mental health status with a score of 50 representing the average of the general U.S. population. While U.S. normative scores provide a useful benchmark to compare our findings, Roberts et al.'s [21] study testing the psychometric properties of the SF-8 among northern Ugandans assists in contextualizing MCS scores with a conflict-affected population, which the authors report MCS scores (M = 39.27, SD = 12.83) to be much lower than the U.S. normative score of 50. The mental health subscale of the SF-8 demonstrated marginal scale reliability (*Cronbach's* α = 0.66) in our sample.

Psychological Distress Symptoms The second measure used was a culturally-grounded measure of mental health developed and validated in Afghanistan, the *Afghan Symptom Checklist* (ASCL) [15]. The ASCL's 23 items include local idioms of distress (e.g. *'jigar khun'*/sadness due to interpersonal loss, *'fishar bala'*/internal agitation) as well as symptoms known to western psychiatry relating to depression (e.g. sadness, appetite loss) and PTSD (e.g. nightmares). Items are based on a two-week recall period and are rated on an ordinal five-point scale of 1 ("never") to 5 ("every day") with scores ranging from 23 to 115 (higher scores indicative of higher distress). The ASCL demonstrated excellent reliability in this sample (Cronbach's α = .914).

Independent Variables

Socio-demographic Characteristics Surveys assessed a number of socio-demographic characteristics such as age, gender, marital status, and ethnicity. Socio-economic characteristics included education (highest level completed ranging from 'less than high school' to 'university degree'), employment status ('unemployed', 'employed'), stability in income ('yes-no' question asking participants whether they are comfortable in covering monthly household expenses with current income).

Physical Health Status We used the four items from the physical health component of the SF-8 [14] to assess physical health status. Items on the physical health component relate to physical functioning as related to performing usual physical activities (walking and climbing stairs), role limitations due to physical health problems, bodily pain, and perceived general health. Items are based on a four-week recall period with each item consisting of a five or six-point response choice. Similar to the MCS score described above, a norm based scoring procedure is used in order to generate a Physical Component Summary (PCS) score. Higher PCS scores indicate better physical health status. Among conflict-affected Ugandans [21], PCS scores were considerably lower (M = 42.21, SD = 11.93) than U.S. normative scores of 50. The PCS subscale demonstrated acceptable reliability in our sample (*Cronbach's* α = 0.70).

Resilience We measured resilience using the Connor-Davidson Resilience Scale (CD-RISC-25) [22]. The CD-RISC-25 includes items that reflect the ability to tolerate experiences such as change, personal problems, illness, painful feelings, etc. Items are based on a one-month recall period and are rated on a scale of 0 ("not true at all") to 4 ("true nearly all the time"). Scores are an equally weighted sum of 25 items that range from 0 to 100 with higher scores being indicative of higher resilience. The CD-RISC-25 demonstrated good reliability in this sample (Cronbach's α = .865).

Hope and optimism For brevity, we assessed *perceived hope* using a single-item measure asking participants whether they believed that they 'would have a better future in Afghanistan as compared to their parents' with a binary 'yes-no' response choice. Similarly, *perceived optimism* was measured using a single item measure asking participants if they were 'optimistic in terms of

Afghanistan's future,' also with binary 'yes-no' response choice. Given their high correlation ($r = 0.53$), we created an index of hope and optimism by summing responses to these questions, scores of which range from 0 to 2 with higher scores indicative of higher perceived 'hope-optimism'. With the exception of the ASCL, which was already available in the Dari language (provided courtesy of the scales developer—Dr. Ken Miller), all scales were translated from English to Dari using a rigorous translation-back-translation process with assistance from the Afghan refugee community in southern California.

Table 1 Socio-demographic Characteristics ($N = 232$)

Variables	n (%)
Age: $M = 23.36$, $SD = 4.64$	–
Gender	
Female	90 (43.2)
Male	117(56.8)
Ethnicity	
Pashtun	73 (36.8)
Tajik	77 (35.9)
Other[a]	59 (27.3)
Marital Status	
Married	80 (38.7)
Not Married[b]	123 (62.3)
Education	
College and beyond	87 (40.3)
HS Diploma and lower	122 (59.7)
Employment	
Employed	87 (42.3)
Unemployed	118 (57.7)
Income	
Comfortable	76 (36.4)
Not comfortable	129 (63.6)
Hope w/re to own future	
Hopeful	119 (57.5)
Not Hopeful	88 (42.5)
Optimism w/re to Afg.'s Future	
Optimistic	134 (65.0)
Not Optimistic	72 (35.0)
CD-RISC-25: Resilience: $M = 60.53$, $SD = 13.86$	–
PCS Score: Physical Health Status: $M = 45.59$, $SD = 7.77$	–

[a]includes Hazaras, Nuristanis, Uzbeks; [b]includes 'never married', and two participants widowed, and four participants divorced/separated

Data analysis

SPSS, version 24.0 [23] was used for all data analyses. We evaluated standard assumptions of parametric tests, which warranted no data transformations; and, handled missing data by imputing the mean score for scales with less than 10% missing items [24]. Statistical significance was considered at $p < .05$ (though we indicate relationships approaching significance: $p < .10$). We calculated means and standard deviations along with percentages for variables where appropriate. Bivariate tests (independent samples *t*-tests, Pearson's '*r*') were used to identify variables significantly associated with our dependent variables, mental health status (MCS scores) and psychological distress (ASCL scores). Variables significantly associated with MCS and ASCL scores at the bivariate level were entered in two separate ordinary least square (OLS) regression models, one for MCS, and another for ASCL. To examine the unique contribution of each type of variable, socio-demographic factors were entered in Step 1 of each model (mainly consisting of risk-factors), followed by protective factors in subsequent steps). Unstandardized and standardized betas along with $R^2_{adjusted}$ and ΔR^2 values are reported in Tables 3 and 4.

Results

Socio-demographic characteristics

Table 1 displays socio-demographic characteristics of our participants. Surveys were completed by 232 participants who were 23.4 ($SD = 4.6$) years of age. The majority were male (56.8%), unmarried (62.3%), of Pashtun ethnicity (36.8%), and unemployed (57.7%) with unstable incomes (63.6%). Unemployment rates observed here are considerably higher than general population rates of 46.2% reported in Kabul, whereas income instability rates mirror perceptions of worsening household financial conditions reported in 2016 [25]. Moreover, the majority indicated being both hopeful (57.7%) and optimistic (65%) about their own future in Afghanistan and their country's socio-political future, respectively. CD-RISC-25 scores ranged from 26 to 92 with an average score of 60.5±13.9, which is approximately 20 points lower than the average score observed in a normative sample in the U.S. [18]. Mean PCS scores were reported at 45.6 ($SD = 7.8$). Further descriptive item responses show 'role limitations due to physical health problems' being rated lowest (43.6±8.9), followed by physical functioning ($M = 44.1$, $SD = 8.3$), perceived general health ($M = 46.6$, $SD = 8.7$), and lastly bodily pain ($M = 50.3$, $SD = 9.2$).

The mean MCS score was 42.5 ($SD = 10.29$), suggesting that participants generally have poor mental health when compared to the U.S. normative score of 50. Only 25% of our sample scored 50 or higher on the MCS. Further descriptive item responses show role limitations owing to personal or emotional problems seemed to affect participants most ($M = 41.8$, $SD = 8.2$), which was closely followed by mental health/emotional problems such as anxiety, depression, or irritability ($M = 42.3$, $SD = 10.4$); social functioning ($M = 45.2$, $SD = 9.1$) was also problematic, while vitality ($M = 49.93$, $SD = 8.98$) was rated highest. ASCL scores ranged from 23 to 94 with a mean of 47.6 ($SD = 16.0$). Some of the most frequently reported symptoms occurring at least once a week included 'thinking too much' (76%), 'trouble concentrating' (72%), 'feeling sad' (72%), becoming 'jigar khun' (70%), and headaches (69%).

Bivariate analyses

Table 2 shows MCS and ASCL scores by our risk and protective factors. Poor mental health status and functional impairment (or lower MCS scores) is significantly associated with higher education, unemployment, and unstable income; whereas, higher physical health status, and being hopeful-optimistic are associated with higher MCS scores. The relationship between ethnicity and MCS scores was marginally significant with Tajiks reporting lower mental health status compared to Pashtuns and all other ethnicities.

However, when ethnicity was correlated with ASCL, we observed that Tajiks reported significantly higher psychological distress as compared to other ethnic groups. In addition, we observed that younger age and female gender were significantly associated with higher ASCL scores. Also, higher ASCL scores were associated with higher education, unemployment, unstable income; whereas lower were associated with good physical health and higher hope-optimism. Strikingly, our measure of resilience demonstrated a weak and non-significant relationship with both MCS and ASCL scores both in its full form and when the measure was divided according to the five constructs (personal competence, high standards, and tenacity; trust in one's instincts, tolerance of negative affect, and strengthening effects of stress; positive acceptance of chance and secure relationships; control; and, spiritual influences). Therefore, the CD-RISC-25 was not included in subsequent (multivariable) analyses.

Multivariable analyses

Factors associated with mental health status (MCS scores)

OLS regressions, shown in Table 3, indicate that demographic variables entered in Step 1 account for 11% of the variance in MCS scores with three variables significantly contributing to the model. Tajik ethnicity and the

Table 2 Bivariate Analyses

Variables	MCS Score *M* (SD)	Statistic and *P*-value	ASCL Score *M* (SD)	Statistic and P-value
Age	–	$r = .070$, $p = .294$	–	$r = -.164$, $\mathbf{p < .05}$
Gender				
Female	42.32 (10.14)	$t(223) = -1.51$, $p = .133$	50.64 (14.96)	$t(205) = 2.40$, $\mathbf{p < .05}$
Male	44.29 (9.36)		45.34 (16.31)	
Ethnicity				
Pashtun	44.06 (8.64)	$F(2,224) = 2.92$, $p = .056$	46.23 (15.01)	$F(2,206) = 5.11$, $\mathbf{p < .01}$
Tajik	41.44 (10.98)		52.01 (16.75)	
Other[a]	45.19 (8.64)		43.75 (15.04)	
Marital Status				
Married	43.56 (9.41)	$t(216) = -.21$, $p = .831$	45.25 (14.04)	$t(201) = 1.96$, $p = .05$
Not Married[b]	43.27 (10.11)		49.56 (17.03)	
Education				
College and beyond	41.21 (10.24)	$t(225) = 2.90$, $\mathbf{p = .004}$	50.93 (17.28)	$t(207) = -2.53$, $\mathbf{p < .05}$
HS Diploma and lower	44.96 (9.11)		45.33 (14.63)	
Employment				
Employed	45.28 (8.64)	$t(221) = -2.61$, $\mathbf{p = .010}$	45.01 (11.90)	$t(203) = 2.44$, $\mathbf{p < .05}$
Unemployed	41.96 (10.33)		50.15 (18.17)	
Income				
Stable	45.99 (9.29)	$t(219) = 3.03$, $\mathbf{p = .003}$	43.71 (13.21)	$t(203) = 3.03$, $\mathbf{p < .01}$
Unstable	41.91 (9.85)		50.18 (17.09)	
Hope-Optimism	–	$r = .319$, $\mathbf{p = .000}$	–	$r = -.279$, $\mathbf{p < .000}$
CD-RISC-25: Resilience	–	$r = -.025$, $p = .732$	–	$r = -.040$, $p = .594$
PCS Score: Physical Health Status	–	$r = .376$, $\mathbf{p = .000}$	–	$r = -.421$, $\mathbf{p < .000}$

[a]includes Hazaras, Nuristanis, and Uzbeks; [b]includes 'never married', and two participants widowed, and four participants divorced/separated

possession of a university degree are associated with poorer mental health status whereas stability in income is significantly associated with better mental health status. Only the significant effect of education remains in Step 2 after adding the physical health status variable to the model, which explains an additional 10% ($\Delta R^2 = .101$, $p < .001$) of the variance in MCS scores. There was a significant positive relationship between physical health status and MCS scores suggesting that higher physical health status is associated with higher mental health status. Interestingly, the beta for physical health demonstrates the strongest effect ($\beta = 0.33$, $p < .001$) on MCS scores and remains this way even after entering hope-optimism in Step 3. Though the hope-optimism variable adds significant variance to the model ($\Delta R^2 = 0.05$, $p < .001$ for a total of 27% of the variance explained) and shows that higher hope-optimism is associated with higher mental health status ($\beta = 0.24$, $p < .001$).

Factors associated with psychological distress symptoms (ASCL scores)

Table 4 shows the regression model for ASCL scores. Here, demographic variables in Step 1 account for approximately 17% of the variance in ASCL scores and parallel the MCS model, such that Tajiks, university graduates, and those reporting unstable incomes report significantly higher distress. In contrast to the MCS model, younger age and female gender approach significance with ASCL ($p < .10$). However, in Step 2 (younger) age emerges as significant, while no significant correlation was detected between gender and ASCL scores after entering the physical health status variable. Physical health status is inversely associated with psychological distress, and similar to the MCS model, possesses the highest beta ($\beta = -0.38$, $p < .001$). In Step 3, hope-optimism adds significant variance to the overall model ($\Delta R^2 = 0.04$, $p < .01$) indicating that higher hope-optimism is associated with lower distress. In addition to hope-optimism, this full model shows that age, ethnicity, education, income, and physical health status contribute significantly to explaining ASCL scores (for a final 34% of variance explained).

Discussion

We conducted a community-based cross-sectional study examining mental health and psychological distress symptoms among young adults residing in Kabul in terms of poor social conditions, rather than primarily war-trauma induced distress in keeping with the findings of Miller and Rasmussen's [7] work. In using two distinct scales, our work shows that the mental health status of young adults is poor when compared to U.S. normative scores, but comparable to other conflict-affected groups such as northern Ugandans [21]. And based on the ASCL, we also found that many endure a number of depressive, anxiety-like, and somatoform symptoms. It is noteworthy that both multivariate models were able to explain high degree of variance with the variables we selected. Our first hypothesis related to demographic variables is partially supported. As expected, we observed that both MCS and ASCL scores were influenced by an array of social factors, namely– ethnicity, unstable income and higher education, the latter consistently maintaining a significant relationship with poorer outcomes in each multivariate model. This relationship reflects the pervasive disillusionment that a broken economy has given rise to, one which does not provide jobs for the surplus of university graduates. This aligns with Panter-

Table 3 OLS Regression Analysis of Factors Associated with Mental Health Status (MCS scores)

	Step 1***		Step 2***		Step 3***	
Variables	B (*SE*)	β	B (*SE*)	β	B (*SE*)	β
Age	.076 (.159)	.034	.068 (.150)	.031	.063 (.145)	.029
Gender: *female*ᵃ	−.908 (1.398)	−.046	−.417 (1.323)	−.021	−.430 (1.280)	−.022
Ethnicity: *Tajik*ᵇ	−3.06 (1.377)	−.149*	− 2.579 (1.303)	−.126†	− 2.353 (1.262)	−.115†
Education: *university degree*ᶜ	−2.96 (1.364)	−.147*	− 2.975 (1.287)	−.147*	−2.594 (1.249)	−.128*
Employment: *employed*ᵈ	2.312 (1.472)	.116	2.365 (1.389)	.118†	2.235 (1.344)	.112†
Income: *stable*ᵉ	3.985 (1.379)	.194**	2.132 (1.351)	.104	1.795 (1.310)	.087
Physical Health Status			.415 (.081)	.331***	.379 (.079)	.302***
Hope-Optimism					2.715 (.703)	.236***
R^2	.116		.216		.270	
Adjusted R^2	.090		.189		.241	
ΔR^2			.101***		.054***	
F statistic for change in R^2			26.053		14.916	

N = 211 as 21 cases omitted by *listwise* deletion; Reference groups: [a]males, [b]Pashtuns and other ethnicities; [c]HS Diploma, [d]Unemployed, [e]Unstable income; †$p < .10$; *$p < .05$; **$p < .01$; ***$p < .001$

Table 4 OLS Regression Analysis of Factors Associated with Psychological Distress Symptoms (ASCL scores)

	Step 1***		Step 2***		Step 3***	
Variables	B (*SE*)	*β*	B (*SE*)	*β*	B (*SE*)	*β*
Age	−.522 (.265)	−.139†	−.550 (.244)	−.156*	−.537 (.237)	−.152*
Gender: *female*[a]	−2.857 (2.34)	.138†	−1.498 (2.17)	−.046	−1.586 (2.11)	−.049
Ethnicity: *Tajik*[b]	6.507 (2.27)	.196**	5.008 (2.11)	.150*	4.835 (2.05)	.145*
Education: *university degree*[c]	5.199 (2.27)	.147*	6.140 (2.10)	.186**	5.616 (2.05)	.170**
Employment: *employed*[d]	−.911 (2.46)	.024	−.649 (2.27)	−.020	−.585 (2.21)	−.018
Income: *stable*[e]	−7.872 (2.28)	−.236**	−4.805 (2.17)	−.143*	−4.292 (2.12)	−.128*
Physical Health Status			−.785 (.135)	−.375***	−.723 (.133)	−.346***
Hope-Optimism					−3.910 (1.15)	−.208**
R^2	.167		.295		.337	
Adjusted R^2	.140		.268		.308	
ΔR^2			.128***		.042**	
F statistic for change in R^2			33.765		11.665	

N = 197 as 35 cases omitted by *listwise* deletion; Reference groups: [a]males, [b]Pashtuns and other ethnicities; [c]HS Diploma, [d]Unemployed, [e]Unstable income; †$p < .10$; *$p < .05$; **$p < .01$; ***$p < .001$

Brick et al.'s [11] observations of educated, young adults in Kabul.

The hypothesis related to demographic variables was shown more strongly in the ASCL scale than the MCS scale. Younger age only contributed to the ASCL model (potentially highlighting a stage of life uncertainty and lack of opportunity). Importantly, women, while shown to be more distressed in bivariate analyses, were no more likely than men to report poorer outcomes in multivariate analyses, which does not support our hypothesis and contrasts with prior research in Afghanistan [6, 11]. Men and women inhabit unique social and emotional spaces in Afghanistan, according to Rasmussen et al. [16], and likely perceive and experience stress differently partly due to men's higher levels of social interaction in the public sphere. Therefore, observing this non-significant relationship was surprising, especially in light of using the ASCL, a culturally-salient scale able to tap into locally-relevant dimensions of mental health that may be more salient for women (e.g. maintaining harmonious family relationships) [15], which we would have expected to more likely be able to identify distress, if it was indeed different from patterns seen in men. Nevertheless, these results extend our knowledge of the impact that daily stressors have on mental health, as originally hypothesized by Miller et al. [6], and to some degree coincides with mental health risk-factors reported in a systematic review of conflict-affected populations in low- and middle-income countries [26].

The correlation between Tajik ethnicity and poor outcomes is noteworthy, particularly in the ASCL model. Similarly, in their household survey, Scholte et al. [5] found that PTSD symptomatology was higher among Tajiks as compared to other ethnicities, but provide no further insight as to why. We speculate that their perceived stress may be a result of feeling disadvantaged or marginalized in a Pashtun-dominated society, or perhaps that Pashtuns may be more guarded and less expressive of their disclosure of symptoms, though further research is needed to replicate and better understand this pattern.

Moreover, the physical health status of our participants was poor when compared to U.S. normative scores while being comparable to PCS scores observed among conflict-affected Ugandans [21]. PCS scores were significantly associated with both the MCS and ASCL models, having a protective effect on mental health and distress symptoms. This result is reasonable given that physical health is widely understood to be significantly related to mental health. Strikingly, our hope-optimism variable emerged as an important coping mechanism in this context, so much so that it added substantial explained variance when added last to both MCS (5.4%) and ASCL (4.2%) models. The concept of hope, according to Eggerman and Panter-Brick's [27] qualitative study is a critical component of resilience in Afghanistan, which is rooted in moral and social order embodied through the expression of Afghan cultural values that include their (Islamic) faith, family unity, service to society, effort, moral behavior, and upholding family honor. In considering this, we assert that our measure of hope-optimism likely provides an indication of "collective" resilience, which explains why higher hope-optimism here is associated with improved mental health status and lower distress symptoms.

This also explains why scales assessing "individual resilience" such as the CD-RISC-25, used here, may lack content validity in a collectivistic society, in which individuals possess a communal sense of self and view themselves inseparable from the social context [28]. The lack of correlation between our hope-optimism variable and our measure of resilience further validates our position. We noticed that our CD-RISC-25 scores ranged from 26 to 92 with an average score of 60.53 (*SD* = 13.86). This is approximately 20 points lower than the average score observed in normative U.S. samples [22, 29]. Our findings on CD-RISC are congruent with studies of other non-Western, collectivistic cultures: 66.8 mean score in Korea [30], 65.4 in China [31], and 60.0 in Hong Kong [32]. Interestingly, a CD-RISC-25 survey [33] of resilience in refugees from Africa (mean 60), Middle East (mean 67), and former Yugoslavia (mean 69) suggests a linear distribution of the resilience scores along a cultural spectrum between individualistic cultures at one end, and collectivistic cultures, at the other, as hypothesized in a 2011 Kyrgyz study [34]. Importantly, this Kyrgyz study found that the correlation between measures of PTSD and an abridged version of the CD-RISC were poor. The authors infer that one reason for the associations between CD-RISC and distress could be a cultural difference in item interpretation and test settings [35]. This coincides with Suarez' [36] results using this measure of resilience alongside cultural idioms of distress in a sample of conflict-affected Peruvian girls, where resilience was found to be more deeply rooted in community and cultural realms and CD-RISC scores were not associated with lower levels of distress.

This suggests that risk and individual resiliency cannot be understood apart from context; self-conceptualizing in relationship to traumatic experiences varies widely across cultures constructing resilience as a cultural phenomenon [37]. Indeed, communities are vital sources of resilience by making needed resources available for individuals with much needed material, emotional, and cognitive reframing support. However, when traumatic events disrupt these vital support networks at most critical times, communities can actually add more turmoil and distress [38]. Therefore, future Kyrgyz, or in our case, Afghan studies, should investigate more closely the relationship between community and individual resilience, and develop community resilience instruments that are culturally-grounded using inductive techniques. This could have important clinical applications in community psychiatry interventions to shift the current traditionally targets of cognitive-behavior, and cognitive-processing therapies for disorders such as PTSD, from "I" and "self-image", to "Us". Such instruments could then be applied to evaluations of interventions that consider an array of psychosocial factors, especially building one's capacity to access resources needed to create social and economic opportunities for one's family [39].

Moreover, public health professionals and policy makers alike should consider how such interventions ought to be delivered. Patel et al. [12] suggests that interventions (reducing risk-factors and strengthening protective factors) could be disseminated through community-based channels, educational settings such as colleges, the internet, and through trained primary care practitioners – the latter being a viable approach given that public mental health services have been formally integrated into the primary care sector in Afghanistan [40]. Additionally, given the highly somatic nature of distress in our sample, the primary care sector provides a realistic avenue for help seeking in a society where mental health problems are highly stigmatized. In addition to formal health services, interventions could be delivered through the informal care sector, perhaps through clergy and herbalists, both of which young people may be inclined to seek help from, which is an area that our future work will concentrate on.

Our work clearly has some limitations. The cross-sectional design does not allow for causal inferences, and there may have been a potential for selection bias due to the convenience sampling technique used. Also, the present study does not adjust for exposure to traumatic experiences, which may have influenced our findings. Another important factor not adjusted for here is one's engagement in civic life or political activity, which has been shown to be both protective and promotive in several studies of conflict-affected children in low- and middle-income countries [41]. Nevertheless, the strength of this contribution lies in the use of etic and emic scales for mental health and psychological distress, respectively, and the fact that our sample represents wide variation across a number of socio- demographic and -economic characteristics, lending credence to the generalizability of our findings within urban Kabul and perhaps other urban regions of Afghanistan, but certainly not to other social and cultural groups outside the country.

Conclusions

In conclusion, our research shows that young adults in Kabul present with poor mental health status and distress symptoms as a result of a number of social factors rooted in the country's current conditions. The evidence from this study suggests that while mental health problems are widely present, possessing good physical health and hope-optimism serve as protective factors. This has important implications for tailoring context-specific policy and programmatic interventions for young adults. Interventions could, at least in part, focus on addressing the less stigmatizing issues young people may face related to physical health, while building up hope and optimism. To support the physical health of young people and their aspirations for realizing a better future, policy and structural changes such as improving access to employment are important to not only strengthen the economy and their living conditions, but to help them deal with their current distress and social functioning issues. Interventions aimed at improving hope and optimism could very well be community based and include aspects of Afghan cultural values related to strengthening family unity and faith, serving society, as well as maintaining moral behavior and upholding honor [27].

Abbreviations

ASCL: Afghan symptom checklist; CD-RISC-25: Connor-davidson resilience scale; MCS: Mental component summary; OLS: Ordinary least squares; PCS: Physical component summary; PTSD: Post-traumatic stress disorder; SF-8: Short-form; U.S.: United States

Acknowledgements

We thank our data collectors, Mr. Musa Gul Zadran and another individual, wishing to remain anonymous for their effort. The authors also wish to gratefully acknowledge the participants of this study.

Funding

Seed Grant from Behavioral Health Institute at Loma Linda University. The funder played no role in the design and conduct (i.e. data collection, analysis, interpretation) of this study.

Authors' contributions

QA conceived the study, managed and analyzed data, and wrote the initial draft of the paper; CS and PMK assisted with data interpretation and wrote parts of the literature review and discussion; SM, VS, and JR contributed to the literature review and discussion sections; GS and BV assisted with data analysis; all authors read and approved the final manuscript.

Consent for publication

Not applicable.

Competing interests

The authors declare that they have no competing interests.

Author details

[1]Department of Social Work & Social Ecology, School of Behavioral Health, Loma Linda University, 1898 Business Center Drive, San Bernardino, CA 92408, USA. [2]Department of Sociology and Social Services, California State University, East Bay, 25800 Carlos Bee Blvd, Hayward, CA 94542, USA. [3]Department of Public Health Sciences, UCD School of Medicine, University of California, One Shields Avenue, Med Sci 1-C, Davis, CA 95616, USA. [4]Department of Health Sciences, California State University, East Bay, 25800 Carlos Bee Blvd, Hayward, CA 94542, USA. [5]Department of Epidemiology, School of Public Health, Loma Linda University, 24951 North Circle Drive, Loma Linda, CA 92350, USA.

References

1. Murthy R, Lakshminarayana R. Mental health consequences of war: a brief review of research findings. World Psychiatry. 2006;5:25–30.
2. United Nations Development Program. (2016). Afghanistan. Human development report 2016. Retrieved from hdr.undp.org/sites/all/themes/hdr_theme/country-notes/AFG.pdf.
3. World Health Organization. (2017). Afghanistan. Mental Health. Retrieved from http://www.emro.who.int/afg/programmes/mental-health.html.
4. Cardozo BL, Bilukha OO, Crawford CAG, Shaikh I, Wolfe MI, Gerber ML, Anderson M. Mental health, social functioning, and disability in postwar Afghanistan. JAMA. 2004;292:575–84.
5. Scholte WF, Olff M, Ventevogel P, de Vries GJ, Jansveld E, Cardozo BL, Crawford CAG. Mental health symptoms following war and repression in eastern Afghanistan. JAMA. 2004;292:585–93.
6. Miller KE, Omidian P, Rasmussen A, Yaqubi A, Daudzai H. Daily stressors, war experiences, and mental health in Afghanistan. Transcult Psychiatry. 2008;45:611–38.
7. Miller KE, Rasmussen A. War exposure, daily stressors, and mental health in conflict and post-conflict settings: bridging the divide between trauma-focused and psychosocial frameworks. Soc Sci Med. 2010;70:7–16.
8. Panter-Brick C, Eggerman M, Gonzalez V, Safdar S. Violence, suffering, and mental health in Afghanistan: a school-based survey. Lancet. 2009;374:807–16.
9. Maley W. Challenges of political development in Afghanistan: mass, elite and institutional dimensions. Int Stud. 2011;48:21–41.
10. Petrillo ER. The securitization of the EU external borders and the rise of human smuggling along the eastern Mediterranean route. Migration in the Mediterranean: socio-economic perspectives. London: Routledge; 2016. p. 105.
11. Panter-Brick C, Eggerman M, Mojadidi A, McDade TW. Social stressors, mental health, and physiological stress in an urban elite of young afghans in Kabul. Am J Human Biol. 2008;20:627–41.
12. Patel V, Flisher AJ, Hetrick S, McGorry P. Mental health of young people: a global public health challenge. Lancet. 2007;369:1302–13.
13. Galea S, Uddin M, Koenen K. The urban environment and mental disorders: epigenetic links. Epigenetics. 2011;6:400–4.
14. Ware JE, Kosinski M, Dewey JE, Gandek B. How to score and interpret single-item health status measures: a manual for users of the SF-8 health survey. Lincoln, RI: QualityMetric Incorporated; 2001a. p. 5.
15. Miller KE, et al. The afghan symptom checklist: a culturally grounded approach to mental health assessment in a conflict zone. Am J Orthopsychiatry. 2006;76:423–33.
16. Rasmussen A, Ventevogel P, Sancilio A, Eggerman M, Panter-Brick C. Comparing the validity of the self reporting questionnaire and the afghan symptom checklist: dysphoria, aggression, and gender in transcultural assessment of mental health. BMC Psychiatry. 2014;14:206.
17. United Nations Fund for Population Activities. Young People. 2016. Retrieved from http://afghanistan.unfpa.org/topics/young-people-0 (Accessed 12 Jan 2017).
18. Petrillo ER. 6 the securitization of the EU external borders and the rise of human smuggling along the eastern Mediterranean route. Migration in the Mediterranean: Socio-economic Perspectives. 2016;105–25.
19. Lavender L. The youth bulge in Afghanistan: challenges and opportunities. Civil Military Fusion Centre. 2011. Retrieved from http://www.operationspaix.net/DATA/DOCUMENT/6394~v~The_Youth_Bulge_in_Afghanistan__Challenges_and_Opportunities.pdf. Accessed 12 Jan 2017.
20. Maruish ME, DeRosa MA. A guide to the integration of certified short form survey scoring and data quality evaluation capabilities. Lincoln, RI: Quality Metric Incorporated; 2009.
21. Roberts B, Browne J, Ocaka KF, Oyok T, Sondorp E. The reliability and validity of the SF-8 with a conflict-affected population in northern Uganda. Health Qual Life Outcomes. 2008;6(1):108.
22. Connor KM, Davidson JR. Development of a new resilience scale: the Connor-Davidson resilience scale (CD-RISC). Depress Anxiety. 2003;18:76–82.
23. IBM Corp IBM SPSS statistics for windows, version 24.0. Armonk: IBM Corp.
24. Cohen J, Cohen P, West SG, & Aiken LS. Applied multiple regression/correlation analysis for the behavioral sciences. Mahwah: Routledge; 2013.
25. The Asia Foundation. (2016). Afghanistan in 2016. A survey of the Afghan people Retrieved from http://asiafoundation.org/where-we-work/afghanistan/survey/
26. Roberts B, Browne J. A systematic review of factors influencing the psychological health of conflict-affected populations in low-and middle-income countries. Global Public Health. 2011;6:814–29.
27. Eggerman M, Panter-Brick C. Suffering, hope, and entrapment: resilience and cultural values in Afghanistan. Soc Sci Med. 2010;71:71–83.
28. Splevins K, Cohen K, Bowley J, Joseph S. Theories of posttraumatic growth: cross-cultural perspectives. J Loss Trauma. 2010;15:259–77.
29. Lamond AJ, et al. Measurement and predictors of resilience among community-dwelling older women. J Psychiatry Res. 2008;43:148–54.
30. Baek HS, Lee KU, Joo EJ, Lee MY, Choi KS. Reliability and validity of the Korean version of the Connor-Davidson resilience scale. Psychiatry Invest. 2010;7:109–15.
31. Yu XN, Lau JT, Mak WW, Zhang J, Lui WW. Factor structure and psychometric properties of the Connor-Davidson resilience scale among Chinese adolescents. Compr Psychiatry. 2011;52:218–24.
32. Ni MY, Li TK, Yu NX, Pang H, Chan BHY, Leung GM, Stewart SM. Normative data and psychometric properties of the Connor-Davidson resilience scale

and the abbreviated version (CD-RISC-2) among the general population in Hong Kong. Qual Life Res. 2015;25:111–6.
33. Ziaian T, de Anstiss H, Antoniou G, Baghurst P, Sawyer M. Resilience and its association with depression, emotional and behavioural problems, and mental health service utilisation among refugee adolescents living in South Australia. Int J Popul Res. 2012;
34. Molchanova ES, Panteleeva L, Nelubova TE, Polkov M, Koga PM. Epidemiological peculiarities of PTSD in Osh and Jalalabad, Kyrgyzstan, during the post conflict period October 2010-February 2011. Slavic Univ J Bishkek Kyrgyzstan. 2011;4:127–41.
35. Bezdjian S, Schneider KG, Burchett D, Baker MT, Garb HN. Resilience in the United States air Force: psychometric properties of the Connor-Davidson resilience scale (CD-RISC). J Psychol Assess. 2017;29:479–85.
36. Suarez EB. Two decades later: the resilience and post-traumatic responses of indigenous Quechua girls and adolescents in the aftermath of the Peruvian armed conflict. Child Abuse Negl. 2013;37:200–10.
37. Hobfoll S, Jackson A, Hobfoll I, Pierce C, Young S. The impact of b communal-mastery versus self-mastery on emotional outcomes during stressful conditions: a prospective study of native American women. Am J Community Psychol. 2002;30:853–71.
38. Harvey M. An ecological view of psychological trauma and trauma recovery. J Trauma Stress. 1996;9:3–23.
39. Ventevogel P, Jordans MJ, Eggerman M, van Mierlo B, Panter-Brick C. Child mental health, psychosocial well-being and resilience in Afghanistan: a review and future directions. In: Handbook of resilience in children of war. New York: Springer; 2013. p. 51–79.
40. Ventevogel P, Nassery R, Azimi S, Faiz H. Psychiatry in Afghanistan. Int Psych. 2006;3:36–8.
41. Tol WA, Song S, Jordans MJ. Annual research review: resilience and mental health in children and adolescents living in areas of armed conflict–a systematic review of findings in low-and middle-income countries. J Child Psychol Psychiatry. 2013;54:445–60.

13

An evaluation of functional mental capacity in forensic mental health practice: the Dundrum capacity ladders validation study

Gearoid Moynihan[1], Ken O'Reilly[1,2], Jane O'Connor[1] and Harry G. Kennedy[1,2*]

Abstract

Background: Because of the potential gravity of finding a person incompetent, assessment of mental capacity is challenging for clinicians. We aimed to test validity of a new structured professional judgement tool designed to assess functional mental capacity in three domains – finances, welfare and healthcare.

Methods: Fifty-five male forensic psychiatric patients with Schizophrenia were interviewed using the Dundrum Capacity Ladders – a new semi-structured interview, and scores were assigned on a stratified scoring system, measuring ability to understand, reason, appreciate the personal importance of the decision at hand and communicate a decision. Data were also gathered pertaining to level of therapeutic security at the time of interview, diagnosis, neurocognitive function and a validated measure of real world function.

Results: The results show that internal consistency and inter-rater reliability were high for all items. There were correlations between higher scores of functional mental capacity, neurocognitive function and measures of real world function in this population. Correlations were in the range 0.358 to 0.693, effect sizes that were moderate to high.

Conclusions: The DUNDRUM Capacity Ladders appear to be a valid measure of functional mental capacity in this population. Further prospective studies of functional mental capacity as a measure of recovery are now required.

Keywords: Schizophrenia, Mental illness, Functional capacity, Neurocognitive ability, Real world function

Background

Functional Mental Capacity refers to neurocognitive and legal constructs concerning an individual's ability to make and communicate decisions in an autonomous fashion. Its assessment has become increasingly important with the move away from paternalistic practises in healthcare provision towards an increased emphasis on an individual's own treatment decisions (Schneider, 1998) [1]. It should also be considered as part of the assessment of functional outcomes in treating mental illnesses such as schizophrenia (Kahn & Keefe 2013) [2].

The evolution of functional capacity

Functional Mental Capacity evolved first as a legal concept, arising from the interplay of expert evidence by clinicians and legal judgements and precedents, followed in some jurisdictions by legislation. The law identifies different competencies e.g. testamentary capacity, competency to marry, fitness to plead and stand trial. Decision-making capacity is but one element in the legal classification of competence. Decisional Capacity relates to a person's ability to perceive, retain and understand information pertaining to the choices at hand, and to use this information to reason about and appreciate the consequences of the choice they may make. Capacity relates to a decision about a person's capability to carry out a specific act or set of acts. Legal Competency relates to a decision made by a judge about whether a person, under the law, has or does not have the capability to carry out a specific act or set of acts. In this instance

* Correspondence: kennedh@tcd.ie
[1]National Forensic Mental Health Service, Central Mental Hospital, Dundrum, Dublin 14, Ireland
[2]Department of Psychiatry, Trinity College Dublin, Dublin 2, Ireland

the clinician will provide the court with information summarising the person's decision-making skills and offer an opinion on how these findings may affect the person's abilities in a specific area. The judge then uses this information, together with legal factors to arrive at a finding of competence or incompetence.

A review of case law literature by Grisso and Appelbaum (1998) [3] resulted in the so-called 'four abilities' model in the assessment of functional mental capacity, namely; the ability to understand the information pertinent to the decision at hand, in keeping with the relevant facts of the decision; the ability to reason with this relevant information so as to engage in a logical weighing and comparison of the positive and negative consequences; the ability to appreciate the significance of the information for one's own situation; and the ability to make and communicate a decision relating to the decision at hand.

Historically, legislative approaches to incapacitated persons were paternalistic. These approaches have been criticised as not being in keeping with the spirit of the Universal Declaration of Human Rights [4] and more explicitly in the United Nations' Convention on the Rights of Persons with Disabilities, Article 3 (a) [5] which states: "*The principles of the present Convention shall be: Respect for inherent dignity, individual autonomy including the freedom to make one's own choices, and independence of persons.*"

In most jurisdictions, modern legislation now includes specific statutory means of protecting the rights of people with mental disabilities, as seen in New Zealand, Ontario, Scotland and England and Wales. All assume presence of mental capacity unless established otherwise. However, all have slightly different definitions for the test of mental incapacity – some require the presence of mental disorder as a first step to define incapacity – as seen in Scottish law [6], and others view capacity under separable domains [7–9]. Newly published Irish legislation has also changed to a functional approach for capacity assessments [10]. In this article, we are primarily concerned with the clinical assessment of functional mental capacity. We regard this as a continuum from fully capable to seriously impaired, like any other neurocognitive mental ability or any physical ability. We are not primarily concerned with legal standards or thresholds for competence or incompetence.

Difficulties in assessment of functional mental capacity

The assessment of functional mental capacity is one of the most ethically complex tasks which clinicians are called upon to perform on a routine basis. In every case a patient's autonomy and right to self-determination must be weighed against a clinician's judgment that as a consequence of illness, mental disorder or intellectual disability, they may not be capable of acting in their own best interest. Clinicians have an ethical and legal responsibility to demonstrate how an illness, mental disorder or intellectual disability may compromise an individual's right to autonomy and self-determination when faced with a specific situation. However the reasons for doing this go beyond the assessment of legal competence. Clinicians must assess responses to treatment for many purposes. It is increasingly recognised that functional abilities are the most important outcomes of treatment for mental disorders such as schizophrenia [2], and functional outcomes are for practical purposes more important than symptomatic improvement. Neurocognitive abilities, social cognition and metacognition all play a part in influencing symptoms and functional outcomes (Fett et al. [11], Lam et al. [12], Gallagher & Varga [13], Lysaker et al. [14]). Indeed deficits in metacognition may be one of the distinguishing features between schizophrenia and other debilitating physical illnesses (Lysaker et al. [15]).

In practice the assessment of functional mental capacity can be complex and challenging. The complexity arises not only because of the balancing of responsibilities, but because functional mental capacity is inextricably linked with contextual and situational factors, and also because it is underpinned by a number of sequential cognitive process. In contrast to illnesses, mental disorders or intellectual disabilities, all of which may be static in nature, functional capacity is dynamic and refers to the extent to which patients can apply their abilities to a particular situation and context independently as well as when offered assistance. The cognitive processes which underpin functional capacity include comprehension, appreciation, reasoning, and judgment and difficulties may occur at any step of this process (Grisso and Appelbaum) [3].

The potential gravity of recommending that a court find a person incompetent – i.e. denying that person the right to an autonomous choice, means that assessments of functional mental capacity can be lengthy and onerous. In such an assessment, the clinician must take account of the patient's mental illness (or otherwise), cognitive function and social attitudes, as well as collateral information from a reliable informant where possible. Furthermore, the information shared by the clinician during the assessment of functional capacity should be such that it is easily understood by the person whose mental capacity is being assessed. This holds true even when the assessment is not for a medico-legal purpose.

Although psychological science has produced objective measures of cognitive capabilities, which can be usefully applied to capacity evaluations, it would be wrong to determine capacity solely on the basis of cognitive testing.

This is because cut-off scores for a particular individual faced with a particular competency question can never be determined in advance. Moreover, the results of cognitive assessments are proxies and thus one step removed from the ultimate issue of whether a patient can understand, reason, appreciate and make and communicate a decision based on the unique demands of a particular situation. All of these factors can be more holistically and directly assessed using clinical interviews with the patient and informants. However, in contrast to cognitive assessments which have established psychometric properties, the reliability and validity of unstructured clinical interviews is unknown and unmeasurable.

Research by Volicer and Ganzini [16] showed that psychiatrists, psychologists and geriatricians do not adhere to a uniform approach for the purpose of assessments of functional capacity. Their work supports the idea that physicians' competence assessments are often subjective and inconsistent (Marson, McInturff et al.) [17].

Case law [18, 19] internationally has increasingly placed emphasis on the patient's right to all material information pertaining to a particular proposed treatment, in order to make an informed decision. However, if a person is suffering from a psychotic illness, it is foreseeable that sharing too much information about treatment options may overburden the person's capacities to make an informed treatment decision, as demonstrated by Kennedy, Dornan et al. [20]. It follows that decision-making in other domains would be similarly affected. Furthermore, other illnesses such as dementia would have similar deleterious effects on decision-making ability.

There are a number of structured professional judgement tools which have been developed for assessment of functional mental capacity, the majority of which are based in Decision Theory [21]; that is identifying the values, uncertainties and other issues relevant in a given decision, its rationality, and the resultant optimal decision. Perhaps the best-known of these in a forensic arena are the MacArthur Competence Assessment Tools for Consent to Treatment [22] and Fitness to Plead [23]. In a psycho-geriatric setting, other tools have also been devised, e.g. The Hopkins Competence Assessment Tool [24]. Fazel, Hope and Jacoby [25] have also published a structured approach to the assessment of mental capacity to complete advance directives, emphasising a patient centred approach. A key feature of these assessment tools is that they provide clinicians with a structure for carrying out their own interviews thus improving transparency, reliability and objectivity. For example, in addition to using a validated functional capacity interview in a complementary and concurrent fashion, clinicians can use capacity instruments as a template to structure their own judgment by substituting the specific idiosyncratic question facing their patient into the structure of the instrument. Used in this manner a structured professional judgement approach to assessing functional mental capacity capacities could facilitate clinician's ability to communicate their opinions in legal settings and to reduce the potential for idiosyncratic differences between experts. More importantly, the assessment of functional mental capacity as a treatment outcome can become a reliable and valid measure. One recent study employed the MacArthur instruments as outcome measures in a controlled trial of cognitive remediation therapy for psychosis (Naughton et al. 2012) [26]. In addition to improved transparency of clinical decision-making, functional capacity instruments are useful to identify targets for treatment and to measure change. The extent to which functional mental capacities change over time is of great importance when considering the legal and human rights protections necessary for mentally incapacitated patients, including those detained and treated under mental health legislation.

Although functional capacity assessments are often specific to the decision in hand, in practice clinicians are most often required to make decisions regarding a patient's capacity to manage their finances, to consent to medical treatment and to make welfare decisions concerning living independently. Currently there is no single instrument to assist clinicians when assessing functional capacity in these three domains. No single instrument has a framework that is readily transferable to idiosyncratic situations. Because of the routine nature of these tasks a valid and reliable functional capacity assessment in these domains would be particularly useful to help clinicians structure their judgments.

In examining these tools, we noted the need for a different form of rating of functional mental capacity, in order to take account of its continuous rather than binary form.

Methods

Objectives

We aimed to establish validity for a structured professional judgement tool to assess functional mental capacity in three domains – finances, welfare and healthcare. In this paper we present results of inter-rater reliability, construct validity (in the form of internal consistency) and criterion validity as compared to neurocognitive function. We wanted to rate each of these using a common decision-making structure for understanding, reasoning, appreciation and decision-making. We wanted these to be structured in such a way that even the most severely ill could be rated and that ratings were on a continuous scale rather than a dichotomous one. We have also examined the relationships between this measure of functional mental capacity, real world function and neurocognitive function.

We hypothesised that patients currently cared for in more highly structured and supportive hospital environments of higher therapeutic security would score lower in terms of functional mental capacity than those who had progressed further along the therapeutic recovery pathway within the hospital. We also hypothesised that scores of functional mental capacity would correlate with scores of occupational, social and symptomatic function; and neurocognitive function.

Setting

The Central Mental Hospital provides high, medium and low therapeutic security and community follow-up mental health services for a population of 4.6 million [27]. At the time of the study there were eighty-two male inpatient beds at varying levels of therapeutic security, and sixteen patients under community supervision. Patients can be admitted to the hospital from prisons under the Criminal Law (Insanity) Act 2006 [28], if medically certified. They can also be admitted from the courts if found unfit to stand trial or not guilty by reason of insanity. Additionally, the service provides a tertiary referral and assessment service for local community mental health teams and admits patients under the civil Mental Health Act 2001 [29] on transfer from local psychiatric hospitals.

Male patients in the Central Mental Hospital are admitted to a high secure admission ward. From there they can move to a series of medium secure units and finally to low secure and pre-discharge units (Pillay et al. 2008) [30]. This is a patient-centred approach, as each service-user is placed at an appropriate level of therapeutic security according to their individual need. These placements correspond to levels of risk, symptom severity and the patient's overall level of functioning. Location at the time of assessment was ranked according to the level of therapeutic security – high, medium or low. This is an ordinal ranking according to the staff-to-patient ratio, and the ranking system matches the position of each unit along the therapeutic pathway as service-users progress from admission to discharge. The units are arranged in clusters by level of therapeutic security – acute cluster (high secure), medium cluster (medium secure) and rehabilitation and recovery cluster (low secure) [30].

Study design

Three vignettes were drafted in simple language to assess functional mental capacity in three domains – finances, welfare and healthcare. The vignettes were designed to assess patients' abilities to: understand and retain the information relevant to the dilemma in each vignette, reason through the dilemma, appreciate the need for a decision and make and communicate a decision in each vignette.

A stratified scoring system from zero to one hundred was designed for each of the four domains understanding, reasoning, appreciation and ability to make and communicate a decision with definitions tethering the ratings at every ten points so that scores could be assigned for each of the three vignettes.

The vignettes were then reviewed by three focus groups, including senior nursing staff, senior social work staff, occupational therapy, consultant forensic psychiatrists, clinical psychologists and patient advocates, and suggested alterations were made accordingly.

Ethical approval for the study was sought from and granted by the Research Ethics, Audit and Effectiveness Committee of the Central Mental Hospital.

Patients were given written information about the study, and all participants who were assessed by their treating psychiatrists as capable of giving consent gave written informed consent to participate.

Inclusion & Exclusion Criteria

All male patients with a diagnosis of schizophrenia or schizoaffective disorder using Structured Clinical Interview for Schizophrenia (Structured Clinical Interview for DSM-IV (SCID; First et al. 2002 [31]). resident in the Central Mental Hospital or under community supervision by the forensic recovery and rehabilitation service during the study period (January 2013 – January 2015) were considered eligible to participate. Female patients were excluded as this group makes up a very small proportion of forensic mental health service-users in this jurisdiction. Male patients who did not have English as a first language were excluded, as were those who were deemed too behaviourally disturbed to participate or unable to give consent as assessed by their treating consultant psychiatrists.

Data collection

In order to rate the Dundrum Capacity Ladders (DCL), GM interviewed all patients who met inclusion criteria and consented to participate. Their responses were recorded in writing, and assigned a score on the ladder scoring system. For measures of inter-rater reliability, GM and JOC took a random sample of completed interviews and scored them using the DCL system. Data regarding contemporaneous level of therapeutic security, diagnosis as confirmed by treating consultant psychiatrist, and a validated measure of function, scored by the patients' treating consultant psychiatrist, the MIRECC-GAF [32] was also recorded by the primary researcher. GM and JOC were blind to the ratings of the MIRECC-GAF and MCCB.

As the MIRECC-GAF and Dundrum Capacity Ladders have different maximum scores (300 and 1200 respectively), the total mean scores of each were corrected to a common total, 100.

Cognitive assessment

Cognitive functioning was assed using the MATRICS Consensus Cognitive Battery [33] (MCCB) by Masters level assistant psychologists trained in its use. The MATRICS battery covers seven cognitive domains: processing speed; attention/ vigilance; working memory; verbal learning; visual learning; reasoning and problem solving and social cognition (assessed using social reasoning tasks for understanding and managing emotions taken from the 'managing emotions' subtest of the Mayer-Salovey-Caruso Emotional Intelligence Test (MSCEIT) which is a social reasoning test). The test comprises of vignettes of various situations, and options for coping with the emotions depicted in these vignettes. Participants are required to indicate the effectiveness of each solution ranging from one (very ineffective) to five (very effective). Overall performance on the MCCB is measured using a composite score which is the preferred outcome for treatment studies. Because there is growing awareness that non-social and social cognition are separable dimensions, the MCCB scoring system now provides an option for a neurocognitive composite that does not include the social cognition sub-scale. In validation studies, and in antipsychotic trials of stable patients, the MCCB demonstrated excellent reliability, minimal practice effects and significant correlations with measures of functional capacity. Those rating the MCCB were blind to the ratings of the Dundrum Capacity Ladders and also blind to the ratings of the MIRECC-GAF.

Statistics

All data was entered using SPSS-22. Internal Consistency was assessed using Cronbach's Alpha. Inter-rater Reliability was assessed using Spearman's Rho and the Intra-class Correlation Coefficient. The relationships between Capacity Scores, function (MIRECC-GAF), Level of Therapeutic Security, age, length of stay and neurocognitive ability were assessed using Spearman's Rho for non-parametric correlations. We took r values of 0.1 to 0.3 as small effect sizes, 0.3 to 0.5 as moderate effect sizes and r values greater than 0.5 as large effect sizes [34]. The relationship between Dundrum Capacity Ladder scores, MCCB scores and GAF scores was examined using regression analysis.

Results

Fifty-five patients gave written consent to participate and completed the interviews with the primary researcher. The mean age of participants was 40.5 years (range 22–73 years). The mean length of stay from admission to the hospital to date of assessment was 2029 days (range 2–14,638 days). Using SCID-I, Forty-eight patients met DSM-IV-TR criteria for Schizophrenia, and seven for Schizoaffective Disorder. The corrected mean MIRECC-GAF was 51.43.

Validity measures

Internal consistency

Cronbach's alpha measures the internal consistency of a scale, the extent to which each item of a scale correlates with the overall score. Cronbach's alpha was high for each of the three domains: Finances 0.960, Welfare 0.973 and Healthcare 0.973. It was similarly high for each of the four abilities measured: Understanding 0.964, Reasoning 0.979, Appreciation 0.968 and Decision 0.961.

Table 1 shows that when omitted, only the Appreciation items on each of the vignettes lead to a small increase in the Cronbach's alpha score. No item, if omitted, lead to a significant increase in the alpha statistic. When comparing abilities across the vignettes, no item if omitted lead to a significant increase in alpha score.

Inter-rater reliability

Thirteen interview transcripts were chosen at random and scored independently by the primary and secondary researchers on the Dundrum Capacity Ladders. Inter-rater reliability was assessed using Spearman's rho and the Intra-class Correlation Coefficient. These results are shown in Table 2.

Relationship between measured capacity scores and neurocognitive ability

Forty-one patients' neurocognitive and social cognitive abilities were assessed using the MATRICS Consensus Cognitive Battery. Spearman's rho was assessed for non-parametric correlation between subscales of the neurocognitive battery, length of stay, age, MIRECC-GAF, and the three subscales of the DUNDRUM Capacity Ladders in a post-hoc analysis. Length of stay did not correlate with cognitive function. Age was found to correlate inversely with processing speed and reasoning. The GAF and all its sub-scales correlated with each of the domains of neurocognitive function. This relationship is shown in Table 3.

There were significant correlations between the Dundrum Capacity Ladders sub-scales and those in the MATRICS battery. This finding was replicated when examining the relationship between the MIRECC-GAF, its sub-scales and the Dundrum Capacity Ladders, as shown in Table 4. All correlations significant at the 0.01

Table 1 Internal Consistency for the subscales of each of the three domains, and for the abilities across the Dundrum Capacity Ladders, $N = 55$

Across Domains	Subscale total alpha	Corrected item – Total Correlation	Cronbach's Alpha if item deleted	Across Abilities	Subscale Alpha	Corrected item – Total Correlation	Cronbach's Alpha if item deleted
Finances	0.960	–	–	Understanding	0.964	–	–
FU	–	0.948	0.933	FU	–	0.892	0.970
FR	–	0.926	0.942	WU	–	0.951	0.928
FA	–	0.812	0.974	HU	–	0.931	0.943
FD	–	0.941	0.935	Reasoning	0.979	–	–
Welfare	0.973	–	–	FR	–	0.934	0.983
WU	–	0.950	0.959	WR	–	0.967	0.960
WR	–	0.941	0.962	HR	–	0.962	0.960
WA	–	0.892	0.976	Appreciation	0.968	–	–
WD	–	0.953	0.958	FA	–	0.893	0.981
Healthcare	0.973	–	–	WA	–	0.959	0.933
HU	–	0.949	0.960	HA	–	0.947	0.942
HR	–	0.937	0.963	Decision	0.961	–	–
HA	–	0.900	0.975	FD	–	0.883	0.967
HD	–	0.956	0.957	WD	–	0.922	0.938
–	–	–	–	HD	–	0.946	0.920

level were in the range $r = 0.358$ to 0.693, effect sizes that were moderate to large.

Relationship between measured capacity scores, level of therapeutic security and scores of function

The relationship between current place on the recovery pathway from acute / high security to medium security and minimum security was tested using ANOVA (Table 5). Post-hoc Bonferroni corrections showed that the mean GAF for the minimum security rehabilitation and recovery cluster patients was significantly better than the acute cluster patients, while for the DCL, each cluster differed significantly from each of the other clusters. Age did not differ significantly, but length of stay did differ as expected. The mean total GAF score and mean total DCL scores differed significantly, with mean DCL scores differing significantly at each step. It is notable that in the acute cluster, patients were severely impaired (GAF mean = 47.3 S.D. =16.2, DCL mean = 18.6 S.D. =26.1) while those in the minimum security / rehabilitation and recovery stage functioned significantly better (GAF mean = 72.7 S.D. =14.2, DCL mean = 78.8 S.D. =21.1).

Discussion

The findings of this study demonstrate the reliability and validity of a new measure of functional capacity, the Dundrum Capacity Ladders, in a national cohort of male forensic mental health patients with schizophrenia or schizoaffective disorder. Within this sample consisting of patients at different levels of therapeutic security as well as differing stages of treatment, the Dundrum Capacity Ladders showed excellent internal consistency and inter-rater reliability. Specifically, Cronbach's alpha for the total score on all three domains was greater than 0.9, and the Inter-class correlation coefficient for the total scores was also greater than 0.9. Moreover, Dundrum Capacity Ladders demonstrated excellent convergent validity with the MATRICS Consensus Cognitive Battery (MCCB) for cognitive deficits in schizophrenia. The correlations between the composite score of the MCCB and the total scores for finance, welfare and health domain where are all significant and large. Significant and large correlations were also observed between Dundrum Capacity Ladders and the Global Assessment of Functioning (GAF) in relation to its occupational, social and symptomatic domains. In other words, amongst forensic patients with schizophrenia and schizoaffective disorder, those who had higher levels of functional capacity, performed better on a separate assessment of occupational and social functioning and were judged to be less symptomatic. Finally, and as would be expected, patient performance on the Dundrum Capacity Ladders was significantly different across three levels of therapeutic security, with those patients in lower levels of therapeutic security possessing greater levels of functional capacity.

The size of the correlations between the Dundrum Capacity Ladders and the MCCB highlights the fundamental relationship between cognitive ability and

Table 2 Inter-rater reliability: Spearman's rho and Intra-class Correlation Coefficients for each subscale. $N = 13$ patients, two raters

Domain	Spearman's Rho	Intra-Class Correlation Coefficient (95% CI)
Finances		
FU	0.930	0.975 (0.921–0.992)
FR	0.969	0.998 (0.992–0.999)
FA	0.957	0.977 (0.925–0.993)
FD	0.928	0.922 (0.765–0.975)
FT	0.979	0.989 (0.966–0.997)
Welfare		
WU	0.967	0.991 (0.972–0.997)
WR	0.963	0.995 (0.985–0.999)
WA	0.991	0.991 (0.971–0.997)
WD	0.938	0.983 (0.946–0.995)
WT	0.974	0.998 (0.992–0.999)
Healthcare		
HU	0.917	0.988 (0.960–0.996)
HR	0.950	0.985 (0.952–0.995)
HA	0.973	0.972 (0.910–0.991)
HD	0.938	0.983 (0.945–0.995)
HT	0.914	0.992 (0.973–0.997)
DCL Total	0.964	0.995 (0.982–0.998)

All correlations significant at the 0.01 level (2-tailed)

functional capacity in the areas of understanding, appreciation, reasoning and judgment. In the cases of the financial, welfare, and health domain the MCCB composite score could account for approximately 40% of the variance. This finding suggests that functional mental capacity which is typically considered to be a dynamic construct may not be as separable from cognitive functioning, typically considered a static construct, as previously believed. The magnitude of these correlations are considerably greater than what has previously been observed (Moser et al.) [35]. But consistent with previous research psychiatric symptoms as measured by the GAF were also strongly correlated with functional capacity (Dornan et al.) [36]. However, whereas psychiatric

Table 3 Relationship between MATRICS Sub-scales, Length of stay, age and GAF MIRECC, independently rated. Spearman's rho. $N = 41$

	Length of Stay	Age	GAF OCC	GAF Soc	GAF Sym	GAF Tot
PS	−0.018	−0.375 *	0.494 **	0.317 *	0.326 *	0.429 **
An	− 0.206	−0.274	0.539 **	0.416 **	0.442 **	0.508 **
WM	− 0.020	−0.137	0.640 **	0.471 **	0.453 **	0.575 **
VeL	0.018	−0.244	0.626 **	0.462 **	0.394 *	0.546 **
ViL	0.142	−0.185	0.529 **	0.399 **	0.320 *	0.469 **
Rg	− 0.024	−0.401 **	0.506 **	0.318 *	0.332 *	0.442 **
SC	− 0.269	−0.107	0.558 **	0.508 **	0.599 **	0.619 **
MC	− 0.056	−0.274	0.673 **	0.515 **	0.503 **	0.626 **
NCC	− 0.037	−0.251	0.631 **	0.472 **	0.430 **	0..567 **

**Correlation is significant at the 0.01 level (2-tailed)
*Correlation is significant at the 0.05 level (2-tailed)

symptoms can be treated effectively with appropriate medication and a therapeutic environment, the cognitive deficits experienced by patients with schizophrenia are less easily ameliorated (Keefe et al.) [37]. Although some improvement may be possible using psychological approaches like cognitive remediation therapy, and by pharmacological approached such as minimising anticholinergic burden (O'Reilly et al. [38]; O'Reilly et al. [39]).

The Dundrum Capacity Ladders are likely to have a number of practical applications. To begin with, the ladders provide clinicians with a useful platform to structure their judgments when determining functional mental capacity to manage finances, to consent to treatment, and to choose to live independently. Clinicians can choose to administer the vignettes or also to use the ladders to structure their own professional judgment regarding patient capacity. The Dundrum Capacity Ladders can also be used as routine outcome measure for psychiatric and psychological interventions, which is in keeping with the current emphasis on functional outcomes with schizophrenia research and treatment [40, 41]. As a measure of recovery the Dundrum Capacity Ladders may also be useful for guiding psychological interventions. A focus on measuring an improving patient capacity is particularly important within contexts where patients are involuntary detained and whether their human rights are by necessity compromised.

The study has a number of strengths as well as limitations. To begin with the study consisted of a national forensic mental health cohort with schizophrenia and

Table 4 Relationship between MATRICS sub-scales, MIRECC-GAF, and sub-scales of Dundrum Capacity Ladders, independently rated. Spearman's rho

Domain	PS	An	WM	VeL	ViL	Rg	SC	MC	NCC	GAF Occ	GAF Soc	GAF Sym	GAF Tot
N	41	41	41	41	41	41	41	41	41	55	55	55	55
Finances													
FU	0.473 **	0.505 **	0.509 **	0.545 **	0.564 **	0.516 **	0.381 *	0.610 **	0.600 **	0.594 **	0.540 **	0.463 **	0.589 **
FR	0.439 **	0.474 **	0.518 **	0.538 **	0.578 **	0.460 **	0.418 **	0.603 **	0.587 **	0.641 **	0.586 **	0.500 **	0.630 **
FA	0.210	0.333 *	0.338 *	0.373 *	0.322 *	0.357 *	0.145	0.363 *	0.374 *	0.541 **	0.491 **	0.358 **	0.498 **
FD	0.418 **	0.491 **	0.525 **	0.507 **	0.507 **	0.450 **	0.339 *	0.574 **	0.579 **	0.616 **	0.521 **	0.418 **	0.560 **
FT	0.444 **	0.518 **	0.540 **	0.550 **	0.560 **	0.486 **	0.368 *	0.610 **	0.606 **	0.618 **	0.569 **	0.418 **	0.611 **
Welfare													
WU	0.505 **	0.510 **	0.532 **	0.549 **	0.569 **	0.603 **	0.458 **	0.644 **	0.632 **	0.626 **	0.528 **	0.460 **	0.612 **
WR	0.494 **	0.512 **	0.558 **	0.522 **	0.514 **	0.548 **	0.482 **	0.631 **	0.615 **	0.670 **	0.625 **	0.526 **	0.663 **
WA	0.285	0.300	0.336 *	0.349 *	0.404 **	0.386 *	0.240	0.405 **	0.410 **	0.567 **	0.529 **	0.371 **	0.530 **
WD	0.483 **	0.512 **	0.561 **	0.534 **	0.463 **	0.578 **	0.433 **	0.615 **	0.604 **	0.687 **	0.577 **	0.468 **	0.631 **
WT	0.503 **	0.503 **	0.547 **	0.548 **	0.529 **	0.586 **	0.449 **	0.634 **	0.625 **	0.664 **	0.620 **	0.492 **	0.648 **
Healthcare													
HU	0.498 **	0.514 **	0.550 **	0.561 **	0.599 **	0.570 **	0.489 **	0.656 **	0.638 **	0.661 **	0.581 **	0.480 **	0.635 **
HR	0.485 **	0.509 **	0.529 **	0.535 **	0.549 **	0.534 **	0.506 **	0.637 **	0.620 **	0.663 **	0.601 **	0.496 **	0.642 **
HA	0.294	0.426 **	0.503 **	0.476 **	0.501 **	0.361 *	0.329 *	0.505 **	0.500 **	0.667 **	0.575 **	0.448 **	0.613 **
HD	0.442 **	0.500 **	0.521 **	0.533 **	0.527 **	0.481 **	0.450 **	0.598 **	0.589 **	0.637 **	0.573 **	0.492 **	0.623 **
HT	0.501 **	0.533 **	0.570 **	0.572 **	0.558 **	0.562 **	0.504 **	0.659 **	0.642 **	0.693 **	0.610 **	0.506 **	0.660 **

** Correlation is significant at the 0.01 level (2-tailed)
*Correlation is significant at the 0.05 level (2-tailed)

Table 5 Distribution of patient characteristics, GAF total score and DUNDRUM Capacity Ladder total score across the recovery pathway

Variable	Acute high secure		Medium secure		Minimum secure R&R		ANOVA	
n	17		27		11			
	mean	SD	mean	SD	mean	SD	F	p
Age (years)	38.6	10.3	40.6	10.7	43.1	14.2	0.5	0.6
Length of stay (days)	590.7	1686.9	2201.9	2715.6	3990.0	3767.9	5.4	0.008
GAF total (0–100)	47.3	16.2	46.5	11.1	72.7	14.2	16.4	0.001
DCL total (0–100)	18.6	26.1	50.9	20.3	78.8	21.1	25.3	0.001

schizoaffective disorder. In addition, convergent validity was also established with a consensus measure of cognitive ability the MCCB whose psychometric properties are established. The participants in this study were at different stages of treatment and under different levels of therapeutic security, demonstrating that the Dundrum Capacity Ladders are applicable to a range of patients. Weaknesses of the study include that the sample consisted entirely of male patients, hence generalisability to female patients may be questioned. Additionally, no attempt was made to determine concurrent validity using established measures of functional capacity such as the MacArthur scales, or criterion validity such as predicting the outcome of legal processes. Also it remains unclear the extent to which the Dundrum Capacity Ladders are sensitive to change. Future research should concentrate on addressing these limitations.

Conclusions

We have concluded that the Dundrum Capacity Ladders are a valid tool for measuring functional mental capacities in a severely ill population with schizophrenia. Furthermore, we believe that our results highlight the interrelated connections between occupational, social and symptomatic function; neurocognitive ability and functional mental capacities. We argue that it logically follows that evidence of restoration of functional mental capacity itself can be viewed as a measure of recovery. When one considers the results shown by Naughton et al. [26], these findings highlight the need for future research into the relationship between mental capacity and recovery, along with informing potential directions for future therapeutic interventions. We now propose that this measure should be tested for sensitivity to change and as a treatment outcome measure. We plan to examine these hypotheses.

Abbreviations

An: Attention; CI: Confidence Interval; DCL: Dundrum Capacity Ladders; FA: Finances Appreciation score; FD: Finances Decision score; FR: Finances Reasoning score; FT: Finances Total score; FU: Finances Understanding score; GAF Occ: GAF Occupational score; GAF Soc: GAF Social score; GAF Sym: GAF Symptom score; HA: Healthcare Appreciation score; HD: Healthcare Decision score; HR: Healthcare Reasoning score; HT: Healthcare Total score; HU: Healthcare Understanding score; MC: Matrics Composite; MIRECC-GAF: Mental Illness Research, Education and Clinical Center Global Assessment of Functioning; NCC: Neurocognitive Composite; PS: Processing Speed; Rg: Reasoning; SC: Social Cognition; SPSS: Statistical Package for the Social Sciences; VeL: Verbal Learning; ViL: Visual Learning; WA: Welfare Appreciation score; WD: Welfare Decision score; WM: Working Memory; WR: Welfare Reasoning score; WT: Welfare Total score; WU: Welfare Understanding score

Acknowledgements

The authors would like to thank the patients and staff who facilitated, cooperated with and part-took in this project.

Funding

This project was undertaken without funding.

Author's contributions

GM was involved in conception and design of the study, composed the vignettes, ran the focus groups to review the vignettes, interviewed the study participants, was involved in the design of the stratified scoring system, gathered data, was involved in statistical analysis and drafted the manuscript. KO'R was involved in data collection for neurocognitive function and contributed to drafting of the manuscript. JO'C was involved in data collection for inter-rater reliability. HGK was involved in conception and design of the study, design of the stratified scoring system and statistical analysis. All authors read and approved the final manuscript.

Consent for publication

N/A.

Competing interests

The authors declare that they have no competing interests.

References

1. Schneider C. The Practice of Autonomy. New York, NY; Oxford university press; 1998.
2. Kahn RS, Keefe RS. Schizophrenia is a cognitive illness: time for a change in focus. JAMA Psychiatry. 2013;70(10):1107–12.
3. Grisso T, Appelbaum PS. Assessing Competence to Consent to Treatment: A Guide for Physicians and Other Health Professionals. New York, NY; Oxford university press; 1998.
4. UN General Assembly, *Universal Declaration of Human Rights*, 10 December 1948, 217 A (III).
5. UN General Assembly, Convention on the Rights of Persons with Disabilities: resolution / adopted by the General Assembly, 24 January 2007, A/RES/61/106.
6. Adults with Incapacity (Scotland) Act 2000 (2000 asp 4).
7. Mental Capacity Act 2005 (2005 c 9).
8. Health Care Consent Act, 1996, S.O. 1996, c 2. Sched. A
9. New Zealand Bill of Rights Act 1990.
10. Assisted Decision Making (Capacity) Act, 2015.
11. Fett AK, Viechtbauer W, Dominguez MD, Penn DL, van Os J, Krabbendam L. The relationship between neurocognition and social cognition with functional outcomes in schizophrenia: a meta-analysis. Neurosci Biobehav Rev. 2011;35(3):573–88. https://doi.org/10.1016/j.neubiorev.2010.07.001. Epub 2010 Jul 8. Review. PMID: 20620163.
12. Lam BY, Raine A, Lee TM. The relationship between neurocognition and symptomatology in people with schizophrenia: social cognition as the mediator. BMC Psychiatry. 2014, 13;14:138. doi: https://doi.org/10.1186/1471-244X-14-138.
13. Gallagher S, Varga S. Social cognition and psychopathology: a critical overview. World Psychiatry. 2015;14(1):5–14. https://doi.org/10.1002/wps.20173.
14. Lysaker PH, Shea AM, Buck KD, Dimaggio G, Nicolò G, Procacci M, Salvatore G, Rand KL. Metacognition as a mediator of the effects of impairments in neurocognition on social function in schizophrenia spectrum disorders. Acta Psychiatr Scand. 2010;122:405–13.
15. Lysaker PH, Vohs J, Hammd JA, Kukla M, Minor KS, de Jong S, van Donkersgoed R, Pijnenborg MHM, Kent JS, Matthews SC, Ringer JM, Leonhardt BL, Francis MM, Buck KD, Dimaggio G. Deficits in metacognitive capacity distinguish patients with schizophrenia from those with prolonged medical adversity. J Psychiatr Res. 2014;55(2014):126–32. https://doi.org/10.1016/j.jpsychires.2014.04.011
16. Volicer L, Ganzini L. Health professionals' views on standards for decision-making capacity regarding refusal of medical treatment in mild Alzheimer's disease. J Am Geriatr Soc. 2003;51(9):1270–4.
17. Marson DC, McInturff B, Hawkins L, Bartolucci A, Harrel LE. Consistency of physician judgements of capacity to consent in mild Alzheimer's disease. J Am Geriatr Soc. 1997;45(4):453–7.
18. Canterbury v Spence (464 F.2d 772, 782 D.C. Cir. 1972)
19. Geoghegan v Harris 2000 3 IR 536
20. Kennedy M, Dornan J, Rutledge E, O'Neill H, Kennedy HG. Extra information about treatment is too much for the patient with psychosis. Int J Law Psychiatry. 2009;32(6):369–76.

21. Gigerenzer G, Selten R. Bounded Rationality: The adaptive toolbox. Cambridge, MA; the MIT Press; 2001.
22. Grisso T, Applebaum PS, Hill-Fotouhi C. The MacCat-T: a clinical tool to assess patients' capacities to make treatment decisions. Psychiatr Serv. 1997; 48(11):1415–9.
23. Akinkunmi AA. The MacArthur competence assessment tool – fitness to plead: a preliminary evaluation of a research instrument for assessing fitness to plead in England and Wales. J Am Acad Psychiatry Law. 2002;30(4):476–82.
24. Janofsky JS, McCarthy RJ, Folstein MF. The Hopkins competency assessment test: a brief method for evaluating patients' capacity to give informed consent. Hosp Community Psychiatry. 1992;43(2):132–6.
25. Fazel S, Hope T, Jacoby R. Assessment of competence to complete advance directives: validation of a patient centred approach. BMJ. 1999;318(7182):493–7.
26. Naughton M, Nulty A, Abidin Z, Davoren M, O'Dwyer S, Kennedy HG. Effects of group meta-cognitive training (MCT) on mental capacity and functioning in patients with psychosis in a secure forensic psychiatric hospital: a prospective-cohort waiting list controlled study. BMC Research Notes. 2012;5:302.
27. Census 2016 Results. Government of Ireland 2017. Available from http://www.cso.ie/en/csolatestnews/presspages/2017/census2016summaryresults-part1/.
28. Criminal Law (Insanity) Act, 2006.
29. Mental Health Act, 2001.
30. Pillay SM, Oliver B, Butler L, Kennedy HG. Risk stratification and the care pathway. Ir J Psychol Med. 2008;25(4):123–7.
31. First MB, Spitzer RL, Gibbon M, Williams JBW. Structured Clinical Interview for DSM-IV-TR Axis I Disorders, Research Version, Patient Edition. (SCID-I/P). New York: Biometrics Research, New York State Psychiatric Institute; 2002.
32. Niv N, Cohen AN, Sullivan G, Young AS. The MIRECC version of the global assessment of functioning scale: reliability and validity. Psychiatr Serv. 2007; 58(4):529–35.
33. Nuechterlein KH, Green MF, Kern RS, et al. The MATRICS consensus cognitive battery, part 1: test selection, reliability, and validity. Am J Psychiatry. 2008;165(2):203–13.
34. Cohen J. A Power primer. Psychol Bull. 1992;112(1):155–9. https://doi.org/10.1037/0033-2909.112.1.155. PMID 19565683.
35. Moser DJ, Schultz SK, Arndt S, et al. Capacity to provide informed consent for participation in schizophrenia and HIV research. Am J Psychiatry. 2002; 159(7):1201–7.
36. Dornan J, Kennedy M, Garland J, Rutledge E, Kennedy HG. Functional mental capacity, treatment as usual and time: magnitude of change in secure hospital patients with major mental illness. BMC Res Notes. 2015(14); 8:566.
37. Keefe RS, Bilder RM, Davis SM, et al. Neurocognitive effects of antipsychotic medications in patients with chronic schizophrenia in the CATIE trial. Catie investigators; neurocognitive working group. Arch Gen Psychiatry. 2007;64: 633–47.
38. O'Reilly K, Donohoe G, O'Sullivan D, et al. Study protocol: a randomised controlled trial of cognitive remediation for a national cohort of forensic mental health patients with schizophrenia of schizoaffective disorder. BMC Psychiatry. 2016;16:5.
39. O'Reilly K, O'Connell P, Donohoe G, et al. Anticholinergic burden in schizophrenia and ability to benefit from psychosocial treatment programmes: a 3-year prospective cohort study. Psychol Med. 2016;46(15):3199–211.
40. Karow A, Moritz S, Lambert M, Schöttle D, Naber D. On behalf of the EGOFORS initiative. Remitted but still impaired? Symptomatic versus functional remission in patients with schizophrenia. Eur Psychiatry. 2012;27:401–5.
41. Schennach-Wolff R, Jäger M, Seemüller F, et al. Defining and predicting functional outcome in schizophrenia and schizophrenia spectrum disorders. Schizophr Res. 2009;113(2–3):210–7.

Development and validation of a mental health screening tool for asylum-seekers and refugees: the STAR-MH

Debbie C. Hocking[1,2,4*], Serafino G. Mancuso[3] and Suresh Sundram[2,3,4,5]

Abstract

Background: There is no screening tool for major depressive disorder (MDD) or post-traumatic stress disorder (PTSD) in asylum-seekers or refugees (ASR) that can be readily administered by non-mental health workers. Hence, we aimed to develop a brief, sensitive and rapidly administrable tool for non-mental health workers to screen for MDD and PTSD in ASR.

Methods: The screening tool was developed from an extant dataset ($n = 121$) of multiply screened ASR and tested prospectively ($N = 192$) against the M.I.N.I. (Mini International Neuropsychiatric Interview) structured psychiatric interview. Rasch, Differential Item Functioning and ROC analyses evaluated the psychometric properties and tool utility.

Results: A 9-item tool with a median administration time of six minutes was generated, comprising two 'immediate screen-in' items, and a 7-item scale. The prevalence of PTSD &/or MDD using the M.I.N.I. was 32%, whilst 99% of other diagnosed mental disorders were comorbid with one or both of these. Using a cut-score of ≥2, the tool provided a sensitivity of 0.93, specificity of 0.75 and predictive accuracy of 80.7%.

Conclusions: A brief sensitive screening tool with robust psychometric properties that was easy to administer at the agency of first presentation was developed to facilitate mental health referrals for asylum-seekers and new refugees.

Keywords: Asylum-seekers, Refugees, Mental health screening, Tool development, Post-traumatic stress disorder, Depression

Background

The world currently has the largest number of displaced persons at any time in history [1]. This has seen increasing numbers of forced migrants entering industrialised countries [1], intensifying the challenge to efficiently screen health conditions. In most countries asylum-seekers are not screened for mental health problems at any point during the asylum process [2], which is similarly the case for a large proportion of newly resettled refugees [3–7].

Compounding this is the knowledge that forced migrant populations have high rates of mental disorders, with major depressive disorder (MDD) and post-traumatic stress disorder (PTSD) in particular being many fold higher than in host [8] and non-forced migrant populations [9]. A large meta-analysis of refugees and other conflict-affected persons reported adjusted weighted prevalence rates of 30% for MDD and PTSD [10], suggesting these to be the most widespread mental disorders in this population with even higher rates reported in asylum-seekers [11–14].

The burgeoning number of displaced persons globally and their disproportionately high rates of mental disorders have prompted the World Health Organisation (WHO) to call upon treatment services to be responsive to the needs of asylum-seekers and refugees [15]. Yet, utilisation of mental health services is comparatively low in this population [16] for reasons including lack of accessibility, poverty, poor language comprehension, lack of knowledge of services, cultural factors and stigma [4]. Furthermore, increasingly time-constrained agencies have to contend with increasing need whilst grappling with limited human resources. Several of these issues could be addressed by the availability of a brief, sensitive and rapidly administrable screening tool by

* Correspondence: debbie.hocking@florey.edu.au
[1]Cabrini Institute, 154 Wattletree Road, Malvern, VIC 3144, Australia
[2]Florey Institute of Neuroscience and Mental Health, 30 Royal Parade (Cnr Genetics Lane), Parkville, VIC 3052, Australia
Full list of author information is available at the end of the article

non-mental health workers which would facilitate triaging of asylum seekers and refugees with mental health problems to be referred to an appropriate health service.

Extant mental health screening tools do not fully meet these aforementioned criteria with several well-utilised tools having a number of drawbacks. These include not being validated in forced migrant populations (e.g., K10, K6, BAI, DASS-21, PTSD-8, GHQ-12) [17, 18]; too prolonged to facilitate rapid screening of large populations (e.g., DASS-21, RHS-15; HSCL-25; HTQ); screening for distress rather than disorder and lacking predictive validity against a standardised psychiatric interview (e.g., K10; RHS-15; WHO-5; SRQ-20) [19]; or screening for either MDD or PTSD – not both [20, 21].

Despite being one of the more commonly used screening tools for depression and anxiety, a recent review raised concerns about the lack of evidence for the validity and cultural equivalence of the K10, including variation between ethnic/linguistic groups for studies with multicultural samples [17]. The SRQ-20 was developed to screen for psychiatric disturbance, but primarily for those in developing countries, and has not established its predictive validity against a standardised psychiatric interview [19]. Whilst the RHS-15 [3] was developed for refugee populations, it was designed to be administered in clinical settings, and has not been validated in asylum-seeker populations or against an acceptable gold standard [3].

A high proportion of mental disorders in the general population go undetected by healthcare professionals in the course of their routine work [22–24] and it would be predicted that non-mental health trained workers would be even less likely to identify possible mental disorders in their forced migrant clients. Consequently, we strove to develop a screening instrument that could be utilised by non-mental health workers across a variety of contexts, to minimise administrator-burden whilst increasing the likelihood of client uptake. To maximise the utility of such an instrument, it also would need to have efficacy in linguistically diverse and potentially under-resourced settings, using interpreters rather than undertaking multiple translations.

The present paper reports on the development and validation of a brief screening tool for PTSD and MDD in adult asylum-seekers and refugees (STAR-MH) that is suitable for use by non-mental health workers.

Methods

Procedure

A visual overview of the data sampling process is presented in Fig. 1 which comprise a derivation sample – from which the initial 12-items scale was derived, and two pilot samples (for the initial 12-item version, and subsequent 10-item versions). The final version was a 9-item scale, which forms the basis of the Results section.

All administrators of the STAR-MH were briefed prior to each pilot study on the importance of adhering to the research protocol (such as delivering each item neutrally, without elaboration; providing written feedback on the process) and instructed about risk management processes should the need arise. Administrators were accustomed to working with interpreters. The tool itself was designed to be sufficiently simple to not require specific training to administer.

Given the purpose was to develop a mental health screening tool for forced migrants, participants were unselected by country of origin. Hence, the tool was not translated, but instead utilised in situ translation by professional telephone or face-to-face interpreters in the language required by participants as they consecutively presented to the recruiting agency.

The STAR-MH items were derived from scales considered to be gold standard instruments for measuring symptoms of depression, anxiety and PTSD in individuals of refugee-like background.

Community leaders from the cultural and linguistic communities with the greatest numbers of forced migrants in Australia (Sri Lankan/Tamil; Iranian/Farsi and Afghan/Dari) were consulted to ascertain the cultural appropriateness and utility of the tool.

Derivation sample

The initial 12-item version of the STAR-MH [25], was derived from a sample of 56 ASR from a previous study [14] whom had completed four self-report questionnaires (Harvard Trauma Questionnaire-R, Parts I – trauma experiences & IV – PTSD and refugee-specific symptoms, and Hopkins Symptom Checklist-25 [26]; Post-Migration Living Difficulties Checklist [27]; and Psychiatric Epidemiology Research Interview—Demoralization Scale [28]) and the M.I.N.I. (Mini International Neuropsychiatric Interview) [29]. Scaled items from the four questionnaires were dichotomised, with values ≥3 designating clinical relevance. All 153 items were then entered into chi-square analyses to establish the sensitivity (SN) and specificity (SP) of each item against M.I.N.I diagnoses of PTSD and MDD. Only statistically significant items (Kappa statistic) were retained, resulting in 66 items.

Spearman's Rho correlations were then performed between the 66 items and PTSD and MDD diagnoses. All items with a correlation ≥0.7 and a predictive accuracy of ≥0.85 for PTSD and/or MDD were retained and after two items were discarded due to redundancy nine items remained. Three 'immediate screen-in' items were included on clinical grounds, resulting in an initial 12-item version of the screening tool. A quantitative and qualitative administrator feedback section was also included to inform the second iteration of the tool (data not shown).

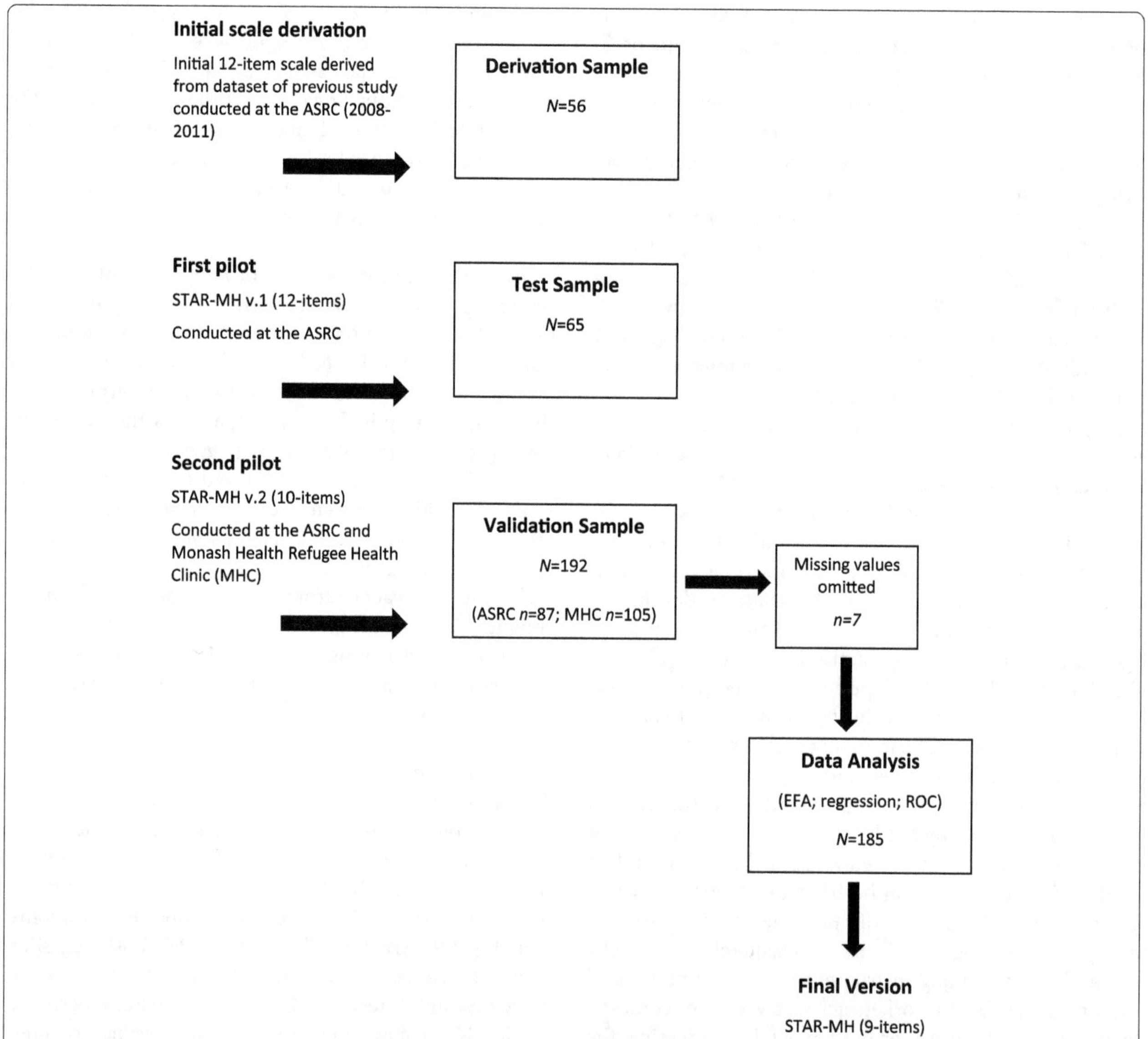

Fig. 1 Sampling and iterative development of the STAR-MH

Test sample

The initial 12-item version was evaluated at a community based asylum seeker welfare centre (Asylum Seeker Resource Centre, ASRC), with a consecutive sample of asylum-seekers ($N = 65$) being recruited through the (non-health) casework program. The sample was inclusive of adults (≥18 years) recently engaged with the ASRC (≤ 6 months) who had not been diagnosed with or treated for a psychiatric disorder since arriving in Australia. Eight ASRC casework program volunteers from a range of non-mental health backgrounds, such as university students, administration, nurses and general practitioners (GP) were briefed on the research protocol for the tool. All screened participants were subsequently administered the M.I.N.I by a researcher (DH), who was blind to the screening results. During the validation interview, demographic information was collected and participants were administered the HTQ-R (Part IV) and HSCL-25. Interpreters were utilised as necessary for both the screening and the validation interview.

Receiver operating characteristic (ROC) curve analyses were conducted on the 12 items with the test sample, resulting in five items being retained.

Given the objective was to identify likely caseness of either MDD or PTSD and because of the substantial co-morbidity, both diagnoses were treated as a single outcome variable for the chi-square analyses below.

The statistical power was increased by pooling the derivation and test sample data. Hence, all 65 HTQ-R and HSCL-25 items were entered into chi-square analyses ($N = 121$) to ascertain the SN and SP of each item against M.I.N.I diagnoses of PTSD and MDD. Items with

≥85% SN and ≥ 75% SP were retained, resulting in 10 items in addition to those retained from the ROC analysis. Classification and Regression Tree (CART) analyses were then conducted for these 15 items with the total dataset (N = 121). This resulted in eight items being retained in addition to two of the original three 'immediate screen in items' from the chi-square analyses. The third 'immediate screen in' item was discarded due to poor predictive accuracy.

The resulting second iteration was a 10-item STAR-MH, the items of which are presented in Table 1, including the scales from which the items were derived.

Validation sample

The 10-item screening tool was piloted with consecutive sample populations of ASR at two sites in Victoria, Australia: the ASRC (n = 87), and Monash Health Community (MHC) (i.e., Refugee Health Clinic; Monash Health Dental Clinic) (n = 105). In addition, a representative sample of administrators was enlisted to test the external validity of the tool.

ASRC participants were recruited through the casework and health programs. The recruitment strategy from the casework program involved screening tool administrators contacting all ASRC 'general access-listed' clients to ascertain eligibility and conduct face-to-face screening with consenting individuals. Consecutive 'walk in' patients presenting to the health program (non-mental health) who were eligible and consented were variously screened by a nurse, GP or untrained ASRC volunteer. Similarly, eligible consecutive patients presenting to the MHC were screened by a bicultural worker, nurse, GP or interpreter. All administrators were briefed on the research protocol for the tool and interpreters were utilised as required.

All screened participants were subsequently administered the M.I.N.I by a research team member (DH), who was blind to all screening results, using interpreters as required.

Instruments

The mini international neuropsychiatric interview (M.I.N.I. 6.0)

The Mini International Neuropsychiatric Interview 6.0 (M.I.N.I) [29] is a brief, structured psychiatric interview developed in the United States and Europe for assessing the presence of DSM-IV and ICD-10 psychiatric disorders. It has been found to have sound SN (i.e., ≥ 0.70 for all but three of the modules), SP, negative predictive values and efficiency (i.e., ≥ of 0.85 across all diagnoses) when measured against the SCID [30]. Additionally, the majority of kappa values have been reported above 0.75, indicating good test-retest reliability, with inter-rater reliability also found to be high when validated with the SCID (i.e., 0.79–1.00) [30].

The M.I.N.I was chosen as the diagnostic instrument by which to validate the STAR-MH due to its brevity of administration compared to the SCID and CIDI [30, 31]; and its application within forced migrant populations [2, 32–34]. All MINI modules were applied, with the exception of Antisocial Personality disorder and Anorexia and Bulimia Nervosa due to i) focusing on prevalence of mental illness and ii) eating disorders being exceedingly uncommon in adult refugee populations.

Self-report measures

Items from the above measures (Harvard Trauma Questionnaire-R; Hopkins Symptom Checklist-25; Post-Migration Living Difficulties Checklist; and Psychiatric Epidemiology Research Interview—Demoralization Scale)

Table 1 Screening tool for asylum-seeker and refugee mental health (STAR-MH) items

	STAR-MH Item	Scale derivation
1.[a]	Have you ever seen a doctor or health worker, gone to hospital, or taken medicines for your 'nerves'? (i.e. *mental or emotional health*)	
2.[a]	Have you ***often*** wished you were dead, wanted to kill yourself or ever attempted suicide or harmed yourself?	
3.[b]	Have you felt ***very*** restless, like you can't keep still?	HSCL-10 (anxiety item)
4.	Have you lost interest in things? (i.e. *things you usually enjoy*)	HSCL-23 (depression item)
5.	Have you worried about going crazy or 'losing your mind'?	PERI-D-11 (also HTQ-24 [d]; trauma item)
6.[c]	Have you had ***a lot*** of trouble sleeping?	HSCL-16 & HTQ-8 (depression and trauma item)
7.	Have you felt ***very*** fearful? (i.e. *scared or afraid*)	HSCL-2 (anxiety item)
8.	Have you felt ***very*** trapped or caught? (e.g. *like you are trapped in a situation you cannot get out of*)	HSCL-21 (depression item)
9.	Have you had ***a lot*** of pain in your body?	HTQ-20 (refugee-specific trauma item)
10.	Have you felt ***very*** worthless? (i.e. *like you have no worth or value*)	HSCL-25 (depression item)

[a]Immediate screen-in item
[b]Items 3–10 timeframe is the last 4 weeks
[c]Excluded from final 9-item scale
[d]Item from the original HTQ (Original Version)

contributed a pool of responses for potential inclusion in iterations of the STAR-MH.

Hopkins symptom Checklist-25 (HSCL-25)

The HSCL-25 [26] is divided into two parts: anxiety symptoms (Part I, 10 items, questions 1–10) and depression symptoms (Part II, 15 items, questions 11–25), with the Total Scale measuring 'nonspecific emotional distress'. All items are coded 1 *(not at all)*, 2 *(a little)*, 3 *(quite a bit)* and 4 *(extremely)* indicating the degree of distress within the previous seven days.

The HSCL-25 has been translated into several languages [26] and used in many studies with forced migrant populations [35]. It was one of only two instruments adapted for refugee populations (the other was the Beck Depression Inventory) which met all five criteria (i.e., Purpose, Construct definition, Design, Developmental process, Reliability and validity) in a critical review of the validity and reliability of psychometric tools to measure mental health status in forced migrants [35]. Demonstrating very good predictive validity for diagnosed depression (SN = 0.88; SP = 0.73) [35], empirical studies have determined the depression items to be consistent with the DSM-IV diagnosis of major depression [26]. Furthermore, the HSCL-25 was found to have high SN (0.93) and SP (0.76) in detecting the presence of any major DSM-III-R-defined Axis I disorder in three Indochinese populations [36].

The HSCL-25 has demonstrated sound reliability in clinical refugee samples [35, 37, 38], having exhibited excellent test-retest reliability ($r = 0.89$) and internal consistency, which has been found to exceed 0.88 in refugee samples [37, 39].

Harvard trauma questionnaire – Revised (HTQ-R)

The Harvard Trauma Questionnaire (HTQ) [26] was designed to assess trauma related to mass violence and its sequelae, and has been used in numerous studies with forced migrant populations. It has been validated in several non-Western populations (e.g., Cambodian, Japanese, Vietnamese, Lao, Bosnian and Croatian) and met four of five criteria in a critical evaluation of instruments used to measure refugee trauma and health status [35].

The HTQ-R comprises four parts: Part 1: trauma events; Part 2: personal description; Part 3: head injury; Part 4: trauma symptoms. Only parts I and IV were included in the protocol, to assess previous traumatic events and PTSD symptoms, respectively, as both are established predictors of PTSD and are associated with other mental disorders, such as depression. Part IV comprises 40 items of trauma symptoms using a scale of 1 *(not at all)*, 2 *(a little)*, 3 *(quite a bit)*, and 4 *(extremely)* indicating the degree of distress within the previous seven days. The first 16 items (PTSD subscale) were derived from the DSM-IV criteria for post-traumatic stress disorder [26]. The remaining 24 items constitute a 'refugee-specific' subscale which measure self-perceived level of functioning and social disability, and which may be more highly correlated with trauma-related distress than the symptoms of PTSD [26].

The HTQ has demonstrated excellent statistical properties, including high interrater reliability (K = 0.93), scale test-retest reliability (1 week, $r = 0.89$); and internal scale consistency ($\alpha = 0.90$) for the traumatic events sale (Part I). The trauma symptoms scale (Part IV) has demonstrated high interrater reliability (K = 0.98), scale test-retest reliability (1 week, $r = 0.92$); and internal scale consistency ($\alpha = 0.96$). The PTSD items (Part IV, 1–16) have exhibited reasonable SN (0.78) and SP (0.65) as a screening instrument for PTSD, however, the additional 'refugee specific' items (Part IV) increased the SP to 0.78 (SN remained unchanged).

Both the HSCL-25 and HTQ are considered to be gold standard self-report measures of psychiatric symptomatology in forced migrant populations, having demonstrated robust psychometric properties [26, 35], and are among the most widely used self-report measures for psychological distress in forced migrants.

Psychiatric epidemiology research interview–demoralisation scale (PERI-D)

The PERI-D [28] demoralisation scale comprises 27 items which measure nonspecific distress using a five-point scale ranging from 0 ('never') to 4 ('very often') with a composite score calculated by dividing the total score by the number of items completed. It has been employed in a conflict-affected population [40], clinical [41] and community [42] populations, and with Jewish and Middle Eastern immigrants [43–46].

Post-migration living difficulties checklist (PMLDC)

The PMLDC [47] is a 23-item checklist to assess current life stressors of asylum-seekers, having been developed from an ad hoc checklist of a range of typical problems reported by asylum-seekers [48]. Hence, it is an important instrument to measure life experiences other than war [35]. Each item is rated on a 5-point scale from 'no problem' to 'very serious problem', with a composite score determined. The PMLDC has been used [47, 49, 50] or adapted for use [51, 52] in forced migrant populations internationally.

Statistical analysis

All data were analysed using *R* version 3.2.2 [53]. The *eRm* [54] and *ltm* [55] packages were used to conduct the Rasch modelling.

Rasch analysis

Rasch analysis was conducted to examine the construct validity of the STAR-MH at instrument, person, and item levels. Rasch modelling is a probabilistic approach to estimate the difficulty of questionnaire items, which assumes that a single latent construct accounts for item responses [56]. The probability of a person endorsing an item is a logistic function of the item difficulty and person ability [57]. This logistic function is an interval scale with a midpoint of 0. The items are ordered on the scale in descending order according to their difficulty level. Items on the top of the scale are considered more difficult and have lower probabilities that a person endorses it, whereas items at the bottom of the scale are deemed less difficult and have a high probability of being endorsed [57]. In the present context, the latent variable is psychological distress and a high item score indicates higher levels of psychological distress. Therefore, the interpretation of item difficulty is such that a high item difficulty estimate relates to fewer people endorsing the symptom of psychological distress. Conversely, individuals achieving a lower score on the STAR-MH items experience lower psychological distress and are assigned a lower person ability.

Dimensionality and local item dependence

The Rasch model assumes that a set of items are unidimensional, with items being locally independent from each other. The procedure of Drasgow and Lissak [58] was used to check the dimensionality of the dichotomously scored STAR-MH responses using modified parallel analysis with 2000 Monte Carlo samples. The test is implemented in the *ltm* [55] package and a non-significant p-value is indicative of unidimensionality.

Local dependency detection was conducted by using Ponocny's "T1" test [59] for local dependence assessing increased inter-item correlations for all 21 possible item pair combinations. This test is implemented by the *NPtest* function in the *eRm* package [54] and a statistically significant test at $p < .05$ is indicative of local dependence.

Item fit

The information-weighted fit (*infit*) and the outlier-sensitive fit (*outfit*) were used to test whether the items fit the expected model. The infit statistic is more sensitive to unexpected responses to items closest to the person's ability level, whereas outfit statistic is more sensitive to unexpected responses to items further away from the person's ability [60]. Items with respective infit and outfit values between 0.60 and 1.40 are considered a good fit to the Rasch model [61]. In addition, standardized infit (*infit-t*) and outfit (*outfit-t*) statistics and an associated chi-squared statistic were calculated. Items with standardized infit and outfit values of between – 2.50 and 2.50 are deemed to indicate adequate fit to the model. To account for multiple testing using Bonferroni corrections, the chi-squared p-value was multiplied by the number of items in the Rasch model. For this series of analyses, an adjusted p-value of less than 0.05 was considered statistically significant.

Differential item functioning (DIF)

DIF or item bias can occur when different groups within a sample, despite having the same levels of the latent trait (i.e., psychological distress), respond in a different manner to an individual item [57, 62]. There should be no differences in the probability to endorse a certain item based on the subgroups. The logistic regression method [63] implemented by the *difLogistic* function in the *difR* package [64] was used to assess DIF for subgroups based on sex, age, interpreter use, support agency, country of origin, marital status, travel mode, and post-migration detention status. Age was dichotomised based on the median age (18–33 vs. 34+), while country of origin was dichotomised into Southern Asia or other. An effect size based on Nagelkerke's R^2 statistic [65] provides a quantification of DIF [66]. The effect sizes are classified as "negligible" ($R^2 < 0.035$), "moderate" ($0.035 \leq R^2 \leq 0.07$), "large" ($R^2 > 0.07$) [67]. Given the multiple comparisons for each item, the Benjamini and Hochberg (BH) false discovery rate was applied to control for Type I error. This is the recommended adjustment when assessing DIF using logistic regression [68].

Internal consistency

The Person Separation Index (PSI) provides an indication of the internal consistency of the scale and is interpreted in the same manner as the Cronbach alpha coefficient [62]. While a PSI of 0.70 is considered a minimal value for group or research use and 0.85 for individual or clinical use [69], it can be influenced by the number of items in the scale. For scales with few items, it is recommended to report the mean inter-item correlation, with an optimal range of between 0.20 and 0.40 [70].

Receive operating characteristic (ROC) analyses

A receiver operating characteristics (ROC) plot was used to assess the sensitivity and specificity of the STAR-MH in discriminating between participants with caseness for PTSD/MDD and those without. Sensitivity is the proportion of true positives that is correctly identified by the test, while specificity is the proportion of true negatives that is correctly identified by the test [71]. A ROC plot is obtained by calculating the sensitivity and specificity of every observed data value and plotting sensitivity against 1 – specificity. The area under the ROC curve (AUC) is the most used measure of the accuracy of a diagnostic test and ranges between 0.5 and 1, with 0.5 indicating poor accuracy and 1 representing perfect accuracy. Furthermore, a ROC analysis is independent of disease prevalence [71].

The bootstrapped optimism-corrected AUC was calculated to estimate the deterioration that the model will have when applied to new participants using the algorithm of Harrell et al. [72]. This approach outperforms split-sample validation, particularly when the sample size is limited [72, 73]. If the bootstrap optimism-corrected AUC shows acceptable predictive accuracy, then the model is validated [72]. As recommended by Harrell et al. [72], 200 resamples with replacement were drawn from the original data ($N = 185$).

Youden's J statistic [74] was used to determine the optimal cut-off score for the STAR-MH. This was calculated as the sum of sensitivity and specificity for each cut-off value to indicate the test score at which the greatest proportion of individuals is correctly identified as being cases and non-cases. The positive and negative likelihood ratios (PLR/NLR), positive and negative predictive values (PPV/NPV), and predictive accuracy were also calculated for each cut-off score. The *R* package *pROC* [75] was used to conduct the ROC analyses.

Results

The final pilot ('validation sample') screened and psychiatrically evaluated 192 participants from 36 countries and 27 different language groups. Eighty-seven participants were recruited through the ASRC, whilst 85 declined, and 105 individuals were recruited through the MHC whilst 10 declined. Overall, this represents a participation rate of 66.9%.

The STAR-MH was deemed to be culturally appropriate by community leaders of the three largest language groups represented in the sample (i.e., Farsi, Dari and Tamil, comprising 43% of the sample). All confirmed the cultural validity of the tool and believed the tool would be a useful resource in their respective communities.

Participants ranged from 19 to 82 years, with a median age of 33 years (IQR 36–43), and median time in Australia of 2 years (IQR 0.70–3.11). Demographic and clinical characteristics of the sample ($N = 192$) are presented in Additional file 1: Table S1.

Twenty-eight non-mental health workers administered the screening tool, with a median administration time of six minutes ($IQR = 5–7$), irrespective of whether an interpreter was used (i.e., $Md = 5$, $IQR = 4–7$ without interpreter; $Md = 6$, $IQR = 5–7$ with interpreter). The M.I.N.I validation interview took place a median of 5.50 (IQR 0–9) days post-screen and identified rates of MDD and PTSD at 29.7% and 19.9% respectively, with the prevalence of PTSD and/or MDD being 32.3%. Sixty-four participants (33.3%) met criteria for at least one mental disorder and there were only two cases (both of whom were diagnosed with substance use disorder [SUD]; one was nil current) that were not comorbid with PTSD or MDD. Hence for 99% of the total sample, other diagnosed mental disorders (i.e., GAD 3%; panic disorder 2%; SUD 1.5%; psychosis 1%; OCD 0.5%; agoraphobia 0.5%) were comorbid with PTSD or MDD. Suicidality was 6.8%.

Preliminary analyses

Cases with missing responses ($N = 7$, 3.6%) to the STAR-MH were omitted from further analyses. Thus, the resulting sample size was 185 participants (Table 2). Table 3 presents the response frequencies for the eight items which comprised the prospectively tested scale (see *Validation Sample*), excluding the two immediate screen-in items. Item 9 had two missing values and item 10 had five. The response frequencies for the eight items for the total sample ($N = 192$) can be found in Additional file 2: Table S2.

The plot of the total score versus the proportion of endorsed responses for each item (see Fig. 2) revealed low variance for item 6 (sleep), demonstrating a 30% chance that individuals would endorse this item even if they did not endorse other items. Furthermore, the probability of endorsing the sleep item increased as respondents endorsed other items (i.e., higher total score). Based on these findings of unacceptably low specificity item 6 was dropped from subsequent analyses.

Rasch analysis

Item fit

Table 4 presents the item fit statistics from the Rasch analysis. All items had an infit statistic between 0.91 and 1.20, and an outfit statistic between 0.85 and 1.27. Similarly, the outfit-t statistic ranged from – 1.09 to 1.97, and the infit-t statistic ranged from 0.89 to 1.20. The chi-squared test for each item was not statistically significant. This pattern of results indicated that none of the items were misfitting.

Dimensionality and local dependence

The unidimensionality test was not statistically significant ($p = 0.785$), suggesting that the STAR-MH was unidimensional. Ponocny's "T1" test indicated that there were no locally dependent items (all p-values > 0.05).

Differential item functioning (DIF)

The analyses indicated that there was a moderate effect of DIF ($R^2 = 0.04$, $p = 0.023$) for item 4 (*Have you felt very fearful?*) caused by support agency. The ARC group were less likely to endorse this item. No other instances of DIF were detected for sex, age, interpreter use, country of origin, marital status, travel mode, and post-migration detention status.

Internal consistency

The PSI for the 7-item STAR-MH scale was 0.75, which indicated good usability at the group levels, but a lack of sensitivity for individual analyses. However, the average

Table 2 Demographic and clinical variables of participants ($N = 185$)

	N [a] (%) [b]
Gender	
Male	129 (69.7)
Age group	
18–24	24 (13.0)
25–34	75 (40.5)
35–44	48 (25.9)
45–54	27 (14.6)
55+	11 (5.9)
Marital status	
Partnered	111 (60.0)
Mode of Arrival	
Irregular maritime arrival	98 (53.0)
Continent of Origin (UN geoscheme)	
Africa	
East Africa	17 (9.2)
North Africa	10 (5.4)
West Africa	6 (3.2)
Asia	
South Asia	98 (53.0)
South-East Asia	37 (20.0)
West Asia	8 (4.3)
Other	9 (4.9)
Interpreter required	
Yes (screening)	113 (61.1)
Yes (interview)	119 (64.3)
Pre-migration camp/detention	
Yes	26 (14.3)
Post-migration Immigration Detention	
Yes	99 (53.5)
Years in Australia	
< 1 year	34 (18.6)
1–2 years	34 (18.6)
2–3 years	75 (41.0)
> 3 years	40 (21.9)
Residency status	
Temporary Visa (Asylum-seeker)	187 (97.3)
Permanent Residency (Refugee)	5 (2.7)
Mental health diagnosis (Australia)	
Yes	8 (4.6)
MINI-assessed Post-traumatic stress disorder (PTSD)[c]	
Yes	38 (20.7)
MINI-assessed Major depressive disorder (MDD)	
Yes	56 (30.3.7)
Either PTSD or MDD (MINI)	
Yes	61 (33.0)

[a]Total *ns* may be less than 185 due to missing data
[b]Refers to valid percentage, excluding missing data
[c]$n = 184$

inter-item correlation ($r = 0.46$) suggested adequate internal consistency given the small number of items [70].

ROC analyses

Figure 3 presents the ROC plot for participants with caseness for PTSD/MDD compared to those without. The AUC for this analysis was 0.912 (95% CI = 0.868–0.956). Using bootstrap validation, the optimism-corrected AUC was 0.911, which represents the predictive ability of the model in future forced migrants.

Table 5 shows that a STAR-MH cut-off score of 3 produced the best balance of sensitivity and specificity based on Youden's *J*. While a cut-off score of ≥2 for the 7-item scale gave a lower positive predictive value than a score of ≥3, it provided higher negative predictive value, which was a desirable requisite for the screening tool. A cut-off score of three rather than two resulted in a greater PLR, with moderate utility (~ + 20–30% change in probability) whilst the NLR was in the moderate to high range (~ – 30– 45% change in probability) for both cut points [76]. Similarly, the overall diagnostic accuracy was above 80% for both.

Discussion

This paper presents the psychometric properties and utility of a screening tool for use by non-mental health practitioners to screen for mental disorders in asylum-seekers and new refugees (ASR). Our aim was to develop a brief, highly sensitive and easily administrable tool which would alert non-mental health workers of the need to refer a positively screened individual for a mental health evaluation.

The resultant STAR-MH is a psychometrically robust 9-item screening tool comprising two 'immediate screen-in' items and a 7-item scale with a cut-off score of ≥2. The administration time was six minutes, with or without an interpreter, whilst noting in routine use that a positive response to either immediate screen-in item (Items 1 or 2) would obviate the need to continue the screen. Therefore, based on our findings, those who screened positive (22.7%; $n = 42$) to one of the first two items would have been effectively screened in less than 3 min.

Given the small number of items comprising the STAR-MH, internal consistency was sound, and the

Table 3 Response frequencies for STAR-MH items

	Item	Yes *n* (%)[a]	No *n* (%)[a]
3.	Have you felt very restless, like you can't keep still?	55 (29.7%)	130 (70.3%)
4.	Have you lost interest in things?	55 (29.7%)	130 (70.3%)
5.	Have you worried about going crazy or 'losing your mind'?	48 (25.9%)	137 (74.1%)
6.	Have you had a lot of trouble sleeping?	62 (33.5%)	122 (66.5)
7.	Have you felt very fearful?	62 (33.5%)	123 (66.5%)
8.	Have you felt very trapped or caught?	59 (31.9%)	126 (68.1%)
9.	Have you had a lot of pain in your body?	61 (33.0%)	124 (67.0%)
10.	Have you felt very worthless?	54 (29.2%)	131 (70.8%)

Note. [a]Percentages based on $N = 185$

Rasch analyses confirmed the unidimensionality of the 7-item scale and goodness-of-fit of all items. It performed well in the latent construct of psychological distress according to the differential item functioning (DIF) across all subgroups apart from one pilot site for item 7 (*Have you felt very fearful*?). A possible explanation may lie in differing ecological influences between the ASRC and MHC that were not accounted for by the pilot. Further post hoc analyses would need to be conducted to elucidate this, particularly the relationship between fear and psychological distress for this population. However, a putative explanation may lie in the high degree of psychosocial support received by ASRC participants. The protective role of social-emotional support in the mental health of forced migrant populations has been well-established [14, 77].

The ROC curve indicated the STAR-MH to be performing in the excellent range, with a diagnostic accuracy of between 81 and 84%, depending on the cut-off score. The empirically derived cut point suggested an optimum cut-off score of ≥3, however privileging sensitivity to minimise screening out 'true' cases of PTSD or MDD indicated a cut-off score of ≥2. It is anticipated that field testing in a larger ASR sample population will clarify the optimal cut-off score, however, ≥ 2 is most consistent with the aim of optimising sensitivity. In depth testing within specific language and ethnic groups would be justified to confirm the validity of these findings. However, the findings from the bootstrap validation analyses suggest that the diagnostic accuracy of the STAR-MH will not likely be diminished when used with other forced migrant populations.

Notwithstanding the inadequacies of the Western diagnostic lens, PTSD is the most 'robust' epidemiological diagnostic construct that we have for assessing and treating trauma-related symptomatology. However, it is important

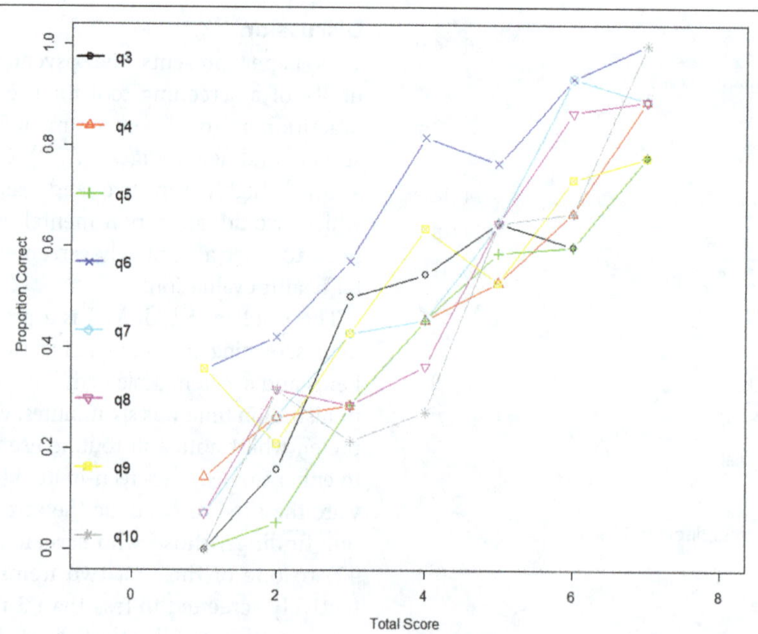

Fig. 2 Total score versus proportion of endorsed (correct) responses for items 3–10

Table 4 STAR-MH item difficulty estimates, chi-squared test, outfit, and infit statistics, and standardised outfit and infit statistics

Item	Difficulty	*SE*	χ^2	*df*	*p*	Outfit	Infit	Outfit-*t*	Infit-*t*
Have you felt very restless, like you can't keep still?	0.06	0.20	98.6	94	1	1.05	1.06	0.41	1.06
Have you lost interest in things?	0.06	0.20	99.4	94	0.269	1.06	1.02	0.47	1.02
Have you worried about going crazy or 'losing your mind'?	0.40	0.21	80.2	94	1	0.85	0.95	−0.99	0.95
Have you felt very fearful?	−0.27	0.20	81.8	94	1	0.87	0.91	−0.99	0.91
Have you felt very trapped or caught?	− 0.13	0.20	90.5	94	1	0.96	0.97	−0.24	0.97
Have you had a lot of pain in your body?	−0.22	0.20	119.6	94	1	1.27	1.20	1.97	1.20
Have you felt very worthless?	0.11	0.20	80.5	94	1	0.86	0.89	−1.09	0.89

to note that diagnostic criteria for disorders such as PTSD and depression are limited in their ability to predict distress and impairment across diverse linguistic and cultural groups. Hence, the items resulting in the final version of the STAR-MH were derived inductively, exploiting measures from scales that have been adapted for use in a range of cultural groups to maximise cultural sensitivity. It is therefore reasoned that the items comprising the STAR-MH reflect trauma manifestations of forced migrant populations rather than corresponding directly to the Western construct of symptoms.

Study limitations included the relatively small sample, consistent with sampling difficulties characteristic of asylum-seeker populations in general [78]. Despite this, the prevalence of PTSD and/or MDD found in this population (32%) was consistent with rates of these disorders found in other ASR populations internationally [10]. Nonetheless, field testing will need to be undertaken to confirm the validity and reliability of the STAR-MH in larger ASR sample populations. Whilst we endeavoured to recruit both a representative and heterogeneous group of administrators and ASR participants (i.e., culturally and linguistically diverse sample), until field studies have been undertaken, the external validity of the tool must be interpreted with caution.

Although administrators were instructed to read the STAR-MH items faithfully and neutrally, no systematic administrator observation was undertaken. In situ translation with different interpreters also presents an increased risk to the fidelity of administration. This raises the critical

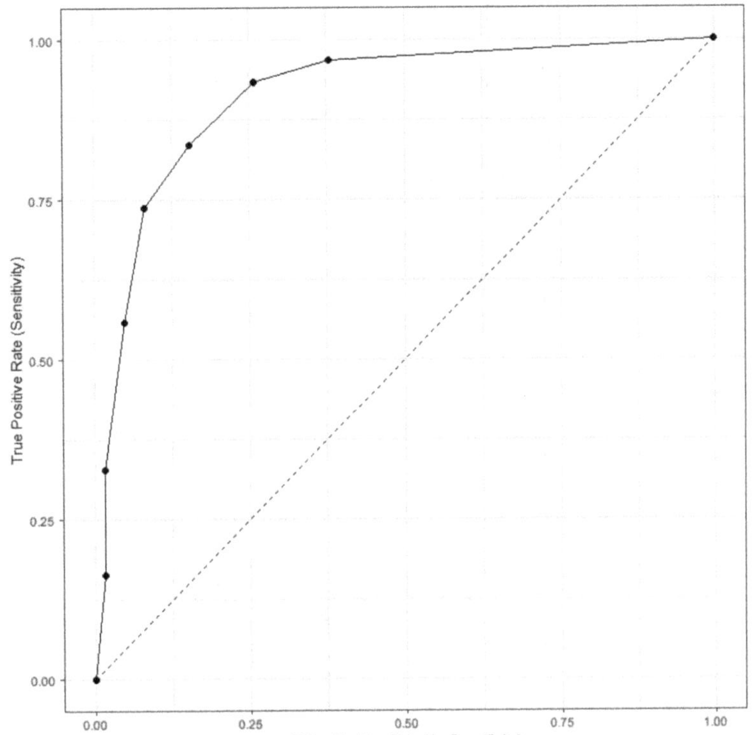

Fig. 3 Receiver operating characteristic plot of STAR-MH scores of participants with caseness for PTSD/MDD and those without

Table 5 Receiver operating curve analysis, likelihood ratios and predictive values of the STAR-MH

Score	Sensitivity % (95% CI)	Specificity % (95% CI)	PLR (95% CI)	NLR (95% CI)	PPV % (95% CI)	NPV % (95% CI)	Efficiency (95% CI)	Youden's *J*
1	96.7% (88.7, 99.6)	63.1% (54.2, 71.4)	2.6 (2.1, 3.3)	0.1 (0.0, 0.2)	55.6% (45.7, 65.1)	97.6% (91.7, 99.7)	74.0% (67.1, 80)	1.60
2	93.4% (84.1, 98.2)	74.6% (66.2, 81.8)	3.7 (2.7, 5)	0.1 (0.0, 0.2)	63.7% (53, 73.6)	96% (90.2, 98.9)	80.7% (74.4, 86.1)	1.68
3	83.6% (71.9, 91.8)	84.6% (77.2, 90.3)	5.5 (3.6, 8.3)	0.2 (0.1, 0.3)	72.2% (60.4, 82.1)	91.7% (85.2, 95.9)	84.4% (78.5, 89.2)	1.69
4	73.8% (60.9, 84.2)	91.5% (85.4, 95.7)	8.8 (4.9, 15.7)	0.3 (0.2, 0.4)	80.7% (68.1, 90)	88.1% (81.5, 93.1)	85.9% (80.2, 90.5)	1.66
5	55.7% (42.4, 68.5)	95.4% (90.2, 98.3)	12.2 (5.4, 27.5)	0.5 (0.3, 0.6)	85.4% (70.8, 94.4)	82.1% (75.1, 87.9)	82.8% 76.7, 87.9)	1.52
6	32.8% (21.3, 46)	98.5% (94.6, 99.8)	21 (5.1, 86.9)	0.7 (0.6, 0.8)	90.9% (70.8, 98.9)	75.3% (68.1, 81.6)	77.1% (70.5, 82.8)	1.31
7	16.4% (8.2, 28.1)	98.5% (94.6, 99.8)	10.5 (2.4, 46.4)	0.9 (0.8, 1.0)	83.3% (51.6, 97.9)	71.1% (63.9, 77.6)	71.9% (64.9, 78.1)	1.15

Note. PLR positive likelihood ratio, *NLR* negative likelihood ratio, *PPV* positive predictive value, and *NPV* negative predictive value

issue of how items were verbally translated by interpreters into culturally valid idioms. However, the STAR-MH is an amalgam of items from gold standard measures of PTSD and MDD symptomatology in ASR populations [35, 79]. Furthermore, leaders from several ethnic communities were consulted about the cultural sensitivity and utility of the STAR-MH and endorsed it for use in their respective communities.

Whilst the brevity and simplicity of the tool means that administrator training is not necessary (i.e., the worker need only follow the instructions on the form itself), the STAR-MH is not designed for self-administration or for lay administration but rather for a worker in the field. This is to ensure that a referral processes can be instigated in the event of a positive screen result and/or an abreaction during the screening process, although none of the latter were noted in this study.

The STAR-MH differentiates itself from related tools in its screening breadth and predictive validity. Hence, in comparison to other widely used screening tools (e.g., K10 and PTSD-8), the STAR-MH screens for both PTSD and MDD. The high comorbidity of PTSD and depression in forced migrant populations [80–82], necessitates a tool that can efficiently screen for both disorders. Unlike the K10 and RHS-15, the STAR-MH has clinical predictive validity, having been validated against a diagnostic instrument in both primary health and community settings. In contrast, relatively high rates of misclassified true cases and non-cases in studies that utilised the K10 in culturally diverse populations have raised questions about its suitability for non-Western groups [17].

Conclusion

The STAR-MH is a simple, sensitive screening tool to facilitate mental health referrals for asylum-seekers and new refugees at the agency of first presentation. The pilot of a 9-item version has demonstrated promising results ahead of field testing to ascertain its external validity in community-dwelling asylum-seeker and new refugee populations in industrialised host nations.

Abbreviations

ASR: Asylum seekers and refugees asylum-seekers; ASRC: Asylum Seeker Resource Centre; AUC: Area under the curve; CI: Confidence intervals; DIF: Differential Item Functioning; GP: General Practitioner; HSCL-25: Hopkins Symptom Checklist-25; HTQ: Harvard Trauma Questionnaire; M.I.N.I.: Mini International Neuropsychiatric Interview; MDD: Major depressive disorder; MHC: Monash Community Health; NLR: Negative likelihood ratio; NPV: Negative predictive value; PERI-D: Psychiatric Epidemiology Research Interview–Demoralisation Scale; PLR: Positive likelihood ratio; PMLDC: Post-migration Living Difficulties Checklist; PPV: Positive predictive value; PSI: The Person Separation Index; PTSD: Post-traumatic stress disorder; ROC: Receiver operating characteristic; SN: Sensitivity; SP: Specificity; STAR-MH: Screening tool for asylum seeker and refugee mental health; WHO: World Health Organisation

Acknowledgements

The authors would like to acknowledge the patients and staff at the Monash Health Refugee Health and Dental services, and the members, staff and volunteers at the Asylum Seeker Resource Centre for theirassistance throughout the pilot and validation studies.

Funding

This project was funded by Cabrini Health and supported by the B.B & A Miller Fund.
Funding bodies had no role in the study design, collection and analysis of data, or writing of the manuscript.

Authors' contributions

DH and SS conceived and designed this study. DH and SS secured funding for the study. DH conducted the study. DH and SM undertook the statistical analysis. All authors drafted, read and approved the final manuscript.

Consent for publication

Not applicable

Competing interests

The authors declare that they have no competing interests.

Author details

[1]Cabrini Institute, 154 Wattletree Road, Malvern, VIC 3144, Australia. [2]Florey Institute of Neuroscience and Mental Health, 30 Royal Parade (Cnr Genetics Lane), Parkville, VIC 3052, Australia. [3]Department of Psychiatry, Faculty of Medicine, Dentistry and Health Sciences, University of Melbourne, Parkville, VIC 3010, Australia. [4]Department of Psychiatry, School of Clinical Sciences, Monash University, Clayton, VIC 3168, Australia. [5]Adult Psychiatry, Monash Medical Centre, Clayton, VIC 3168, Australia.

References

1. UNHCR: Global Trends: the world at war. In.; 2014.
2. Heeren M, Mueller J, Ehlert U, Schnyder U, Copiery N, Maier T. Mental health of asylum seekers: a cross-sectional study of psychiatric disorders. BMC Psychiatry. 2012;12:114-21.
3. Hollifield M, Verbillis-Kolp S, Farmer B, Toolson EC, Woldehaimanot T, Yamazaki J, Holland A, St. Clair J, SooHoo J. The refugee health Screener-15 (RHS-15): development and validation of an instrument for anxiety, depression, and PTSD in refugees. Gen Hosp Psychiatry. 2013;35(2):202–9.
4. Shannon PJ, Im H, Becher E, Simmelink J, Wieling E, O'Fallon A. Screening for War Trauma, Torture, and Mental Health Symptoms Among Newly Arrived Refugees: A National Survey of U.S. Refugee Health Coordinators. Journal of Immigrant & Refugee Studies. 2012;10(4):380–94.
5. Shannon PJ, Vinson GA, Wieling E, Cook T, Letts J. Torture, war trauma, and mental health symptoms of newly arrived Karen refugees. Journal of Loss and Trauma. 2015;20(6):1–14.
6. Hvass AMF, Wejse C. Systematic health screening of refugees after resettlement in recipient countries: a scoping review. Ann Hum Biol. 2017; 44:1–9.
7. Barnes DM. Mental health screening in a refugee population: a program report. J Immigr Health. 2001;3(3):141–9.
8. McMahon J, MacFarlane A, Avalos G, Cantillon P, Murphy AW. A survey of asylum seekers' general practice service utilisation and morbidity patterns. Ir Med J. 2007;100(5):461–4.
9. Porter M, Haslam N. Predisplacement and postdisplacement factors associated with mental health of refugees and internally displaced persons. JAMA. 2005;294(5):602–12.

10. Steel Z, Chey T, Silove DM, Marnane C, Bryant RA, van Ommeren MH. Association of torture and other potentially traumatic events with mental health outcomes among populations exposed to mass conflict and displacement: a systematic review and meta-analysis. JAMA. 2009;302(5):537–49.
11. Gerritsen AA, Bramsen I, Devillé W, van Willigen LH, Hovens JE, van der Ploeg HM. Physical and mental health of afghan, Iranian and Somali asylum seekers and refugees living in the Netherlands. Soc Psychiatry Psychiatr Epidemiol. 2006;41(1):18–26.
12. Toar M, O'Brien KK, Fahey T. Comparison of self-reported health & healthcare utilization between asylum seekers and refugees: An observational study. BMC Public Health. 2009;9:214–24.
13. Heeren M, Wittmann L, Ehlert U, Schnyder U, Maier T, Müller J. Psychopathology and resident status–comparing asylum seekers, refugees, illegal migrants, labor migrants, and residents. Compr Psychiatry. 2014;55(4):818–25.
14. Hocking DC, Kennedy GA, Sundram S. Social factors ameliorate psychiatric disorders in community-based asylum seekers independent of visa status. Psychiatry Res. 2015;230(2):628–36.
15. World Health Organization. Mental health action plan 2013–2020. In: Geneva: world health organisation; 2013.
16. Laban CJ, Gernaat H, Komproe IH, De Jong JTVM. Prevalence and predictors of health service use among Iraqi asylum seekers in the Netherlands. Soc Psychiatry Psychiatr Epidemiol. 2007;42(10):837–44.
17. Stolk Y, Kaplan I, Szwarc J. Clinical use of the Kessler psychological distress scales with culturally diverse groups. Int J Methods Psychiatr Res. 2014;23(2): 161–83.
18. Dowling A, Enticott J, Russell G. Measuring self-rated health status among resettled adult refugee populations to inform practice and policy – a scoping review. BMC Health Serv Res. 2017;17(1):817.
19. Beusenberg M, Orley JH, Organization WH: A User's guide to the self reporting questionnaire (SRQ-20). 1994.
20. Hansen M, Andersen TE, Armour C, Elklit A, Palic S, Mackrill T. PTSD-8: a short PTSD inventory. Clin Pract Epidemiol Ment Health. 2010;6:101–8.
21. Kroenke K, Spitzer RL, Williams JB. The PHQ-9: validity of a brief depression severity measure. J Gen Intern Med. 2001;16(9):600–13.
22. Liebschutz J, Saitz R, Brower V, Keane T, Lloyd-Travaglini C, Averbuch T, Samet J. PTSD in Urban Primary Care: high prevalence and low physician recognition. J Gen Intern Med. 2007;22(6):719–26.
23. Ehlers A, Gene-Cos N, Perrin S. Low recognition of post-traumatic stress disorder in primary care. London Journal of Primary Care. 2009;2(1):36-42.
24. Rodriguez BF, Weisberg RB, Pagano ME, Machan JT, Culpepper L, Keller MB. Mental health treatment received by primary care patients with posttraumatic stress disorder. The Journal of Clinical Psychiatry. 2003;64(10):1230–6.
25. Hocking DC, Sundram S. Screening tool for asylum-seeker mental health (STAMH): a pilot study. Eur Psychiatry. 2016;33:S231.
26. Mollica RF, LS MD, Massagli MP, Silove DM. Measuring Trauma, Measuring Torture: Instructions and guidance on the utilization of the Harvard Program in Refugee Trauma's versions of the Hopkins Symptom Checklist-25 (HSCL-25) & the Harvard Trauma Questionnaire (HTQ). Cambridge, MA: Harvard Program in Refugee Trauma; 2004.
27. Momartin S, Steel Z, Coello M, Aroche JR, Silove D, Brooks R. A comparison of the mental health of refugees with temporary versus permanent protection visas. In: Med J Aust, vol. 185; 2006. p. 357–61.
28. Dohrenwend BP, Shrout PE, Egri G, Mendelsohn FS. Nonspecific psychological distress and other dimensions of psychopathology: measures for use in the general population. Arch Gen Psychiatry. 1980;37(11):1229–36.
29. Sheehan DV, Lecrubier Y, Sheehan KH, Amorim P, Janavs J, Weiller E, Hergueta T, Baker R, Dunbar GC. The mini-international neuropsychiatric interview (M.I.N.I.): the development and validation of a structured diagnostic psychiatric interview for DSM-IV and ICD-10. J Clin Psychiatry. 1998;59(Suppl 20):22–33.
30. Sheehan D, Lecrubier Y, Sheehan KH, Janavs J, Weiller E, Keskiner A, Schinka J, Knapp E, Sheehan M, Dunbar G. The validity of the MINI international neuropsychiatric interview (MINI) according to the SCID-P and its reliability. Eur Psychiatry. 1997;12(5):232–41.
31. Lecrubier Y, Sheehan DV, Weiller E, Amorim P, Bonora I, Harnett Sheehan K, Janavs J, Dunbar GC. The MINI international neuropsychiatric interview (MINI). A short diagnostic structured interview: reliability and validity according to the CIDI. Eur Psychiatry. 1997;12(5):224–31.
32. Bogic M, Njoku A, Priebe S. Long-term mental health of war-refugees: a systematic literature review. BMC Int Health Hum Rights. 2015;15(1):29.
33. Jankovic J, Bremner S, Bogic M, Lecic-Tosevski D, Ajdukovic D, Franciskovic T, Galeazzi GM, Kucukalic A, Morina N, Popovski M, et al. Trauma and suicidality in war affected communities. Eur Psychiatry. 2013;28(8):514–20.
34. Priebe S, Bogic M, Ajdukovic D, Franciskovic T, Galeazzi GM, Kucukalic A, Schutzwohl M. Mental disorders following war in the Balkans: a study in 5 countries. JAMA Psychiatry. 2010;67(5):518–28.
35. Hollifield M, Warner TD, Lian N, Krakow B, Jenkins JH, Kesler J, Stevenson J, Westermeyer J. Measuring trauma and health status in refugees: a critical review. JAMA. 2002;288(5):611–21.
36. Mollica RF, Wyshak G, de Marneffe D, Khuon F, Lavelle J. Indochinese versions of the Hopkins symptom Checklist-25: a screening instrument for the psychiatric care of refugees. Am J Psychiatry. 1987;144(4):497–500.
37. Lhewa D, Banu S, Rosenfeld B, Keller A. Validation of a Tibetan translation of the Hopkins symptom checklist–25 and the Harvard trauma questionnaire. Assessment. 2007;14(3):223–30.
38. Khuon F, Lavelle J. Indochinese versions of the Hopkins symptom Checklist-25: a screening instrument for the psychiatric care of refugees. Am J Psychiatry. 1987;144(4):497–500.
39. Tinghög P, Carstensen J. Cross-cultural equivalence of HSCL-25 and WHO (ten) wellbeing index: findings from a population-based survey of immigrants and non-immigrants in Sweden. Community Ment Health J. 2010;46(1):65–76.
40. Levav I, Kohn R, Billig M. The protective factor of religiosity under terrorism. Psychiatry: Interpersonal and Biological Processes. 2008;71(1):46–58.
41. Shrout PE, Dohrenwend BP, Levav I. A discriminant rule for screening cases of diverse diagnostic types: preliminary results. J Consult Clin Psychol. 1986;54(3):314–9.
42. Gilboa S, Levav I, Gilboa L, Ruiz F. The epidemiology of demoralization in a kibbutz. Acta Psychiatr Scand. 1990;82(1):60–4.
43. Ritsner M, Rabinowitz J, Slyuzberg M. The Talbieh brief distress inventory: a brief instrument to measure psychological distress among immigrants. Compr Psychiatry. 1995;36(6):448–53.
44. Ritsner M, Ponizovsky A, Chemelevsky M, Zetser F, Durst R, Ginath Y. Effects of immigration on the mentally Ill—does it produce psychological distress? Compr Psychiatry. 1996;37(1):17–22.
45. Dohrenwend BP, Levav I, Shrout PE. Screening scales from the psychiatric epidemiology research interview (PERI). In: Weissman A, Myers JK, Ross CE, editors. Community Surveys of Psychiatric Disorders. New Jersey: Rutgers University Press; 1986.
46. Lerner Y, Kertes J, Zilber N. Immigrants from the former soviet union, 5 years post-immigration to Israel: adaptation and risk factors for psychological distress. Psychol Med. 2005;35(12):1805.
47. Silove DM, Steel Z, McGorry P, Mohan P. Trauma exposure, postmigration stressors, and symptoms of anxiety, depression and post-traumatic stress in Tamil asylum-seekers: comparison with refugees and immigrants. Acta Psychiatr Scand. 1998;97(3):175–81.
48. Silove DM, Sinnerbrink I, Field A, Manicavasagar VL, Steel Z. Anxiety, depression and PTSD in asylum-seekers: associations with pre-migration trauma and post-migration stressors. Br J Psychiatry. 1997;170:351–7.
49. Schweitzer RD, Melville F, Steel Z, Lacherez P. Trauma, post-migration living difficulties, and social support as predictors of psychological adjustment in resettled Sudanese refugees. Aust N Z J Psychiatry. 2006;40(2):179–88.
50. Steel Z, Silove D, Brooks R, Momartin S, Alzuhairi B, Susljik I. Impact of immigration detention and temporary protection on the mental health of refugees. Br J Psychiatry. 2006;188:58–64.
51. Laban CJ, Gernaat H, Komproe IH, van der Tweel, I.,, De Jong JTVM: Post-migration living problems and common psychiatric disorders in Iraqi asylum seekers in the Netherlands. J Nerv Ment Dis 2005, 193(12):825–832.
52. Ryan DA, Benson C, Dooley B. Psychological distress and the asylum process: a longitudinal study of forced migrants in Ireland. J Nerv Ment Dis. 2008;196(1):37–45.
53. R Core Team: R: A language and environment for statistical computing. Version 3.2.2. Vienna, Austria: R Foundation for Statistical Computing; 2015.
54. Mair P, Hatzinger R. Extended Rasch modeling: the eRm package for the application of IRT models in R. J Stat Softw. 2007;20(9):1–20.
55. Rizopoulos D: ltm: An R package for latent variable modeling and item response theory analyses.

56. Rasch G. An item analysis which takes individual differences into account. The British journal of mathematical and statistical psychology. 1966;19(1):49–57.
57. Bond TG, Fox CM. Applying the Rasch model: fundamental measurement in the human sciences, vol. 2. New Jersey: Lawrence Erlbaum Associates; 2007.
58. Drasgow F, Lissak RI. Modified parallel analysis: a procedure for examining the latent dimensionality of dichotomously scored item responses. J Appl Psychol. 1983;68(3):363–73.
59. Ponocny I. Nonparametric goodness-of-fit tests for the rasch model. Psychometrika. 2001;66(3):437–59.
60. Linacre JM. What do infit and outfit, mean-square and standardized mean. Rasch Measurement Transactions. 2002;16(2):878.
61. Wright BD, Linacre JM, Gustafson J, Martin-Lof P. Reasonable mean-square fit values. Rasch measurement Transactions. 1994;8(3):370.
62. Wright BD, Stone MH. Measurement essentials. 2nd ed. Wide Range Inc: Wilmington; 1999.
63. Swaminathan H, Rogers HJ. Detecting differential item functioning using logistic regression procedures. J Educ Meas. 1990;27(4):361–70.
64. Magis D, Béland S, Tuerlinckx F, De Boeck P. A general framework and an R package for the detection of dichotomous differential item functioning. Behav Res Methods. 2010;42(3):847–62.
65. Nagelkerke NJ. A note on a general definition of the coefficient of determination. Biometrika. 1991;78(3):691–2.
66. Gómez-Benito J, Hidalgo MD, Padilla J-L. Efficacy of effect size measures in logistic regression: an application for detecting DIF. Methodology. 2009;5(1):18–25.
67. Jodoin MG, Gierl MJ. Evaluating type I error and power rates using an effect size measure with the logistic regression procedure for DIF detection. Appl Meas Educ. 2001;14(4):329–49.
68. Kim J, Oshima TC. Effect of multiple testing adjustment in differential item functioning detection. Educ Psychol Meas. 2013;73(3):458–70.
69. Tennant A, Conaghan PG. The Rasch measurement model in rheumatology: what is it and why use it? When should it be applied, and what should one look for in a Rasch paper. Arthritis Care & Research. 2007;57(8):1358–62.
70. Briggs SR, Cheek JM. The role of factor analysis in the development and evaluation of personality scales. J Pers. 1986;54(1):106–48.
71. Zhou XH, Obuchowski NA, DK MC. Statistical methods in diagnostic medicine. New York: Wiley-Interscience; 2002.
72. Harrell FE, Lee KL, Mark DB. Multivariable prognostic models: issues in developing models,evaluating assumptions and adequacy, and measuring and reducing errors. Stat Med. 1996;15(4):361–87.
73. Smith GCS, Seaman SR, Wood AM, Royston P, White IR. Correcting for optimistic prediction in small data sets. Am J Epidemiol. 2014;180(3):318–24.
74. Youden WJ. Index for rating diagnostic tests. Cancer. 1950;3(1):32–5.
75. Robin X, Turck N, Hainard A, Tiberti N, Lisacek F, Sanchez J-C, Müller M. pROC: an open-source package for R and S+ to analyze and compare ROC curves. BMC Bioinformatics. 2011;12(1):1–8.
76. McGee S. Simplifying likelihood ratios. J Gen Intern Med. 2002;17(8):647–50.
77. Silove DM, Steel Z. Understanding community psychosocial needs after disasters: implications for mental health services. In: J Postgrad Med, vol. 52; 2006. p. 121–5.
78. Silove DM, Steel Z, Watters C. Policies of deterrence and the mental health of asylum seekers. JAMA. 2000;284(5):604–11.
79. Kleijn W, Hovens J, Rodenburg J. Posttraumatic stress symptoms in refugees: assessments with the Harvard trauma questionnaire and the Hopkins symptom checklist–25 in different languages. Psychol Rep. 2001;88(2):527–32.
80. Nickerson A, Schick M, Schnyder U, Bryant RA, Morina N. Comorbidity of posttraumatic stress disorder and depression in tortured, treatment-seeking refugees. J Trauma Stress. 2017;30(4):409–15.
81. Karam EG. Comorbidity of posttraumatic stress disorder and depression. In: Fullerton C, Ursano RJ, editors. Posttraumatic stress disorder: Acute and long-term responses to traumas and disaster. Washington DC: American Psychiatric Press; 1997. p. 77–90.
82. Fazel M, Wheeler J, Danesh J. Prevalence of serious mental disorder in 7000 refugees resettled in western countries: a systematic review. Lancet. 2005;365(9467):1309–14.

Understanding the ups and downs of living well: the voices of people experiencing early mental health recovery

Nicola Hancock[1*], Jennifer Smith-Merry[1], Glenda Jessup[1], Sarah Wayland[2] and Allison Kokany[3]

Abstract

Background: The aim of this study was to better understand early-stage mental health recovery experiences of people living with severe and persistent mental illness and complex needs.

Methods: Semi-structured, in-depth interviews were conducted with 13 people engaged in an Australian program specifically designed for people facing complex barriers to their recovery. Interview data were analysed thematically using constant comparative methods.

Results: Participants described engaging with seven interconnecting aspects of early recovery: (1) engaging with the challenge of recovery; (2) struggling for a secure and stable footing; (3) grieving for what was and what could have been; (4) seeking and finding hope; (5) navigating complex relationships; (6) connecting with formal and informal support, and finally, (7) juggling a complexity of health issues.

Conclusions: This study illuminated the complexity of earlier-stage recovery which was characterised both by challenging personal circumstances and a hope for the future. It illustrated that even at an early point in their recovery journey, and amidst these challenging circumstances, people still actively engage with support, draw on inner strengths, source resources and find accomplishments. Stability and security was foundational to the ability of participants to draw on their own strengths and move forward. Stability came when material needs, including housing, were addressed, and an individual was able to connect with a supportive network of workers, carers, friends and family.

Keywords: Early recovery, Recovery, Mental illness, Experience, Severe and complex mental illness

Background

Consistent evidence now refutes previously pessimistic views (e.g., [1, 2]), that severe and persistent mental illnesses such as schizophrenia, are inevitably degenerative and life-long. A multitude of large, longitudinal studies evidence that at least a quarter of people living with severe and persistent mental illnesses such as schizophrenia, will recover in a curative or clinical sense [3]. However, rather than this curative framing or understanding of recovery, mental health systems and policies internationally have adopted a different, personal or consumer-defined, understanding of recovery. This personal recovery is witnessed in published testimonies of consumers or people living with mental illness themselves as well as the analysis and synthesis of first-person qualitative data [4, 5]. These accounts emphasise an individualised, ongoing and non-linear journey towards living a life of personal meaning and value irrespective of whether symptoms of mental illness persist or not (e.g., [6, 7]). This understanding of recovery, is the focus of the current study.

While the language of personal recovery is now visible across mental health policies, system guidelines and plans internationally (e.g., [8–10]), there remain challenges regarding the utility and relevance of dominant discourses and understandings of recovery across the diversity of experiences for those living with mental illness.

* Correspondence: nicola.hancock@sydney.edu.au
[1]The University of Sydney, Sydney, Australia
Full list of author information is available at the end of the article

Critics have also challenged conceptualisations and models developed to operationalise the construct of recovery as too optimistic. The literature lacks a focus upon the more complex process of recovery experiences by many living with severe and persistent mental illness at earlier points in their recovery journey [11]. It is therefore argued that, without a more inclusive conceptualisation or model, recovery is not accessible or considered relevant or relatable to many individuals commencing their recovery journey, or to those supporting them [12, 13].

There has been a call for a more nuanced understanding of recovery which, while focusing on the positive parts of the recovery journey, also acknowledges and respects the perhaps more challenging earlier recovery experiences. This more inclusive conceptualisation would place more emphasis on difficulties and complexity as a valid and normal part of recovery. Authors [14], in a meta-synthesis of 12 qualitative studies of recovery, evidenced that there are indeed complexities and difficulties that are not encapsulated in dominant recovery discourse and models. Comparing the data against the much heralded CHIME (Connectedness, Hope and optimism, Identity, Meaning, Empowerment) recovery model [15], they found that only 70% of data fitted within the relatively optimistic themes of this model. The authors coded the remaining data under four additional themes, one of which they labelled "Difficulties", encompassing: ambivalence and contradiction; disempowerment; financial concerns; loss and negative life changes; stumbling, struggling and suffering and substance use comorbid with mental illness. Difficulties was the second most frequently occurring theme overall, second only to the CHIME theme of Empowerment. They argued for a conceptualisation of recovery in which difficulties and struggles are more prominently considered, so that an overly optimistic view of recovery does not result in professionals' homogenising or blaming individuals [14].

While recovery is understood as an individual and often non-linear journey, numerous authors have proposed that a person's recovery process involves a process of early, mid and later stages. There has been less focus upon recovery's early stages and the literature on stages may thus be less relevant or meaningful to those at this earlier point on their recovery journey. This is perhaps because a staged understanding of recovery is typically informed by those at later stages of recovery reflecting back on their experiences, rather than being informed by in-the moment experiences [14, 16]. It might also be because of a desire, in line with recovery philosophy, to focus upon the positive. For these reasons, and likely others, we have a much poorer understanding of the early-stage recovery experiences and achievements than we do of later stages [14, 17].

With these considerations in mind we sought to understand the early recovery experiences of people engaged in a Sydney-based Partners in Recovery (PIR) program. This national, government-funded, program was established to support individuals with severe and persistent mental illness and complex needs or barriers (e.g. homelessness, drug-use, physical ill-health) to engaging in their recovery. Central to PIR programs are the support facilitators who meets with individuals to understand their needs and goals and then seek out and bring together the services needed. The PIR initiative, including the demographic profile of program participants, their needs and the role of the Support Facilitator is described in further detail elsewhere [18–20]. While the program, as indicated in its name, has a specific orientation to recovery, there was little understanding of who this group were and their specific recovery needs when it was initiated [21]. There was also little literature that spoke directly to this group which could be drawn on to either assist support facilitators in their work or to provide PIR clients with a realistic representation of what recovery may involve for them. For that reason we set out to better understand the recovery experiences of people assessed as currently experiencing a complexity of needs and multiple barriers to engaging in their recovery.

Methods

Aims and study design

This project aimed to better understand the recovery experiences of people with severe and complex mental illness. A qualitative approach built around semi-structured, in-depth interviews was adopted in order to develop a rich understanding of participants' experiences of mental health recovery. Pseudonyms are used to protect participant confidentiality. The study practices were aligned with the consolidated criteria for reporting qualitative research (COREQ) [22].

Participant recruitment

Participants were recruited from a Sydney-based PIR program operating in an area of high social disadvantage. The demographic profile of PIR participants in this program has been reported elsewhere [23]. To be eligible for the study, potential participants needed to be deemed: 1) able to provide informed consent, and 2) able to participate in an interview without the interview being likely to cause significant distress. This was determined by Support Facilitators who identified eligible potential participants. These individuals were sent an invitation to participate by the PIR administration staff. A participant information sheet containing the interview questions was included with the invitation letter so that potential participants understood what would be covered in the interviews. Consumers were asked to contact the research team directly if they wanted to participate in the research. Participants received a $20AUS grocery card as appreciation for their time and stories.

Data collection

Semi-structured, in-depth interviews were facilitated by the use of an interview guide. The guide consisted of broad questions focused around the topic of inquiry such as "What has helped or made you feel good as part of your recovery journey?" and "What has caused difficulties for you on recovery journey?" The guide was designed to ensure all pertinent areas were explored, while providing enough flexibility to ensure participants could elaborate on aspects of recovery that were most pertinent to them.

Each participant's Support Facilitator was present at the interview location (although not in the room unless requested). During the interview, the trained interviewer (SW) checked for participant distress by monitoring each participant's responses and non-verbal cues. If participants became distressed they were asked if they wished to take a break or to stop the interview. Participants were given an opportunity to speak with their support facilitators after the interview to ensure they were not unduly distressed as a result of the interview. Interviews took between 22 and 74 min and were recorded, transcribed verbatim, and summaries sent to each participant for the opportunity to remove any materials that they did not want included in the final study. No data was requested to be removed.

Data analysis

Data were entered into NVivo 10 [24] and analysed using constant comparative analysis [25, 26]. The first stage of analysis involved a process of line-by-line coding to label small segments of data to summarise concepts [26]. A code could be a word, sentence, or paragraph that expressed a single idea, feeling, experience or topic. As this analysis continued, data and codes were constantly compared within and between transcripts. Two authors (GJ and NH) independently coded the first two transcripts, and then came together to discuss, compare, and reach consensus on early coding decisions. Subsequent transcripts were coded by author GJ. The next stage of analysis, focused coding, involved examining the relationship between codes and synthesising or drawing together those that were conceptually overlapping into broader conceptual categories [26]. These categories also included examples of exceptions, contradictions and contrasts. Throughout the analysis, reflexive discussions were conducted between authors (GJ and NH) to ensure emerging codes were representative of the data, enhancing coding rigor [26]. A third author independently reviewed all coding (JSM).

Results

Participants

Thirteen consumers, eleven female and two males, contacted the research team and were interviewed. In keeping with the PIR inclusion guidelines all had a severe and persistent mental illness with a complicating co-morbidity, including physical ill-health or addiction. To mimimise risk of distress, participants were not directly asked about their diagnoses, however through interview data, it was evident that: most had more than one psychiatric diagnosis; five were currently grappling with additional drug and or alcohol addiction, and almost all described a range of physical health co-morbidities, including three who were concurrently grappling with cancer. Six participants were currently in precarious accommodation. All participants were aged between 18 and 65, the criteria for PIR registration. Nine participants described lengthy periods as an inpatient within a psychiatric hospital, with one person having recently spent over 30 years in an inpatient facility (Table 1).

All participants described their experience of mental health recovery as an ongoing, active, challenging, but ultimately positive journey of ups and downs. Our analysis of the data brought to light seven inter-connected, over-arching experiences that patients spoke about as central to their recovery journeys including: (1) engaging with the challenge of recovery; (2) struggling to find safety and security; (3) grieving for what was and what could have been; (4) seeking and finding hope and purpose; (5) navigating complex relationships; (6) connecting with formal and informal support; and finally, (7)

Table 1 Early mental health recovery: themes and sub-themes

1. Engaging with the challenge of recovery
a it needs to be me
b standing up for myself
c fighting the desire to withdraw or give up
d accepting support and that recovery can't be 'done' alone
e struggling with stigma and learning to be king to yourself
2. Struggling to find safety and security
3. Grieving for what was and what could have been
4. Seeking and finding hope and purpose
5. Navigating complex relationships
a managing the impact of illness on others
b separating carer roles from family and friends
c managing and avoiding unhelpful relationships
6. Connecting with formal and informal support
7. Juggling a complexity of health issues

juggling a complexity of health issues. These are detailed below. Quotations are an important part of reporting qualitative research. They provide illustration and evidence that findings and interpretations have arisen from the data [22, 27]. We utilise quotations extensively to demonstrate as much as possible what recovery meant for participants in their own words.

Engaging with the challenge of recovery

Repeatedly participants used the word 'fight' to describe the internal processes involved in their recovery. This internal fight involved: coming to terms that it needs to be me; standing up for myself; fighting the desire to withdraw or give-up; accepting support and that recovery can't be done alone; and struggling against stigma – learning to be kind to yourself.

It needs to be me All participants talked about coming to the realisation that they needed to be active in their own recovery. Lara reflected on this process: *"I believed I could go to a doctor... I believed there was a magic pill. The only magic pill is from within.... you have to make that step, and it's scary."* Some participants were very clear and resolute, for example, Naree said: *"I have to do this for myself. Nobody can do it for me"*. Suzy commented, *"I'm not going to be able to progress....if I don't find a way to deal with... those issues that I now know I have. "* Other participants grappled with this, and their sense of agency fluctuated: *"I feel like sometimes I'm trying to climb up a hill and I just keep getting pushed back down, so I just sit there and think, well, bugger it. But then I find after a day or two... I get back [up]... I get this inner strength"* (Lara).

Standing up for myself Participants repeatedly discussed the difficulty but importance of standing their ground, challenging advice and instructions, and standing up against clinical views and practices that they did not agree with. They talked about the fight to get the right medication and treatment. Most participants felt that they were often not listened to when it came to medication. Ann said, *"They were medicating me, but not listening too... it was horrible."* Similarly, Suzy said *"within 20 minutes [psychiatrist] had given me all these diagnoses, which are true, but the medication - he put me on medication with 20 minutes of meeting me, not even knowing too much about me."* Ryan commented, *"GPs and all that ... after a couple of sessions they just want to prescribe you medication."* Ann challenged the clinical treatment she was receiving: *"...before I saw my current psychiatrist I saw another one. If I said to her I feel a bit anxious [her response was] "have another pill", to the point where I asked in the end for a second opinion whilst I was an inpatient, and ended up seeing my current psychiatrist for a second opinion. He flipped. He* [said] *you are on double the recommended doses of some of this stuff."* Standing up to professionals however, particularly when it came to medication or being believed, was not always easy. As Ann commented, *"It's hard to question professional advice."* At this early stage on their recovery journey participants did not always feel able to stand up for themselves and argue for their needs. Questioning was made easier if participants felt validated by other professionals. Coralyn's counsellor, for example, encouraged her to question treatment decisions, by saying to her *"... stand for your right. When you don't have the answer, when you don't ask... how are you going to find your answer?"*

Fighting the desire to withdraw or give-up Another internal fight repeatedly described by participants was the battle against a desire to give up or withdraw from the process of recovery. Participants talked about fighting against internal negative impulses, thoughts, poor coping habits, or self-doubt. Ann's *"constant fight"* was against negative thoughts, *"they drive me batty"*, while Suzy fought the desire to give up on life, *"At the very last moment before I try to commit suicide I'd be saying... 'What are you doing? Don't stop fighting, don't give up.'"* Julie fought the impulse to isolate herself from others, *"I'm trying to get my life where I shouldn't have to keep myself in my house."* Suzy and Naree spoke about fighting against and sometimes giving in to drugs and alcohol which they had adopted as coping habits.

Accepting support and that recovery can't be 'done' alone Participants described coming to a point of realising, they could not, and did not have to, strive for recovery alone. They described a sometimes challenging process of accepting that they needed help, formal or informal, from others. Dana reflected, *"I do strive for independence, but at the same time, I'm aware that I need a network of support...to be independent."* Lara echoed Dana's sentiment, *"... you need support. Without support, it can't be done."* However, learning to ask for and accept help did not always come easily. Dana, found it *"quite hard."* She commented, *"Three years ago, I could have got all this help... but I don't know if I would have been strong enough to accept all that help at the same time."* Kerry also had difficulty asking for help: *"I've been a proud independent person and I've earned good money over the years.... I hate having to ask for help."*

Struggling with stigma and learning to be king to yourself Participants described struggling against their own and others' judgements and stigma, and the need to learn to be kind to themselves. They repeatedly spoke about encountering stigma from people in their communities. Participants recounted how both their own and others' stigma surrounding mental illness affected their preparedness to disclose, and their relationships with others. Suzy commented, "I *need people to know,... for my growth and my benefit,... I need them to know about mental health. It's not scary and it's not wrong.*" Dana, who initially did not disclose or discuss her mental illness with her family, *"we didn't talk about it very much at all. Yeah, so it pretty much wasn't there"* talked about the value of them ultimately understanding and *"not... pretending... you* [the family] *know"*. Kerry could not disclose to her church friends, *"Mental health within church circles isn't always widely accepted as a 'thing'. They can deal with a broken leg or a broken back but mental illness they don't deal well with."* Another participant (Ann) was cut off from family contact because of her mental illness. Stigma from others compounded the self-judgement participants levelled at themselves. Lara said that she had become, *"antisocial, to protect everyone else from me."* Some participants talked about finding the strength to overcome self- and others' judgement and about starting to be gentler and kinder to themselves. Kerry, for example, reflected on the importance of, *"learning to be kinder to myself on those days when I'm not having a good day."* Yvonne, described her strength in overcoming previously hurtful comments from others: *"you've got a choice either to let it get to you or... use it to... gain your inner strength."*

Struggling to find safety and security

All but one participant described struggling for immediate safety and security in their lives. This included the need for physical safety, secure and stable housing, food and basic daily necessities, and reliable, dependable support services. Malcolm, for example, wanted reassurance, *"that my future is safe."* Naree needed a safe place to live stating that "*stability is the home.... There's a roof. It's very important... Once I have stability I'm fine*" Brenda commented, that *"people don't realise how much [difficult] financial states of things... can add to your mental health and the strain that it puts on you."* Housing stability was emphasised most frequently with lack of money exacerbated participants' housing instability. They described being subject to short rental periods, having nowhere to go when their lease expired, lived in substandard housing, or in neighbourhoods in which they felt unsafe. Eileen for example felt *"terrified"* and unsafe in her public housing, *"You can't walk the streets...you're living around ice addicts and they're always breaking into my backyard.... I get scared for my son."* Participants escaping domestic violence had spent time in refuges, often with their children. Others had spent time being homeless. Yvonne, the only participant who did not express a need for stability, lived in a *"tight-knit family"* and drew on them for stable support.

Desperate attempts to meet these basic needs sometimes led to participants making decisions, actions and choices they later regretted. Sometimes, to fulfil their basic needs, participants put themselves at risk physically or legally. For example, Suzy, *"not thinking very clearly whatsoever, just the desperation of wanting to get somewhere"* agreed to a stranger visiting her home to discuss accommodation. *"He arrived at my place and he sexually assaulted me.... I should have thought about it better."* Naree, who, with her young daughter, had escaped domestic violence, recounted, *"I was falling behind in my rent.... before I know it I'm in mess and it's really hard to catch up."* She tried to sell drugs to make some quick money and was arrested, *"life slapped me so hard.... I thought, that's it, I'm screwed up and now ... I've definitely lost [daughter]."*

The stability of affordable support services was also regarded as a basic need. Lara reflected on unreliable services and *"constantly... getting let down"* with, *"counsellors saying, 'all right, your time is up now,' your file goes there and you'll be okay'."* She contrasted these experiences with her current counsellor who said, *"You belong here whenever you want to belong here."* Stability of support services could be compromised by instability in the individual's own lives. Naree's frequent accommodation changes, for example, impacted on the continuation of her support services: *"every time I had someone calling... to catch up and see me, I was changing location."* She continued, *"By the time they get their arse there I'm [at] a different address. So they go, 'okay, that's out of my area'.... They were not interested in me... Even though I was screaming out for help."* Financial barriers also reduced service stability. Lara said, *"the money gets too high, the cost."*

Grieving for what was and what could have been

Participants described grieving over the losses they experienced due to mental illness. These included: loss of a previous identity, loss of dreams and aspirations, and loss of family and social networks. Kerry said, *"I didn't realise how much...my identity was tied up into being a nurse."* Ann *"cried buckets over the fact that I can't work...I'm no longer the same as everybody else."* Dana lost her job and with it, her social network, *"when I took the work away...there was just me at home with the kids.... there are no networks there."* Suzy also struggles to find her purpose in life, *"I'm trying to find out who I am and what my purpose is here."* Her dream, *"was to have a husband and kids and that's what I've wanted since I was little."* Instead she felt that she had lost *"everything"* because of her heroin use. Ryan's aspirations changed when he went to jail, *"I had everything, I was working, everything."* Coralyn, who took great pride in her appearance, gained weight on her medication. She struggles to reconcile with this new self-image, *"I'm short and the tiny bones, and just getting fatter and fat...and lots of puffiness."*

Seeking and finding hope and purpose

Alongside living with loss, participants described seeking and finding purpose and hope for their future. Lara's recovery defied others' messages of hopelessness: *"I used to think that I wasn't worth helping...that they'd come to the end of the road with me.... I have been told by people that nothing will ever change"* Hopelessness was, *"horrible... I'd just go home and cut myself."* Over time Lara came to new realisations, *"But now I realise, of course there's hope."*

Hope supported people to seek and finding purpose and meaning through doing positive things both for themselves and for others. Life was more meaningful when participants were doing positive things for themselves: *"you have to put yourself first."* (Julie). Yvonne loved long nature walks, *"I go for walks, I sing out loud."* Malcolm wrote poetry, *"My poems [are] something special.... I write unique stuff.... I always remember myself as an inheritor of my own contribution to life on earth."* Participants also valued structure in their day. Ann, for example, needed *"something on each day to try and keep me well and accountable."*

Beyond doing things for themselves, participants found affirmation and purpose in doing things for others. Ann gave her artwork to friends. Suzy helped her neighbour, *"they're struggling. I've got some spare bed frames and stuff, she needs a bed and they need food vouchers. So I ran around and got all the numbers and made appointments for stuff like that."* Kerry is training as a counsellor. She feels her experiences have qualified her to help others, *"I went through all of that for the here and now... for me to help others... you can't look at it any other way."*

Seven participants were parents. This parenting role gave them a sense of being needed by another even when their children were now adults. Supporting, protecting, guiding and seeking to re-gain custody of children was a central life purpose for most participants. Parents described finding purpose and accomplishment in meeting their children's needs and routines. Julie was doing new things for her children which she felt proud of, *"changing eating habits.... Setting them some little goals.... That's new for them."* Naree reflected, *"I came out better because [daughter's] there...You realise how beautiful that little thing has been in your life ... still hugs you and says, 'Mummy I love you.'"* They also found purpose in being good role models for their children, or giving them a better life than they had experienced. Lara commented, *"Everything I do is for [son], because I don't want him to see me as a failure. I want him to understand that... you've got to take a step forward to get somewhere."* Eileen's energies were directed towards her youngest son's future, *"I fought too hard to keep this boy alive. I'm not going to sit back and watch him go down the drain and become a street buck. He's better than that."*

For some participants, religious faith provided hope and purpose in life. Participants however, described needing to reconcile why they had been subjected to deep suffering. Ann found hope in her belief that *"Jesus will come again and there will be no more sadness, no more tears, no more pain, no more suffering."* In contrast, Suzy said *"there's a bit of faith left... I've got some renewed faith"* but *"I'm still finding it hard to believe that there's something out there that wants good things for me, because I've got nothing but pain."* She described being *"envious"* of people who had a strong faith, *"I want something like that."*

Navigating complex relationships

Participants spoke about navigating complex friend and family relationships. They described navigating: a) the impact of their illness on others; b) the need to separate carer roles from friends and family, and c) managing and avoiding unhelpful relationships.

Managing the impact of illness on others Participants expressed concern about the impact their illness might have on friends and family. Suzy for example, felt that her good friend should not have to be *"putting up with my crap."* Lara, described being *"very upfront"* with her young son about her illness, but striving to provide him with age-appropriate explanations for what he witnessed, *"I had to, otherwise he would have been a very screwed up kid."*

Separating carer roles from family and friends Participants also struggled to keep carer roles separate from friend and family relationships. Ann's friends, *"were starting to take over"* as carers. This became a source of tension, *"I like to keep my friends as friends and my carers as carers."* Equally, the adult children of some participants assumed carer roles and participants felt ambivalent about this. While acknowledging its necessity, some described a sadness about this blurring of roles. Julie for example reflected, *"I don't like ... that, because I'm the parent. I'm the one that's supposed to be supporting people, not them supporting me... I shouldn't have to speak to her [daughter] because I'm a parent."* and Lara recounted *"My son had to do everything for me, take me shopping, talk for me, ring up people."* Ann's support services helped her negotiate the tension of friends becoming carers by sourcing personal carers for her.

Managing and avoiding unhelpful relationships For most participants, family relationships were exceedingly complex to negotiate. Family members could support or hinder recovery. Eileen, who had isolated herself from friends who were drug users to live *"a very lonely"* but *"safe"* life, found it more difficult to isolate herself from her brother, a drug user, with whom she shared accommodation, *"I was so angry and disappointed that my brother was using drugs under my roof."* Ann was one of a number of participants whose family had stopped having contact with her. She replaced this loss with her *"church family"*, but still found traditional festive times difficult: *"They're* [biological family] *all together for birthdays, Christmas, Easter...I'm just not welcome there. "* Coralyn needed protection from an emotionally abusive husband, whom she could not afford, financially, to leave. She battled to have her reports of abuse believed and not dismissed as *"a mental person making a story"*. Being vindicated, helped her endure, *"I have someone to talk and believe, and help....my psychologist believes me, my friends believing me... People who can support me and stand behind... me."* Ann and Naree described needing to set boundaries in their relationships with their mothers. Ann commented, *"Probably the best thing that I've done in terms of my wellness journey is really limiting the amount of time I'm with my mother...she's nasty when she drinks."* Naree's *"relapse prevention strategies"* included not depending on her mother because: *"You [mother] just take off.... By the time you come back, I've already done the grieving .... picked myself up ...going stable... then you turn up."*

Connecting with formal and informal support

Participants described two important connections that supported their recovery. These were support workers and informal supports that included peers, helpful friends and family members. Participants highly valued the help they received from their Support Facilitators and other mental health workers or professionals. They valued their: persistence; care in checking on them through the ups and downs; accessibility; ability to facilitate access to resources; belief in them, and their focus on them as individuals. Julie said, *"...ever since I've met [Support Worker]... she's actually made me a little bit stronger... I know that sounds stupid, meeting somebody that you've only known for a few months who's given you the courage and the knowledge to be able to go places."* Kerry, explaining the difference between friends and her Support Worker, stated *"I had my friends, but they didn't understand. They just knew that I was doing things that weren't safe.... If it hadn't been for [Support Worker] walking beside me, just being that strength there for me I wouldn't have got through."*

The personal connection and accessibility of workers was important to participants. Ryan, for example commented, *"...if I get too worried, I'll talk to [support worker], I'll ring her up for support."* Julie said, *"You feel like you can speak to her about anything"*. Naree described feeling valued, *"...the fact that she shouted me coffee and she said, do you want something to eat? It was great because you feel like, wow, you feel important. I haven't felt like that for a long time."* Ann said her psychiatrist, *"...respects me, and he has said to me on numerous occasions 'You're the expert in this, you tell me', and that's good."*

However participants did not feel this connection with all mental health workers. *"I've got that connection to [Support worker] that I can't seem to get with a psychologist. I think it's because I trust her and she knows a lot about what's going on. She's seen me in my ups and she's seen me in my downs, where they haven't."* The support workers that participants described as 'successful' at engaging or connecting were those that were personable, valued them as individuals and were able to connect them with services and supports that facilitated their recovery, such as housing (Kerry; Julie), the Police (Suzy), financial advisors (Dana), the National Disability Insurance Scheme and physical health support (Brenda). Participants spoke of the importance of working in a team with support workers to identify and source services. Brenda enjoyed feeling part of a team when exploring support options and resources, "*[support worker] said," "I don't know a lot about it" and I said, "neither do I." "So we went as like a team together."*

Some participants also described the value of connecting with peers, or others with their own lived experience of mental illness. Lara for example, felt *"inspired"* by peer workshops, *"I take everything I can with me and use it in day to day life...you do go home knowing that you're not alone and you can make friends."* Peer connection was important to Lara as she had isolated herself from other people: *"I find with this illness, most people are like me, they'll hide from the public because they're worried about what people will say. But when you meet likeminded people ....it can do a lot of good."*

Juggling a complexity of health issues

Participants described having to navigate a multitude of health challenges. Most were living with more than one mental illness; five participants additionally managed chronic physical conditions, and five participants spoke about struggling with drug and alcohol addiction. Participants described being overwhelmed by the medication regime required to treat both mind and body. They reported that mental health facilities did not consider or address their physical conditions, and physical health services didn't consider their mental health needs. This siloed approach hindered their recovery. Ann noted, *"My biggest problem with actively seeking out help... at [mental health facility] is they don't look after my physical health there because it's not an acute hospital."*

Stigma associated with mental ill-health also influenced the treatment of physical conditions. A number of participants described barriers to accessing pain medication for physical health needs, especially if they were also experiencing drug addiction. Eileen, who has a back injury, commented, *"I went to the hospital for pain...because I couldn't stand the pain in my spine. They weren't even interested in looking at my spine; just* [saw me as a] *junkie and that stigma sticks."* Similarly Lara, who had cancer, found, *"they [doctors] wouldn't give me pain meds, they'd treat me like a drug addict."* However, some participants, including Lara talk triumphantly of successfully managing the double whammy of physical and mental health issues: *"I've done all that on my own and I've come out the other side.... If I can do this, I can do anything".*

Discussion

While challenges of experiencing mental illnesses, particularly those with illnesses labelled severe and persistent, are well reported, an account of these challenges are absent from much of the recovery-focused literature. Given that recovery and recovery-focused practice are increasingly prominent in policies and mental health service plans internationally [e.g., 8, 9, 10], it is important to ensure that this 'paradigm' is inclusive of and relevant to those at an earlier and more complex point of their recovery journey, and does not un-intentionally exclude them. While the recovery experiences of people in the later stages of recovery have been documented (e.g., [17, 28]), there is a need to better understand the experiences of those who are beginning their recovery. Our research findings facilitate the 'expansion' of our understanding and framing of recovery by focusing on early recovery. This knowledge is important because insights into consumers' perspectives and needs early on in their recovery journey can ensure that support services can be more effectively tailored to meet earlier recovery needs and that both consumers, and those that support them, do not feel discouraged by comparing their recovery experiences to accounts of later stage recovery.

A sense of resilience came through these interviews, of strength amidst adversity and a sense of triumph. In all of the interviews people spoke about their hopes for the future and the steps that they had taken towards recovery. However it was not an easy recovery journey for these participants and there was a sense of vulnerability as they recounted past difficulties and ongoing struggles. The results reveal seven key aspects of early recovery: (1) engaging with the challenge of recovery; (2) struggling to find safety and security; (3) grieving for what was and what could have been; (4) seeking and finding hope and purpose; (5) navigating complex relationships; (6) connecting with formal and informal support; and, (7) juggling a complexity of health issues. These findings align with and extend the CHIME (Connectedness, Hope and optimism, Identity, Meaning, Empowerment) model or framework of recovery [15] by adding a layer of early recovery complexity.

Within the CHIME framework 'connectedness' refers to positive relationships with peers, family, friends and health professionals. Early in recovery, connectedness is central and our results showed that positive human supports were the greatest facilitator of early recovery and this extended to workers. Helpful workers, were those that valued people as individuals, showed kindness and saw them as experts in their own recovery. These accounts emphasised the importance of personal, human connections, a relational approach in which people are individually valued and their agency recognised despite the perceived 'messiness' of their lives at this early stage of recovery. However there are also numerous challenges to overcome for connection. Participants were navigating and learning to 'leave' un-helpful relationships behind. They were struggling with loss of relationships and to keep friend and family relationships distinct from carer roles. They were also learning to stand up against health professional practices, and directives that they did not agree with and to seek second opinions.

A second component of the CHIME model is hope and optimism – a belief that a better life is both possible and attainable. For participants in this study, hope and optimism waxed and waned. What was important was repeatedly re-finding them and fighting the urge to withdraw or give up. Identity and regaining a positive sense of self is the third component of CHIME. Participants in this study described battling with self-stigma and seeing beyond the immediate. They described learning to be kinder to themselves but talked little about longer-term visions for their future. Meaning as defined within the CHIME model was also reflected in participant stories. Participants found meaning through doing things for themselves, doing things for others and for some, through religious faith. Parenting roles provided great meaning for many participants. Importantly, meaning and identity were tempered by grieving for the losses associated with having a mental illness, be that loss of employment, loss of connections and family, or loss of previous life dream or aspirations. Finally, empowerment in the CHIME model refers to control over an individual's life and the decisions about their treatment and supports. Participants were learning and still struggling to assert their views and wishes within the treatment and service context. Some workers facilitated empowerment while others did not. Control over life more broadly was still not in the grasp of most participants. This leads to the aspect of this study that is not captured within the CHIME model: a secure and stable footing. Central to participants' ability to engage in their recovery was material, interpersonal and environmental stability and security.

Stability of material needs provided a basis from which recovery could be prioritised [7]. The struggle for basic physical needs featured prominently in these interviews. Participants spoke about the need for money, food and above all stable accommodation. The lack of stable, affordable and safe accommodation impacted on consumers' decision making capacity and their ability to direct their energies towards recovery. This issue of stable accommodation is not new [29] with its historical roots in de-institutionalisation but compounded in recent years by staggering decreases in housing affordability, particularly in Sydney, where this study took place. Housing prices and rent costs have increased up to 70% in Sydney since 2012. The stock or amount of low cost and social housing has not kept up with population increases. Income supports payments have not kept up with rental price increases. Collectively this has resulted in over 40% of Australians on welfare support experiencing housing-related financial stress [30]. There is a need to prioritise these non-clinical aspects that impact upon recovery. Mental health support programs, need to focus holistically on an individual and ensure that these basic needs such as housing security are met. Stability of support from services, families, friends, peers and carers was important to participants. Families of origin were a source of both hope and difficulty. Children provided a purpose and support, but participants struggled with trying to separate out family and child relationships with carer roles. They were also concerned about the impact of their mental illness on others including their children. This period of recovery can cause significant stress for children and other family members, who need to be supported themselves. Reacting to the one-sidedness of current parenting support programs which focus only on the parent living with mental illness, authors recommend the development of 'family-focused' programs which support both parent and child to ensure a consistent, individualised and collaborative approach to recovery [31]. The predominance of participant focus upon relationships with others, and the positive and negative impacts of these speak directly to the 'relational' approach to recovery recently promoted [32, 33] and calls for extension to the CHIME component of connectedness. A relational approach warns against focusing too heavily on an individual's inner recovery struggle and neglecting the interpersonal aspects of recovery. Instead programs should focus both on the individual and those relationships closest to them, including their families of origin and particularly their children [32].

Limitations

As is the case with all qualitative research, the broader relevance of these findings needs to be considered with reference to characteristics of participants. Participants were all engaged in an Australian Sydney-based PIR program. Voluntary participation also means that experiences of early recovery reported here do not reflect experiences of those likely to be at a similarly early point in their recovery journey who chose not to engage in the study. Participants only received invitations to participate if they were deemed by Support Facilitators to be able to participate without undue distress. Results should be considered in the light of this limitation.

Conclusions

Findings of this study provide further understanding of the early recovery experiences for people living with severe, persistent mental illness and complex needs that align well to, but expand upon the components of the CHIME model. This suggests that a broader conceptualisation is needed within optimistic and aspirational point-of-recovery frameworks if they are to be inclusive of, and relevant to people with severe and persistent mental illness, at an early point of recovery. Recovery at this early stage is not all positive and people described multiple barriers and struggles which impeded their recovery journey. Rather than focusing upon symptoms of illness, participants emphasised relational enablers and barriers. People, and material resources, created physical and emotional safety and support that allowed them to prioritise recovery.

Abbreviation

PIR: Partners in Recovery

Acknowledgements

We would like to acknowledge the participants who generously shared their experiences and wisdom.

Funding

This research was funded by Wentwest through a Partners in Recovery Flexible Funding scheme grant. The grant funder, through the Partners in Recovery program, approved the project design and assisted with participant recruitment to the extent described in the paper. The funding body has had no input into the data analysis and interpretation.

Authors' contributions

NH led the analysis of the data and led on drafting the paper. JSM devised and managed the project, was involved in project design, reviewed the analysis and helped to develop the paper draft. GJ carried out the data analysis and writing of the paper. SW carried out all data collection and was involved in drafting the final paper. AK provided expertise from lived experience within the project development, recruitment and writing stages. All authors read and approved the final manuscript.

Competing interests

AK is employed as a consumer advocate by Wentwest who are the lead consortium partner for the Partners in Recovery program site in which this research took place.

The other authors declare that they have no competing interests.

Author details

[1]The University of Sydney, Sydney, Australia. [2]University of Technology, Sydney, Sydney, Australia. [3]WentWest, Blacktown, Australia.

References

1. Kraepelin E. Dementia praecox. In: Kraepelin E, editor. Clinical Psychiatry: A text book for students and physicians. New York: Macmillan; 1902. p. 152–202.
2. Association AP. Diagnostic and statistical manual of mental disorders, 4 edn. Washington, DC: American Psychiatric Association; 2000.
3. Warner R. Recovery from schizophrenia and the recovery model. Current opinion in psychiatry. 2009;22(4):374–80.
4. Davidson L, Sells D, Sangster S, O'Connell M. Qualitative studies of recovery: what can we learn from the person? In: Ralph RO, Corrigan PW, editors. Recovery in mental illness: Broadening our understanding of wellness. 1st ed. Washington, DC: American Psychological Association; 2005. p. 147–70.
5. Smith-Merry J, Sturdy S. Recovery in Scotland. Soc Ment Health. 2013;3(2):114–32.
6. Mead S, Copeland ME. What recovery means to us: Consumers' perspectives. Community Ment Health J. 2000;36(3):315–28.
7. Onken SJ, Craig CM, Ridgway P, Ralph RO, Cook JA. An analysis of the definitions and elements of recovery: a review of the literature. Psychiatr Rehabil J Summer. 2007;31(1):9–22.
8. Council of Australian Governments. The Roadmap for National Mental Health Reform 2012–2022. Canberra: Australia: Australian Government; 2012.
9. Her Majesty's Government. No Health without Mental Health: A Cross-Government Mental Health Outcomes Strategy for People of All Ages. London: UK: Department of Health; 2011.
10. World Health Organization. Comprehensive Mental Health Action Plan 2013–2020. Geneva: Switzerland: World Health Organisation; 2013.
11. Silverstein SM, Bellack AS. A scientific agenda for the concept of recovery as it applies to schizophrenia. Clin Psychol Rev. 2008;28(7):1108–24.
12. Remington G, Shammi C. Overstating the case about recovery? Psychiatr Serv. 2005;56(8):1022.
13. Slade M, Amering M, Farkas M, Hamilton B, O'Hagan M, Panther G, Perkins R, Shepherd G, Tse S, Whitley R. Uses and abuses of recovery: implementing recovery-oriented practices in mental health systems. World Psychiatry. 2014;13(1):12–20.
14. Stuart SR, Tansey L, Quayle E. What we talk about when we talk about recovery: a systematic review and best-fit framework synthesis of qualitative literature. J Ment Health. 2017;26(3):291–304.
15. Leamy M, Bird V, Le Boutillier C, Williams J, Slade M. Conceptual framework for personal recovery in mental health: systematic review and narrative synthesis. Br J Psychiatry. 2011;199(6):445–52.
16. Andresen R, Caputi P, Oades L. Stages of recovery instrument: development of a measure of recovery from serious mental illness. Aust N Z J Psychiatry. 2006;40(11–12):972–80.
17. Hancock N, Bundy A, Honey A, Helich S, Tamsett S. Measuring the later stages of the recovery journey: insights gained from clubhouse members. Community Ment Health J. 2013;49(3):323–30.
18. Hancock N, Scanlan JN, Gillespie JA, Smith-Merry J, Yen I. Partners in Recovery program evaluation: changes in unmet needs and recovery. Aust Health Rev. 2017; https://doi.org/10.1071/AH17004.
19. Smith-Merry J, Gillespie J, Hancock N, Yen I. Doing mental health care integration: a qualitative study of a new work role. Int J Ment Heal Syst. 2015;9(1):32.
20. Sutton K, Isaacs AN, Dalziel K, Maybery D. Roles and competencies of the support facilitator in Australia's recovery-oriented mental health initiative: a qualitative study from Gippsland, Victoria. Aust Health Rev. 2017;41(1):91–7.
21. Smith-Merry J, Gillespie J. Embodying policy-making in mental health: the implementation of Partners in Recovery. Health Sociol Rev. 2016;25(2):187–201.
22. Tong A, Sainsbnury P, Criag J. Consolidated criteria for reporting qualitative research (COREQ): a 32 item checklist for interviews and focus groups. International J Qual Health Care. 2007;19(6):349–57.
23. Hancock N, Smith-Merry J, Gillespie JA, Yen I. Is the Partners in Recovery program connecting with the intended population of people living with severe and persistent mental illness? What are their prioritised needs? Aust Health Rev. 2016;https://doi.org/10.1071/AH17004.
24. QSR International: NVivo qualitative data analysis software; version 10. In: QSR International Pty Ltd; 2012.
25. Bazeley P. Qualitative data analysis: practical strategies. London: Sage; 2013.
26. Charmaz K. Constructing grounded theory. London: SAGE; 2014.
27. Anderson C. Presenting and evaluating qualitative research. Am J Pharm Educ. 2010;74(8):141.
28. Deegan PE. Recovery as a journey of the heart. Psychiatri Rehabil J. 1996; 19(3):91–7.
29. Rog DJ, Marshall T, Dougherty RH, George P, Daniels AS, Ghose SS, Delphin-Rittmon ME. Permanent supportive housing: assessing the evidence. Psychiatr Serv. 2014;65(3):287–94.
30. Daley J, Coates B, Wiltshire T. Housing affordability: re-imagining the Australian dream. Grattan Institute 2018. https://grattan.edu.au/wp-content/uploads/2018/03/901-Housing-affordability.pdf.
31. Foster K, O'brien L, Korhonen T. Developing resilient children and families when parents have mental illness: a family-focused approach. Int J Ment Health Nurs. 2012;21(1):3–11.
32. Price-Robertson R, Manderson L, Duff C. Mental ill health, recovery and the family assemblage. Cult Med Psychiatry 2017;41(3):407–30.
33. Price-Robertson R, Obradovic A, Morgan B. Relational recovery: beyond individualism in the recovery approach. Advances in Mental Health. 2017; 15(2):108–20.

Predictors of quality of life among inpatients in forensic mental health: implications for occupational therapists

Padraic O' Flynn[1], Roisin O' Regan[1], Ken O' Reilly[1,2] and Harry G Kennedy[1,2*]

Abstract

Background: Optimising quality of life (QOL) for service users in a forensic hospital is an important treatment objective. The factors which contribute to QOL in this setting are currently unclear. The aim of this study was to analyse the predictors of QOL amongst service users within an inpatient forensic mental health hospital.

Methods: This study is a naturalistic, cross-sectional, observational study. Fifty-two male service users with schizophrenia or schizoaffective disorder participated in the study. QOL was measured using the World Health Organisation QOL Bref. We used the Engagement in Meaningful Activity Survey (EMAS), ward atmosphere was measured using the Essen Climate Evaluation Schema (EssenCES), occupational functioning was assessed using the Social and Occupational Functioning Scale (SOFAS). We also collected level of ward security, length of stay and community leave data.

Results: Stepwise regression showed that meaningful activity, level of ward security, and therapeutic hold on the EssenCES significantly predicted QOL on a range of specific QOL domains. These variables accounted for 40% of the variance for total QOL score. Engagement in meaningful activity added the largest contribution to total QOL score accounting for 30% of the variance.

Conclusions: This study shows that provision of meaningful activities, level of ward security and therapeutic hold may contribute to QOL amongst forensic mental health inpatients.

Background

Quality of Life (QOL) is important in forensic mental health inpatient settings [1–6]. There are moral, ethical, clinical and legal reasons for considering QOL as an outcome [2]. Coid [2] argues that 'any discussion on the QOL of a detained person must proceed on the principle that basic or moral rights exist... and that they should be reflected in the law'.

QOL has long been regarded as a core outcome for service users with a diagnosis of schizophrenia in general mental health settings [7–13]. For instance, numerous studies have found that higher levels of clinical symptoms are associated with reduced QOL for patients with schizophrenia [9–13]. In particular, many cross-sectional and longitudinal studies showed that lower depressive symptoms and a higher level of social functioning significantly predicted improved QOL [14]. Multivariate analyses explained 53% of the total variance in one such study where the significant predictors were depressive symptoms and social functioning [14]. Furthermore, a recent meta-analysis confirmed an association between neurocognition and expert reported QOL (i.e daily functioning), but indicated that there is largely no association between neurocognition and self reported QOL [15]. Similarly, recent studies have shown that negative symptoms are associated with expert-related QOL however there are no significant associations with self reported QOL. Moreover, it has been shown that psychosocial interventions are associated with improved QOL [16] and in particular, meaningful and satisfying daily activities were consistently associated with QOL [17, 18].

In recent years greater attention has been given to the concept of QOL in forensic mental health [1–6]. For instance, with the shift towards recovery-focused practice,

* Correspondence: kennedh@tcd.ie
[1]National Forensic Mental Health Service, Central Mental Hospital, Dundrum, Dublin, Ireland
[2]Department of Psychiatry, Trinity College, Dublin, Ireland

QOL and wellbeing are now recognised as important outcomes [1, 3]. Drennan et al. [3], writing on recovery in forensic mental health suggested that from the perspective of service providers, QOL should be an essential outcome. Similarly, the U.K. College of Occupational Therapists [COT] has recommended in a key practice guideline that occupational therapists working on forensic mental health should consider the impact of interventions on QOL [19]. Moreover, the European Union Cooperation in Science and Technology [20] have recently set up an international forum for experts in the area of forensic mental health to gain and share knowledge. One of the primary goals of this forum is to develop a greater understanding of the factors that contribute to QOL for forensic inpatients [20].

Additionally, it is known that QOL is a positive protective factor in reducing both short term and long term criminal recidivism and therefore emphasis on this outcome contributes to public protection [21, 22]. A number of theories associate QOL with reduced recidivism. For example, the conjecture that risk of criminal offending reduces when individuals have a 'good life' is central to the Good Lives Model [23]. In addition, the relationship between social indicators of quality of life and recidivism has been shown in numerous studies. For example, the association between reduced recidivism and engagement in meaningful leisure activities, work and adequate management of finances has been demonstrated [21–27]. Because QOL and subjective wellbeing are associated with reducing recidivism, the concept of QOL is of central importance within forensic mental health.

The World Health Organisation has defined QOL as an 'individual's perception of their position in life in the context of culture and value systems in which they live and in relation to their goals, expectations, standards, and concerns' [28]. Forensic mental health services provide treatment for people with mental illnesses such as schizophrenia who come into contact with law enforcement agencies as a consequence of their mental disorder, or who cannot be safely managed within another service. Admission to a forensic mental health hospital is almost always compulsory and via the courts. Length of stay in a forensic inpatient setting is often greater than 5 years [29–32]. In addition, many civil liberties may be restricted. Because forensic mental health service users are detained within restrictive settings, optimising QOL is an essential component of their care [1–3]. In addition the QOL experienced by forensic mental health service users may be lower than that experienced by service users in a general mental health population and also non- clinical populations [8, 9, 33–35]. This is because the clinical presentation of this patient group is complex [33–36]. For instance, treatment resistant psychopathology and impaired neurocognition are prevalent [33–36]. Because service users may have a longer period of stay within forensic inpatient services and a more complex presentation in comparison to their non-forensic counterparts, maximising their QOL is an essential treatment objective.

To our knowledge, only three studies have explored factors associated with QOL within a forensic mental health setting [37–39]. Factors such as level of ward security, diagnosis, use of atypical antipsychotics, and length of stay were considered in one such study by Long et al. [37]. The findings did not support an association between better QOL and length of hospital stay, a diagnosis of schizophrenia, or the use of atypical antipsychotics. However, this study did report that service users had a significantly higher level of satisfaction on wards with a lower level of security. The authors additionally reported that perceptions of personal control, mastery, freedom of choice and privacy are potential reasons for this association with better QOL. The study also showed an association between better QOL and lower levels of anxiety, depression and hostility. The authors concluded that interventions that enhance service users' perceptions of control and mastery are important [37]. Conversely, Trizna & Adamowski [38] found that there was no significant difference between quality of life scores on medium and low secure wards. The authors highlighted that the differences between unmet needs on medium secure wards as compared to lower secure wards did not translate to improvements in self report quality of life or improved satisfaction with care. Interestingly within this study, service users on lower levels of security had increased psychopathology. The authors reported that service users had been in detention more frequently on lower secure wards hence had a more complex and severe psychopathology. Within this study increased psychopathology on lower security levels may explain the little change in self report QOL scores between wards. Swinton et al. [39] investigated QOL amongst service users with personality disorder and schizophrenia detained within a secure setting. Although environmental conditions and length of stay were similar for both groups the authors reported that service users with personality disorder subjectively reported poorer QOL than service users with schizophrenia. Thus far, research exploring factors associated with QOL in forensic mental health is sparse. Nevertheless findings from these studies indicate that level of ward security, psychopathology and diagnoses are associated with QOL for service users detained within a forensic mental health setting. Despite QOL and wellbeing now being recognised as core outcomes in forensic mental health there remains a paucity of research investigating the predictors of QOL in forensic mental health inpatient settings. Therefore, this study aims to analyse the predictors of QOL from a range of psychosocial factors that are relevant for forensic mental health service users. To our knowledge, no previous research has explored these issues.

Objective/aim of study

We hypothesised that some or all of a range of psychosocial variables would account for a significant proportion of the measured variance in total QOL score and individual scores across specific QOL domains. The psychosocial variables included engagement in meaningful activity, ward atmosphere [therapeutic hold, experienced safety and patient cohesion], social and occupational functioning, community leave, length of stay and level of ward security.

Methods

Study design

This study is a naturalistic, cross-sectional, observational study.

Setting

The national forensic mental health service (NFMHS) provides specialised care for adults who have a mental disorder and are at risk of harming others and themselves. Service users within the NFMHS are cared for in a safe and secure therapeutic hospital. Care is provided for those who are both residing within the hospital and within the community. Stratified care pathways via high, medium and low-secure wards within the hospital enable a safe therapeutic environment to maximise recovery potential.

Participants

This study included male inpatients who were not in an acute stage of illness and who had a diagnosis of schizophrenia or schizoaffective disorder. Participants resided in high and medium secure rehabilitation wards and low secure wards. This study included a national cohort of forensic inpatients. Participants were aged between 20 and 65 years. All participants were diagnosed with schizophrenia or schizoaffective disorder by a consultant psychiatrist. Diagnoses were made in accordance with the Diagnostic and Statistical Manual of Mental Disorders IV-TR [40] using SCID-I based on interview and chart review.

Variables

World Health Organisation QOL assessment (WHOQOL Bref)

The most widely used definition of QOL was provided by the World Health Organization Quality of Life (WHOQOL) Group in 1995. Hence, the most widely used scale for measuring QOL for service users with schizophrenia is the WHOQOL Bref [41]. This measure is deemed to adequately capture the salient QOL concepts for service users in a forensic setting and has been used to validate more specific forensic quality of life measures [5] and is used as an outcome measure in routine clinical practice at the research site. In addition the WHOQOL Bref is a valid, useful and reliable measure of QOL for people with schizophrenia [42, 43]. Psychometric properties were analysed using cross-sectional data obtained from a survey of adults carried out in 23 countries [n = 11,830]. The instrument demonstrated adequate internal consistency [Cronbach's alpha coefficients were higher than 0.7 across the 4 domains and for the total score] and all items had acceptable correlation with the corresponding domain scores [r = 0.32–0.73]. It is regarded as a valid assessment of QOL, which is reflected by its four domains: physical, psychological, social and environment [42, 43]. Each individual domain is scaled in a positive direction. The total score on the four domains combined represents overall QOL and is scaled in a positive direction (i.e. higher scores denote higher QOL) with scores ranging between 0 and 100.

Essen climate evaluation schema (EssenCES)

The EssenCES is a short questionnaire, developed for assessing aspects of the social and therapeutic atmosphere of forensic psychiatric wards [44]. It has three dimensions: 'patient cohesion and mutual support' (PC; e.g. 'service users care for each other'), 'experienced safety' (ES; e.g. 'there are some really aggressive service users in this unit') and 'Therapeutic hold' (e.g. 'staff take a personal interest in the progress of service users'). Each question is scored on a scale between 0 and 4. The total score in each domain (patient cohesion, experienced safety, therapeutic hold) is scored positively on a scale between 0 and 20. Psychometric properties have been validated for UK forensic samples [44–46]. An examination of construct validity with the English EssenCES showed satisfactory internal consistency for all EssenCES scales, and using confirmatory factor analysis the expected three-factor structure was confirmed with residents in secure hospital settings [45].

Engagement in meaningful activity survey (EMAS)

The EMAS [47] assesses aspects of the meaning of activity with a particular emphasis on the synergy between an activity and an individual's value system and needs. The EMAS is regarded as a valid and reliable tool and the instrument measures a unidimensional construct. It measures 12 facets of the meaningfulness of activities. Test-retest reliability and Cronbach Alpha are .69 and .84, respectively [47]. Scoring is conducted by summing the responses [ranging from 1 = Rarely to 4 = Always] of the 12 EMAS items for a possible score range of 12–48. The scale is scored positively and persons may be classified as perceiving the meaningfulness of their activities as being either low (EMAS < 29), moderate (EMAS 29–41) or high (EMAS > 41) [47].

Social and occupational functioning assessment scale (SOFAS)

The SOFAS is a global rating of current functioning which is scored positively on a scale from 0 to 100. Higher scores represent higher levels of functioning. The SOFAS has adequate psychometric properties [48]. A six-month cohort of general adult psychiatric inpatients were followed for up to two years to contrast the validity of *DSM-IV* measures of functioning—the Global Assessment of Functioning (GAF) and the Social and Occupational Functioning Assessment Scale (SOFAS) [48]. SOFAS and GAF scores on admission were found to significantly correlate with duration of hospital admission, and the SOFAS ratings on discharge were significantly correlated with psychiatric outcome at two years. The authors concluded that the SOFAS appeared to have better predictive validity and concurrent validity than the GAF and the SOFAS may be a more clinically useful measure of functioning [48, 49].

Community leave status

Community leave status refers to whether a service user has access to the community or not. Based on risk assessment, selected service users will have access to the community for specified periods to engage with interventions that are intertwined with rehabilitation goals. Typically, service users who have progressed in the care pathway have community leave and are usually accompanied in the community by staff who work wihin the hospital. Risk factors are usually reduced and symptoms stabilised before community leave is recommended. Service users who have access to the community are usually well engaged with hospital rehabilitation programs. Access to the community is used for rehabilitation interventions such as building skills for using public transport and shopping, attending work or education programmes and participating in leisure activities such as going to the cinema, a museum or going to a coffee shop. For the purpose of this analysis service users without community leave were coded as zero and service users with community leave were coded as one.

Length of stay

The length of stay is calculated from the date of admission to the date in which data were captured.

Level of ward security

Service users were residing on high secure, medium secure, low secure wards or within a pre-discharge hostel. All wards are on the site of the Central Mental Hospital. The level of ward security was coded ordinally. The hostel setting (lowest level of security) was coded as one, the low secure rehabilitation ward was coded as two, the medium secure rehabilitation ward was coded as three, the medium secure sub-acute ward was coded as four, and the high secure ward was coded as five.

Data sources/measurement

Participants were invited to participate within the study and each participant completed questionnaires which measured QOL, ward atmosphere, and engagement in meaningful activity. Data on occupational functioning were measured by clinicians who best knew the service users level of functioning. Length of stay and community leave status were also collected on the same day by lead author and co-authors. Participants were provided with questionnaires by clinicians who were not working directly with service users. The data collection tools used were the World Health Organisation QOL Assessment (WHOQOL- Bref) to measure QOL, the 'Essen Climate Evaluation Schema' (EssenCES) to measure ward atmosphere, the Social and Occupational Functioning scale (SOFAS) and the Engagement in Meaningful Activity Survey (EMAS). There were other variables considered such as community leave status, length of stay and level of ward security.

Bias

We considered a national cohort of forensic mental health patients so as to minimise selection bias.

Study size

Eligible participants for this study were recruited from the inpatient population residing in high, medium or low-secure wards ($n = 67$). Of the 67 that were asked if they wanted to participate in the study, 52 (78%) consented and completed all questionnaires. There were 7 service users who originally consented but did not complete all of the questionnaires and withdrew from the study and there were 8 people who did not give consent.

Statistical methods

Data were analysed using Statistical Package for the Social Sciences (SPSS) version 23.

A stepwise multiple regression analysis was conducted to determine the unique contributions of clinical variables to QOL (WHOQOL-Bref total score). In addition a stepwise multiple regression analysis was used to determine the unique contributions of clinical variables to the specific domains within the WHOQOL Bref (physical health, psychological health, social relationships and environment). Due to the range of variables considered within the analysis it was deemed appropriate to use this method in identifying significant predictors of QOL. In the regression models the dependent variable was QOL as measured by the total score of the WHO-QOL Bref across all domains and total score on individual domains. Independent variables were engagement in meaningful activity as measured by the EMAS, social and occupational functioning as measured by the SOFAS, ward atmosphere (therapeutic hold, experienced safety, patient cohesion) as measured by the EssenCES, level of ward security, community leave status and length of stay.

Ethics, consent and permissions

The study was approved by the Research, Ethics and Audit Committee of the National Forensic Mental Health Service (NFMHS). All participants gave informed signed consent. An information sheet was provided to each participant. The information sheet detailed the aim of the study, the potential risks and benefits and the re-assurance that participation was voluntary and that participation could be withdrawn at any time. This study was compliant with the Declaration of Helsinki.

Results

Participants

Of the 67 that were asked if they wanted to participate in the study 52 (78%) consented and completed all questionnaires. There were 7 service users who originally consented but did not complete all of the questionnaires and withdrew from the study and there were 8 people who did not give consent.

Descriptive data

The median length of stay was 5.5 yrs. (SD 6.8) with a minimum of 0.5 yrs. and a maximum of 35.5 yrs. The mean age of participants was 40.3 yrs. (SD 16.4). Participants resided within high security [$n = 6$], medium security ($n = 14$), medium security rehabilitation ($n = 15$), low security rehabilitation ward ($n = 11$) and low security hostel (n = 6). Community leave status was dichotomised between those with no community leave ($n = 16$) or those with community leave ($n = 36$). There were 67 service users who met inclusion criteria. All service users were male and met diagnostic criteria for schizophrenia or schizoaffective disorder ($n = 67$). 8 service users declined to participate. 7 service users did not to complete all questionnaires and withdrew from the study. Data were therefore available for 52 participants which are presented in Table 1.

Outcome data

The mean WHOQOL Bref total QOL score and WHO-QOL Bref individual domain scores (physical health, psychological health, social relationships and environment) are detailed in Table 2. In addition the mean score for the engagement in meaningful activity scale, social and occupational functioning scale and EssenCES constructs (therapeutic hold, patient cohesion and experienced safety) are also detailed.

Main results

Table 3 shows results of stepwise regression analysis for the overall model. Within this model, engagement in meaningful activity, level of ward security and therapeutic hold statistically predicted total QOL score across all domains. Engagement in meaningful activity was automatically entered first into the overall model $R^2 = 0.31$, $F\ (1, 51) = 22.5$, $p < 0.0001$, adjusted $R^2 = 0.30$ and added the largest contribution. Level of ward security was automatically entered second into the overall model $R^2 = 0.37$, $F\ (2, 50) = 14.3$, $p < 0.0001$, adjusted $R^2 = 0.34$ and finally EssenCES therapeutic hold was entered into the overall model $R^2 = 0.43$, $F\ (3, 49) = 12.0$, $p < 0.0001$, adjusted $R^2 = 0.40$. The other variables included in the

Table 1 Describes demographic and clinical characteristics $n = 52$

Patient characteristics				
Mean age	Years 40.3	SD 16.4	Min 27.0	Max 55.0
Median length of stay	Years 5.5	SD 6.8	Min 0.5 yrs	Max 33.5 yrs
Ward location				
Low secure hostel	6 [12%]			
Low secure rehabilitation ward	11 [20%]			
Medium security rehabilitation	15 [29%]			
Medium security sub-acute	14 [27%]			
High secure [long stay]	6 [12%]			
Community leave status				
Community leave	36 [70%]			
No community Leave	16 [30%]			
Primary Diagnosis				
Schizophrenia/ Schizoaffective disorder	52 [100%]			

Table 2 Describes mean and standard deviations of variables [n = 52]

	Mean	Std. Deviation
WHOQOL Bref [QOL] Total	66.0	12.9
WHOQOL Bref Physical Health	73.8	12.9
WHOQOL Bref Psychological Health	64.6	12.6
WHOQOL Bref Social Relationships	57.6	19.3
WHOQOL Bref Environment	67.9	16.4
Engagement in meaningful activity scale [EMAS]	35.4	8.2
Social and occupational functioning scale [SOFAS]	56.2	12.5
EssenCES Therapeutic Hold	13.7	4.3
EssenCES Patient Cohesion	12.1	4.3
EssenCES Experienced safety	16.3	3.4

model did not add significantly to the prediction and were automatically removed. The overall model of engagement in meaningful activity, level of ward security, and therapeutic hold was statistically significant $R^2 = 0.43$, $F(3, 49) = 12.0$, $p < 0.0005$; adjusted $R^2 = 0.40$.

Table 4 shows results of stepwise regression model with significant predictors of the WHOQOL Bref 'physical health' domain detailed. Within this model EssenCES therapeutic hold alone predicted WHOQOL Bref 'physical health' $R^2 = 0.08$, F (1, 51) = 5.6, $p = 0.02$. The other variables included in the model did not add significantly to the prediction and were automatically removed.

Table 5 shows results of stepwise regression model with significant predictors of the WHOQOL Bref 'psychological health' domain. Engagement in meaningful activity was automatically entered first into this model $R^2 = 0.24$, F (1, 51) = 17.1, $p < 0.001$ and level of ward security was entered second $R^2 = 0.30$, F (2, 50) = 11.8, $p < 0.001$. The other variables included in the model did not add significantly to the prediction and were automatically removed.

Table 4 Shows stepwise regression model with significant predictors of the WHOQOL Bref physical domain detailed

Model 1	Unstandardized coefficients		Standardized coefficients	t	Sig.
	B	Std. Error	Beta		
1] Constant	60.94	5.73		10.64	p < 0.0001
EssenCES therapeutic hold	0.945	0.400	0.317	2.36	p = 0.022

Table 6 shows results of stepwise regression model with significant predictors of the WHOQOL Bref 'social relationships' domain. Engagement in meaningful activity was automatically entered into this model $R^2 = 0.12$, F (1, 51) = 8.0, $p = 0.007$. The other variables included in the model did not add significantly to the prediction and were automatically removed.

Table 7 shows results of stepwise regression model with significant predictors of the WHOQOL Bref 'environment' domain. EssenCES therapeutic hold was automatically entered first into this model $R^2 = 0.28$, F (1, 51) = 21.2, $p < 0.001$ and level of ward security was entered second $R^2 = 0.37$, F (2, 50) = 15.7, $p < 0.001$. The other variables included in the model did not add significantly to the prediction and were automatically removed.

Discussion

Key results

We hypothesized that some or all of a range of psychosocial variables would account for a significant proportion of the measured variance in QOL. The psychosocial variables included engagement in meaningful activity, ward

Table 3 Shows stepwise regression model for total WHOQOL Bref score with significant variables entered

Model 1	Unstandardized coefficients		Standardized coefficients	t	Sig.
	B	Std. Error	Beta		
1] Constant	34.99	6.70		5.22	p < 0.0001
Engagement In Meaningful Activity Scale	0.874	0.185	0.557	4.738	p < 0.0001
Model 2	Unstandardized coefficients		Standardized coefficients	t	Sig
	B	Std. Error	Beta		
2] Constant	53.65	10.90		4.927	p < 0.0001
Engagement in meaningful activity survey	0.767	0.185	0.489	4.144	p < 0.0001
Level of ward security	−2.33	1.092	−0.251	−2.133	p = 0.038
Model 3	Unstandardized coefficients		Standardized coefficients	t	Sig.
	B	Std. Error	Beta		
3] Constant	52.99	10.46		5.066	p < 0.0001
Engagement in meaningful activity survey	0.478	0.219	0.305	2.185	p = 0.034
Level of ward security	−2.551	1.053	−0.275	−2.422	p = 0.019
EssenCES Therapeutic Hold	0.902	0.398	0.305	2.264	p = 0.028

Table 5 Shows stepwise regression model with significant predictors of the WHOQOL Bref psychological health domain detailed

Model 1	*Unstandardized coefficients*		*Standardized coefficients*	*t*	*Sig.*
	B	*Std. Error*	*Beta*		
1] Constant	*26.16*	*9.54*		*2.74*	*p = 0.008*
Engagement In Meaningful Activity Scale	*1.08*	*0.262*	*0.505*	*4.133*	*p < 0.0001*
Model 2	*Unstandardized Coefficients*		*Standardized Coefficients*	*t*	*Sig*
	B	*Std. Error*	*Beta*		
2] Constant	*54.08*	*15.40*		*3.51*	*p = 0.001*
Engagement In Meaningful Activity Scale	*0.924*	*0.262*	*0.430*	*3.53*	*p = 0.001*
Level of ward security	*−3.49*	*1.54*	*−0.275*	*−2.26*	*P = 0.029*

atmosphere (therapeutic hold, experienced safety and patient cohesion), social and occupational functioning, community leave, length of stay and level of ward security. Engagement in meaningful activity, level of ward security, and therapeutic hold all significantly accounted for a proportion of the variance for QOL. The three variables together accounted for 40% of the variance of total QOL score across all domains. In addition within specific QOL domains, EssenCES therapeutic hold significantly accounted for a small proportion of the variance (8%) in the 'physical health' domain. Engagement in meaningful activity and level of ward security together significantly accounted for a large proportion of variance (30%) within the 'psychological health' domain. Engagement in meaningful activity significantly accounted for 12% of the variance in the 'social relationships' QOL domain and finally EssenCES therapeutic hold and level of ward security together contributed to a large proportion of the variance (37%) within the QOL 'environment' domain. Length of stay, social and occupational functioning, patient cohesion, experienced safety [EssenCES] and community leave did not make a contribution to the model in this study. This study contributes to an understanding of the predictors of QOL for service users within a forensic hospital.

Interpretation

Meaningful activity and QOL

This study shows a positive association between engagement in meaningful activity and QOL for service users who reside within a forensic mental health hospital. In particular engagement in meaningful activity made a significant contribution to the QOL 'psychological health domain and QOL 'social relationships domain'. The association between engagement in meaningful activity and wellbeing is a well known tenet of occupational therapy theory [50–54]. This present study provides empirical support for this relationship in a forensic mental health inpatient setting. The provision of meaningful activities for service users within this setting is a key recommendation made within the college of occupational therapists 'practice guidelines for forensic mental health' and the 'quality network for forensic mental health standards' [19, 54]. The results of this study provide further support for these recommendations. It has previously been shown that meaningful activity may provide purpose, structure, social connectnedness, routine and pleasure and these factors may contribute to a sense of personal agency and wellbeing [50–54]. Furthermore, the skills and competence developed as a result of participating in meaningful activity may improve functioning and subsequently provide a more seamless reintegration into the community upon discharge. Moreover, engagement in meaningful activity may reduce the person's risk for mental illness relapse. In addition engagement in meaningful activity may prevent readmission to hospital and contact with the criminal justice system [21–27, 55].

Level of ward security and QOL

This present study shows a significant negative association between level of ward security and QOL. In particular, level of ward security makes a significant contribution to the QOL 'psychological health' domain and QOL 'environment' domain. Similarly, Long et al.

Table 6 Shows stepwise regression model with significant predictors of the WHOQOL Bref social relationships domain detailed

Model 1	*Unstandardized coefficients*		*Standardized coefficients*	*t*	*Sig.*
	B	*Std. Error*	*Beta*		
1] Constant	*26.50*	*11.26*		*2.35*	*p = 0.023*
Engagement in Meaningful Activity Scale	*0.877*	*0.310*	*0.372*	*2.83*	*p = 0.007*

Table 7 Shows stepwise regression model with significant predictors of the WHOQOL Bref environment domain detailed

Model 1	*Unstandardized coefficients*		*Standardized coefficients*	*t*	*Sig.*
	B	*Std. Error*	*Beta*		
1] Constant	*39.80*	*6.40*		*6.22*	*p < 0.001*
EssenCES Therapeutic Hold	*2.06*	*0.447*	*0.546*	*4.60*	*p < 0.0001*
Model 2	*Unstandardized coefficients*		*Standardized coefficients*	*t*	*Sig*
	B	*Std. Error*	*Beta*		
2] Constant	*64.15*	*10.76*		*5.95*	*p > 0.001*
EssenCES Therapeutic Hold	*0.924*	*0.262*	*0.430*	*3.53*	*p = 0.001*
Level of ward security	*−3.60*	*1.32*	*−0.305*	*−2.73*	*P = 0.009*

[37] showed that higher levels of security were associated with a lower QOL. The authors additionally reported that perceptions of personal control, mastery, freedom of choice and privacy are potential reasons for this association with better QOL [37]. This present study shows that service users on lower secure wards have increased QOL scores. The particular characteristics of lower secure wards within this setting include increased autonomy, privacy and personal control. In addition, oppurtunities to manage activities of daily living are optimised. For instance, service users can manage their own self catering, shopping, personal care and deploy community living skills regularly as many have access to the community. Additionally increased access to a variety of leisure oppurtunities, vocational projects, education or work, and a greater choice regarding personal routines are other notable differences. An array of factors within the physical, social and therapeutic environment that stem from physical, procedural and relational security hospital policies on lower secure wards may additionally explain associations with better QOL scores. For instance, increased control over one's personal routine and increased privacy may be specific factors that contribute to QOL. Furthermore, there may be other factors which account for this association. Trizna and Adamowski [38] showed that there was no significant difference in QOL between medium and lower secure wards. Within their study psychopathology was increased in those at lower levels of security [38]. Conversely on the site where research data was collected for this study service users on lower levels of security generally have decreased pscyhopathology. A decrease in symptom severity has previously been shown to be associated with improved subjective QOL [9–13]. Thus, there maybe a range of factors that account for this relationship.

Therapeutic relationship and QOL

Additionally, the results of this study show a positive association between therapeutic relationship and QOL. In particular therapeutic hold on the EssenCES significantly contributed to QOL within the 'physical health' domain and 'environment' domain. The results provide further evidence to support the importance of optimising therapeutic relationships. It is well documented in the recovery literature [1, 3, 56] that an optimisation of therapeutic rapport can be achieved primarily through avoiding coercive choices, involving individuals in care planning/service development, identifying and working towards individualised goals and providing a safe and non-judgemental environment. Additionally, a positive therapeutic relationship may reduce symptomatology, increasing engagement with services and medication adherence [56–59]. Hence optimising therapeutic relationships may improve QOL in this setting.

Challenges in secure services

There are multifaceted challenges to providing activities that are meaningful, optimising therapeutic rapport and positive risk taking within forensic inpatient settings [55, 60, 61]. The confined environment of a secure inpatient ward with limited access to the community may present fewer opportunities for engaging in meaningful activities, practicing and applying skills, and providing choice and autonomy which may impact on QOL [55, 60, 61]. Additionally, there can be tension between safety, security and the provision of a therapeutic environment. For instance, features such as secure physical and social environments are required however these features can also result in restricted routines, autonomy and choice which can negatively affect therapeutic relationships [55]. Furthermore the clinical complexities may account for deficits in occupational performance [36]. For instance, neurocognitive deficits associated with schizophrenia contribute to impaired abilities to perform instrumental activities of daily living and engage with meaningful activities [36]. Conversely if abilities to perform instrumental activities of daily living and meaningful activities are intact, opportunities to deploy skills may be limited due to risk management [60–62]. Consequently, optimising the environment to afford service users an opportunity to deploy and retain skills whilst remaining as inpatients is an added complexity within a forensic mental health inpatient environment.

Opportunities to make progress

Optimising ward routines by facilitating autonomy and independence within the context of positive risk taking should be prioritised. However it must be acknowledged that there may be a heterogeneous group of service users with a range of security needs/risk issues residing on a single medium security ward. Hence, adjustments to the ward physical layout, therapeutic and ward operational policies may be necessary to stratify activity provision effectively, to ensure the least restrictive environment and to optimise therapeutic relationships.

In addition, service user participation in the design and delivery of therapeutic programmes should be considered [3, 55]. For instance, this could include participation in planning/governance committees and in the organisation of ward and personal activity timetables. Ward-based forums or community meetings for service users and staff to discuss daily life on a ward and the experiences of those that participate in it may be useful, particularly in making adjustments at a ward operational level. In addition, instilling the recovery principles particularly co-production may enhance therapeutic rapport and improve the quality of service provision.

Finally, it is important that clinicians explore potential factors impacting on 'meaning' within this setting. For instance, meaningful occupation is thought to reflect one's personal values, beliefs, goals, interests, world-view and experiences including pleasure, social connectedness, competency, control and enjoyment [47, 56–59]. Exploration of self identity could be considered at a number of stages throughout the care pathway. Occupational therapists could utilise theories within occupational science to support and guide practice within this area.

Limitations

This study was conducted within a secure forensic setting which may limit the generalisability of the findings to non-forensic settings. In addition the sample size was small with 52 service users participating. Moreover, social desirability, emotional state, psychopathology, neurocognition, insight or co-morbidities were not controlled for at the time of QOL evaluation. These factors may confound the measurement of QOL. There are also limitations with the cross sectional design. This means that the results only show associations and not a direct causal relationship. Repeating the QOL measure on a number of occasions within a prospective design would be beneficial to account for confounding factors.

The use of a self report QOL measure alone has specific limitations. Becker et al. [63] reported that QOL assessments should be carried out not only via the patient, but also via professional helpers and key informants. However the aim of this study was to analyse self- report QOL and Voruganti et al. [64] reported that service users with schizophrenia, while in remission and willing to cooperate, are capable of adequate estimation of their QOL. Future research should consider asking staff members to rate QOL using a proxy measure to get both perspectives.

The present study however combined objective and subjective measures in the model. Level of ward security is an objective measure and did influence the subjective rating of QOL. It is interesting therefore that level of community leave dropped out of this statistical model – possibly because it is confounded with level of ward security. Length of stay however is also an objective measure and did not relate to QOL. Finally, this is a cross-sectional study, so patients who have shorter periods of stay may be underrepresented.

Generalisability

This study was conducted with service users with a diagnosis of schizophrenia and schizoaffective disorder within a secure forensic hospital across a care pathway stratified by levels of security. The results of this study may be generalisable to other forensic mental health settings with a similar model of care.

Conclusion

The purpose of this study was to develop a greater understanding of the predictors of QOL within an inpatient forensic mental health setting. The results show that there is an association between meaningful activity, level of ward security, therapeutic hold and domains of QOL. The results provide support for a central assumption of occupational therapy theory; that there is a relationship between engagement in meaningful activity and well-being/QOL. In addition the results provide support for the least restrictive principle and theories about the importance of therapeutic relationships. Forensic service providers should routinely measure QOL. Furthermore, ensuring the least restrictive environment and optimising therapeutic relationships should be a priority. Occupational therapists are excellently placed and skilled to pioneer initiatives that enrich inpatient forensic environments with meaningful activities. It is anticipated by the authors that the QOL of service users who reside as inpatients within secure environments for many years may be improved by increasing access to meaningful activities, positive risk taking and optimisation of therapeutic relationships. Future studies investigating the effects of occupational therapy interventions on outcomes such as QOL and occupational performance/functioning are needed.

Abbreviations

EMAS: Engagement in Meaningful Activity Survey; ESSENCES: Essen Climate Evaluation Schema; QOL: Quality of life; SOFAS: Social and Occupational Functioning Scale; WHOQOL Bref: World Health Organisation QOL Bref

Acknowledgements

Joanne Fahy, Heather Ni Mhurchu and Emma Carroll were all involved in data collection and clinical ratings.

Funding

There are no funding sources to declare.

Authors' contributions

PO'F lead out on the overall design of the study, data collection methods, data analysis and preparation of the manuscript. RO'R, KO'R & HGK contributed to the overall design of the study, data collection methods and manuscript. All authors read and approved the final manuscript.

Consent for publication

No patient identifiable information has been reported.

Competing interests

All of the authors declare that they have no competing interests.

References

1. Mann B, Matias E, Allen J. Recovery in forensic services: facing the challenge. Adv Psychiatr Treat. 2014;20:125–31.
2. Coid JW. QOL for patients detained in hospital. Brit J Psychiat. 1993;162:611–20.
3. Drennan G, Wooldridge J. Making recovery a reality in forensic settings. ImROC briefing paper. London: Centre for Mental Health and Mental Health Network, NHS Confederation; 2013.
4. Van Nieuwenhuizen CH, Schene MH & Koeter M. QOL in forensic psychiatry: an unreclaimed territory?, Int Rev Psychiatr. 2002; 14:3: 198–202.
5. Vorstenbosch E, Bouman Y, Braun P, et al. Psychometric properties of the forensic inpatient QOL questionnaire: QOL assessment for long-term forensic psychiatric care. Health Psychol Behav Med. 2014;2:1.
6. Mulholland F, Rooney B, Pettigrew J. The hen project: introducing vocational opportunity into a high secure forensic unit. Irish J Occup Therapy. 2015;43:34.
7. Lehman AF, Ward NC, Linn LS. Chronic mental patients: the QOL issue. Am J Psychiat. 1982;139:1271–6.
8. Skantze K, Malm U, Denker SJ, et al. Comparison of QOL with standard of living in schizophrenic out-patients. Brit J Psychiat. 1992;161(6):797–801.
9. Atkinson M, Zibin SH, Chuang H. Characterizing QOL among patients with chronic mental illness: a critical examination of the self-report methodology. Am J Psychiat. 1997;105:99–105.
10. Eack S, Newhill C. Psychiatric symptoms and quality of life in schizophrenia: a meta-analysis. Schizophr Bull. 2007;33:1225–37.
11. Vatne S, Bjorkly S. Empirical evidence for using subjective quality of life as an outcome variable in clinical studies. A meta-analysis of correlates and predictors in persons with a major mental disorder living in the community. Clin Psychol Rev. 2008;28:869–89.
12. Priebe S, McCabe R, Junghan U, et al. Association between symptoms and quality of life in patients with schizophrenia: a pooled analysis of changes over time. Schizophr Res. 2011;133:17–21.
13. Galuppi A, Turola MC, Nanni MG, Mazzoni P, Grassi L. Schizophrenia and quality of life: how important are symptoms and functioning? Int J Ment Health Syst. 2010;4:31.
14. Meesters PD, Comijs HC, de Haan L, et al. Subjective quality of life and its determinants in a catchment area based population of elderly schizophrenia patients. Schizophr Res. 2011;147:275–80.
15. Tolman AW, Kurtz MM. Neurocognitive predictors of objective and subjective quality of life in individuals with schizophrenia: a meta-analytic investigation. Schizophr Bull. 2012;38:304–15.
16. Pitkanen A, Valimaki M, Kuosmanen L, et al. Patient education methods to support quality of life and functional ability among patients with schizophrenia: a randomised clinical trial. Qual Life Res. 2012;21:247–56.
17. Eklund M. Work status, daily activities and quality of life among people with severe mental illness. Qual Life Res. 2009;18:163–70.
18. Goldberg B, Brintnell S, Goldberg J. The relationship between engagement in meaningful activities and quality of life in persons disabled by mental illness. Occup Ther Ment Health. 2002;18(2):17–44.
19. College of Occupational Therapists. Occupational therapists' use of occupation-focused practice in secure hospitals: practice guideline. 2012. London: COT.
20. Braun P. Towards an EU research framework on forensic psychiatric care. 2013.http://www.cost.eu/COST_Actions/isch/IS1302. Accessed 4th January 2018.
21. Bouman Y, Schene AH. Subjective well-being and recidivism in forensic psychiatric outpatients. Int J Forensic Ment Health. 2009;8(4)
22. Abidin Z, Davoren M, Naughton L, et al. Susceptibility [risk and protective] factors for in-patient violence and self-harm. BMC Psychiatry. 2013;13:197.
23. Ward T, Brown M. The good lives model and conceptual issues in offender rehabilitation. Psychol Crime & Law. 2004;10:243–57.
24. Bouman Y, Ruiter C, Schene AH. Social ties and short-term self-reported delinquent behaviour of forensic personality disordered outpatients. Legal Criminol Psychol. 2010;15:357–72.
25. Monahan J, Steadman HJ, Silver E, Appelbaum PS, Robbins PC, Mulvey E, et al. Rethinking risk assessment: the MacArthur study of mental disorder and violence. Oxford, New York: Oxford University Press; 2001.
26. Ogloff JRP, Davis MR. Advances in offender assessment and rehabilitation: contributions of the risk-need-responsivity approach. Psychol Crime & Law. 2004;10:229–42.
27. Webster CD, Martin M, Brink J, Nicholls TL, Middleton C. Short term assessment of risk and treatability [START]. Clinical guide for evaluation risk and recovery. St. Joseph's Healthcare Hamilton: Ontario, Canada; 2004.
28. Saxena S, Orley J. WHOQOL Group. QOL assessment: The world health organization perspective. Eur Psychiatry. 1997;3:263s–6s.
29. Andreasson H, Nyman M, Krona H, et al. Predictors of length of stay in forensic psychiatry: the influence of perceived risk of violence. Int J Law Psychiatry. 2014;37:635–42.
30. Sharma A, Dunn W, O'Toole C, et al. The virtual institution: cross-sectional length of stay in general adult and forensic psychiatry beds. Int J Ment Health Syst. 2015;9:25.
31. Davoren M, Byrne O, O'Connell P, et al. Factors affecting length of stay in forensic hospital setting: need for therapeutic security and course of admission. BMC Psychiatry. 2015;15:301.
32. Shah A, Waldron G, Boast N, et al. Factors associated with length of admission at a medium secure forensic psychiatric unit. J Forens Psychiatry Psychol. 2011;22:496–512.
33. Katschnig H, Freeman H, Sartorius N. QOL in mental disorders. 2nd ed. Chichester: Wiley; 2006.
34. Barry MM, Crosby C. QOL as an evaluative measure in assessing the impact of community care on people with long-term psychiatric disorders. Br J Psychiatry. 1996;168:210–6.
35. Samuli I, Saarni S, Jonna P, et al. QOL of people with schizophrenia, bipolar disorder and other psychotic disorders. Br J Psychiatry. 2010;197:386–94.
36. Reilly K, G O' D, Sullivan D, et al. Study protocol: a randomised controlled trial of cognitive remediation for a national cohort of forensic mental health service users with schizophrenia or schizoaffective disorder. BMC Psychiatry. 2016;16:5.
37. Long CG, McLean A, Boothby AJ. Factors associated with QOL in a cohort of forensic psychiatric in-patients. Br J Forensic Pract. 2008;10:4–11.
38. Trizna M, Adamowski T. Assessment of needs and clinical parameters in forensic patients in low and medium security wards. Archives Psychiatry and Psychother. 2016;3:48–57.
39. Swinton M, Oliver J, Carlisle J. Measuring QOL in secure care: comparison of mentally ill and personality disordered patients. Int J Soc Psychiatary. 1999;45:284–91.
40. American Psychiatric Association. Diagnostic and statistical manual of mental disorders 4th edition, Text Revision. Washington, DC, American Psychiatric Association; 2000.
41. Karow A, Wittman L, Schöttle D, Schäfer I, Lambert M. The assessment of quality of life in clinical practice in patients with schizophrenia. Dialogues Clin Neurosci. 2014;16(2):185–95.

42. The WHOQOL Group. The World Health Organization QOL assessment [WHOQOL]: development and general psychometric properties. Soc Sci Med. 1998;46:1569–85.
43. The WHOQOL Group. Development of the World Health Organization WHOQOL-BREF QOL assessment. Psychol Med. 1998;28:551–8.
44. Schalast N, Redies M, Collins M, et al. EssenCES, a short questionnaire for assessing the social climate of forensic psychiatric wards. Crim Behav Ment Health. 2008;18:49–58.
45. Tonkin M, Howells K, Ferguson E, et al. Lost in translation? Psychometric properties and construct validity of the English Essen climate evaluation schema [EssenCES] social climate questionnaire. Eur J Psychol Assess. 2012;24:573–80.
46. Dickens GL, Suesse M, Snyman P, et al. Associations between ward climate and patient characteristics in a secure forensic mental health service. J Forens Psychiatry Psychol. 2014;25:195–211.
47. Eakman AM. Measurement Characteristics of the Engagement in Meaningful Activities Survey in an Age-Diverse Sample. Am J Occup Ther. 2012;66:e20–e29.
48. Rybarczyk B. Social and occupational functioning assessment scale [SOFAS]. In: Kreutzer J, Deluca J, Caplan B, editors. LXIII, encyclopedia of clinical neuropsychology, vol. 1. New York: Springer Reference; 2011. p. 2313.
49. Hay P, Katsikitis M, Begg J, et al. A two-year follow-up study and prospective evaluation of the DSM-IV Axis V. Psychiat Ser. 2003;54:1028–30.
50. Law M, Sandy S, Leclair L. Occupation, health and well-being. Can J Occup Ther. 1998;65(2)
51. Wilcock AAA. Theory of the human need for occupation. J Occup Sci. 1993;1:17–24.
52. Yerxa EJ, Baum S. Engagement in daily occupations and life satisfaction among people with spinal cord injuries. Occup Ther J Res. 1986;6:272–83.
53. Jackson J, Carlson M, Mandel D, et al. Occupation in lifestyle redesign: the well elderly study occupational therapy program. Am J OccupTher. 1998;52:326–36.
54. Canadian Association of Occupational Therapists. Enabling occupation: an occupational therapy perspective. Ottawa: CAOT; 1997.
55. Quality network for forensic mental health: Standards for medium secure services. Royal College of Psychiatrists Centre for Quality Improvement; 2014.
56. Perkes D, Whiteford G, Charlesworth G, et al. Occupation- focussed practice in justice health and forensic mental health: using a practice-based enquiry approach. World Federation Occup Therapists Bulletin. 2015;71:101–7.
57. Repper J, Ford R, Cooke A. How can nurses build trusting relationships with people who have severe and long term mental health problems? Experiences of case managers and their clients. J Adv Nurs. 1994;19:1096–104.
58. Bjorkman T, Hansson L. Predictors of improvements in QOL of long term mentally ill individuals receiving care management. Eur Psychiatry. 2002;17
59. Weiss K, Smith T, Hull J, et al. Predictors of risk of non-adherence in outpatients with schizophrenia and other psychotic disorders. Schizophr Bull. 2002;28:341–9.
60. Cleary M. The challenges of mental health care reform for contemporary mental health nursing practice: relationship, power and control. Int J Ment Health Nurs. 2003;12:139–47.
61. Farnworth L, Nikitin L, Fossey E. Being in a secure forensic psychiatric unit: every day is the same, killing time or making the most of it. Br J Occup Ther. 2004;67:430–8.
62. O'Connell M, Farnworth L. Occupational therapy in forensic psychiatry: a review of the literature and a call for a united and international response. Br J Occup Ther. 2007;70:184–91.
63. Becker A, Hagenberg N, Roessner V, et al. Evaluation of the self-reported SDQ in a clinical setting: do self-reports tell us more than ratings by adult informants? Eur Child Adolesc Psychiatry 2004;13: 17–24.
64. Voruganti L, Heslegrave R, Awad AG, Seeman MV. QOL measurement in schizophrenia: reconciling the quest for subjectivity with the question of reliability. Psychol Med. 1998;28:165–72.

17

Factors associated with mental health consultation in South Korea

Jieun Jang[1,2], Sang Ah Lee[1,2], Woorim Kim[1,2], Young Choi[1,2] and Eun-Cheol Park[2,3*]

Abstract

Background: The aim of this study was to examine factors associated with the use of mental health consultation for depressive symptoms.

Methods: We used data from the 2013 Community Health Survey, which included responses from 13,269 individuals who reported that they had experienced depressive symptoms for more than 2 weeks in Korea. We investigated associations between mental health consultation rates for depressive symptoms and sociodemographic, socioeconomic, and health-related factors. Logistic regression analysis was used to examine the significance of associations.

Results: Among participants who report depressive symptoms, 16.0% ($n = 2120$) undergo mental health consultation. Respondents with a college education or over are more likely to undergo mental health consultation (odds ratio (OR) = 1.49; 95% CI: 1.21–1.84) than respondents with less education. Individuals aged 70 years or above are less likely to receive mental health consultation than those aged between 19 and 29 years. Females exhibit higher mental health consultation rates than males. Respondents who are divorced show greater odds of receiving mental health consultation than respondents who are married and cohabitate with their spouse.

Conclusions: This study indicates that rates of use of mental health consultation services are lower among older adults and men and higher among divorced people. Educational level shows a significant positive association with mental health consultation among Koreans. The results could have implications for mental health policy in many ways in Korea.

Keywords: Depression, Mental health consultation, Education, Depress, Mental health

Background

Questions about why individuals do not seek mental health services for treatment of their mental illness and how to improve use of mental health consultation services are important topics worldwide [1, 2]. Depression is a common disease, affecting at least 300 million people around world [3]. However, people with depression often still do not receive mental health consultation for depression [4]. People with depression are less likely to obtain continuous treatment for depression due to lack of information on how to manage depression and the stigma associated with the condition [5–7]. The World Health Organization projected for the year 2030 that depression would be a major cause of the disease burden [8]. Depression is a significant public health problem [9].

Depression is an important issue, because it is a major cause of suicide [10]. Mounting evidence suggests that depressive disorder is strongly associated with completed suicide [11, 12]. About 60% of all suicides are estimated to stem from depression and other mood disorders [13–16]. Organisation for Economic Co-operation and Development (OECD) statistics indicate that, in 2013 and 2014, Korea ranked first in suicide rates among OECD countries [17]. Therefore, addressing depression is an important issue for Korea.

Mental health consultation is an effective treatment for depressive symptoms, but many do not seek the help of mental health services [18–20]. The results of the

* Correspondence: ECPARK@yuhs.ac
[2]Institute of Health Services Research, Yonsei University, Seoul, Republic of Korea
[3]Department of Preventive Medicine & Institute of Health Services Research, Yonsei University College of Medicine, 50 Yonsei-ro, Seodaemun-gu, Seoul 120-752, Republic of Korea
Full list of author information is available at the end of the article

2013 Community Health Survey (CHS) indicate that approximately 5.8% of Koreans are affected by depressive symptoms, but only 16% of those depressed receive mental health consultation for their depression symptoms. Mental health consultation for treatment of depression is as important as the use of medications [18]. Despite the fact that mental health consultation is an effective treatment for depression, it is a real problem that people with depressive symptoms do not receive a mental health consultation.

Utilization of mental health services has been found to be related to several factors [18, 19]. Howard et al. noted that mental health services were associated with educational level, marital status, and race [21]. Vessey, John T et al. reported that the most educated people are the most likely to utilize mental health services [22]. Moreover, divorced people are the most likely to consult with mental health services than married, bereaved, and unmarried people [22]. They identified that there was no strong relationship between the utilization of mental health services and income level [22]. In addition, stigma is a barrier to the use of mental health consultation. Stigma has been shown to influence help seeking and consistency with treatment for mental illness [23]. People with suicidal thoughts also may have more severe depressive symptoms than people with no suicidal thoughts. Severe mental disorder is significantly related to the use of mental health services [24]. Demyttenaere K. et al. indicated that people with serious mental disorders show much higher use of mental health treatment than people with moderate mental disorders [24].

Seeking help for mental health problems has been shown to be related with several factors. These include age, gender, and educational level [4, 21]. Educational level, in particular, exhibits several associations with the use of mental health consultation. A higher educational level appears to dispose an individual to greater access to health information [25, 26]. Moreover, individuals who have attained higher educational levels are more likely to actively respond to the information they receive [25, 26]. Meanwhile, negative attitudes towards mental health services and distrust of the effect of treatment also affect the utilization of mental health consultation services [27]. Therefore, education may be essential in improving help-seeking attitudes and willingness to undergo mental health consultation.

The purpose of this study was to identify several factors related to the use of mental health consultation. In Korea, the government supports mental health promotion centers in each city [28]. Since 2005, a mental care health hotline (+82-129) has provided mental health consultations from mental health experts anywhere and anytime [29]. Additionally, the government has proposed policies to address depression rates and recommend mental health consultation for depressive symptoms in Korea. Therefore, it is essential to study factors associated with the use of mental health consultation.

Methods

Study population

Data from the nationwide 2013 Community Health Survey (CHS) were used for this study. The CHS used a cross-sectional study design and was performed in cooperation with the Korea Centers for Disease Control and Prevention and municipalities in Korea. The Korea Centers for Disease Control and Prevention approved the use of data from CHS through the CHS website (https://chs.cdc.go.kr/chs/index.do). A total of 228,781 individuals responded to the survey. Our study population consisted only of those who had depressive symptoms. We selected participants using the question 'Within the last year, did you experience any emotions, such as sadness or despair, continuously for more than 2 weeks, which increased difficulties in daily life?' Respondents who answered 'no' ($n = 215{,}345$) and didn't answer the question ($n = 59$) were excluded from our study population. Respondents who answered 'yes' were classified as individuals with depressive symptoms ($n = 13{,}377$). We excluded individuals with data missing for use of mental health consultation services ($n = 1$), marital status ($n = 11$), educational level ($n = 26$), occupation ($n = 11$), stress level ($n = 16$), smoking status ($n = 3$), suicidal thoughts ($n = 11$), perceived health status ($n = 2$), and physical activity ($n = 27$). Therefore, a final sample population of 13,269 people was included for analysis in this study.

Variables

The dependent variable was participants' use of mental health consultation services. Participants who had depressive symptoms ($n = 13{,}269$) were asked the question, 'Did you receive any mental health consultation (e.g., medical institution, professional consulting institution, local health centre) for these symptoms?' We examined the participants' use of mental health consultation services based on a 'yes' or 'no' answer.

The main independent variable of interest in this study was education level of the participants. We examined education attainment using a survey question. The question asked for the respondents to indicate the last school grade that was completed. In order to compare the educational level from a global perspective, the International Standard Classification of Education (ISCED) was used in the analysis. International Standard Classification is one of the standard frameworks to compare education statistics. Low educational level included ISCED classification of 0–1 (early childhood education and primary education) and medium educational level included

ISCED classification of 2 (lower secondary education). High education was defined as ISCED classification of 3 (upper secondary education), and college or over as ISCED classification of 5 to 8 (short-cycle tertiary education, bachelor or equivalent, master or equivalent, doctoral or equivalent.

Other variables in the analysis included sociodemographic, socioeconomic, health-behaviour, and health-condition variables. The sociodemographic factors were age (19 to 29 years, 30 to 39 years, 40 to 49 years, 50 to 59 years, 60 to 69 years, 70 or above) and gender (male, female). The socioeconomic factors were marital status (married and cohabit, married and non-cohabit, bereaved, divorced, unmarried), region (capital, urban, rural), household income level (divided into quartiles), and occupation (managers, professionals, clerical support workers, service workers, sales worker, skilled agricultural, forestry and fishery workers, craft and related trades workers, plant and machine operators, and assemblers, elementary occupations, armed forces occupations, others).

The capital region included Seoul, which is the capital of Korea, and Gyeonggi province, which surrounds Seoul. About a population of 20 million (about 50% of Korea) live in the capital region. Urban areas included metropolitan cities usually with a population of about 1 million. Rural areas included the remaining geographic areas, excluding capital and urban regions. The standards of dividing house income level per year were less than 8,400,000 won (about 75,350,000 USD), less than 24,000,000 won (about 215,290,000 USD), less than 40,000,000 won (about 358,800,000 USD), and more than 40,000,000 or above (about 358,800,000 USD). Occupation was classified by the Korean Standard Classification of Occupations (KSCO). The KSCO is based on the International Standard Classification of Occupations. The International Standard Classification of Occupations is one of the standard frameworks for classifying jobs according to the tasks and duties undertaken in the job [30]. This classification was simplified as high-skilled white collar, low-skilled white collar, high-skilled blue collar, low-skilled blue collar, and others. The high-skilled white collar group included managers, professionals, and clerical support workers. Low-skilled white collar workers included service workers and sales workers. The high-skilled blue collar group included skilled agricultural, forestry, and fishery workers, as well as craft and related trade workers. Low-skilled blue collar workers included plant and machine operators and assemblers and elementary occupations. Others included armed forces occupations, students, and other job statuses.

Health-behaviour factors included physical activity (inactive and active by metabolic equivalent task), smoking status (never or former, current [within a year]) and alcohol consumption (never or former, current [within a year]). Health-condition factors included stress level (very, little no), suicidal thoughts (yes or no), sleep duration (<7 h, 7 to 8 h, ≥9 h), and perceived health status (good, normal, bad). Participants were asked the question, 'Did you have suicidal thoughts within the last year?' And we examined the participants' suicidal thoughts based on a 'yes' or 'no' answer.

Statistical analysis

Statistical analysis was performed using SAS software, version 9.4 (SAS Institute, Cary, NC, USA). All analyses included the use of weighted variables. Chi-square tests were used to confirm the significant differences between respondents who did and did not obtain mental health consultation for depression symptoms. Logistic regression analysis was used to determine odds ratios (ORs) and 95% confidence intervals (CIs). Subgroup analysis was performed according to age and suicidal thoughts. A p-value <0.05 was considered to indicate a statistically significant result.

Results

Table 1 presents the general characteristics of the study populations. There are 4019 males (30.3%) and 9250 females (69.7%) included in this study. Of the 13,269 participants who have depressive symptoms, 2120 (16.0%) received mental health consultation and 11,149 (84.0%) did not. The rate of use of mental health consultation is the lowest among participants with low educational level (14.6%) relative to among college or over (15.5%). Of the 13,269 participants, the rate of receiving mental health consultation is the lowest among the 70 years or above participants (12.4%). The rate of use of mental health consultation is the highest among divorced people (21.8%). Moreover, females (17.3%) show higher mental health consultation rates than males (13.0%).

Table 2 presents the results for the factors associated with the use of mental health consultation services for depressive symptoms. Educational level shows a significant positive association with the use of mental health consultation. Respondents in the college or over level are more likely to receive mental health consultation for depressive symptoms (OR = 1.49; 95% CI: 1.21–1.84), compared to respondents in the low educational level. Individuals in the 70 years or above age group are less likely to receive mental health consultation (OR = 0.46; 95% CI: 0.33–0.64) than the 19 to 29 years old groups. Females shows higher mental health consultation rates (OR = 1.19; 95% CI: 1.02–1.38) than males. There is no significant association between household income level and utilization of mental health consultation. Respondents who are divorced have greater odds of receiving mental health consultation (OR = 1.32; 95% CI: 1.08–

Table 1 General characteristics of the study population

Variables	Total		Mental health consultation				P-value*
			YES		NO		
	N	%	N	%	N	%	
Total	13,269	100.0	2120	16.0	11,149	84.0	
Educational level - ISCED							0.0005
Low	4832	36.4	704	14.6	4128	85.4	
Medium	1606	12.1	295	18.4	1311	81.6	
High	4119	31.0	700	17.0	3419	83.0	
College or over	2712	20.4	421	15.5	2291	84.5	
Age							<.0001
19–29	1305	9.8	210	16.1	1095	83.9	
30–39	1745	13.2	292	16.7	1453	83.3	
40–49	2144	16.2	365	17.0	1779	83.0	
50–59	2695	20.3	453	16.8	2242	83.2	
60–69	2259	17.0	412	18.2	1847	81.8	
70≤	3121	23.5	388	12.4	2733	87.6	
Gender							<.0001
Male	4019	30.3	523	13.0	3496	87.0	
Female	9250	69.7	1597	17.3	7653	82.7	
Household income level							0.0129
Quartile 1 (lowest)	3518	26.5	536	15.2	2982	84.8	
Quartile 2	3349	25.2	595	17.8	2754	82.2	
Quartile 3	3048	23.0	468	15.4	2580	84.6	
Quartile 4 (highest)	3354	25.3	521	15.5	2833	84.5	
Region							0.7874
Capital (Seoul, Gyeonggi)	4366	32.9	705	16.1	3661	83.9	
Urban	2604	19.6	423	16.2	2181	83.8	
Rural area	6299	47.5	992	15.7	5307	84.3	
Marital status							<.0001
Married-cohabit	7638	57.6	1178	15.4	6460	84.6	
Married-no cohabit	449	3.4	72	16.0	377	84.0	
Bereaved	2440	18.4	364	14.9	2076	85.1	
Divorced	908	6.8	198	21.8	710	78.2	
Unmarried	1834	13.8	308	16.8	1526	83.2	
Occupation							<.0001
High-skilled white collar	1756	13.2	215	12.2	1541	87.8	
Low-skilled white collar	1499	11.3	234	15.6	1265	84.4	
High-skilled blue collar	1528	11.5	194	12.7	1334	87.3	
Low-skilled blue collar	1469	11.1	193	13.1	1276	86.9	
Others	7017	52.9	1284	18.3	5733	81.7	
Physical activity							0.0265
Inactive	8932	67.3	1471	16.5	7461	83.5	
Active	4337	32.7	649	15.0	3688	85.0	
Smoking status							0.3816
Never or former	10,807	81.4	1741	16.1	9066	83.9	

Table 1 General characteristics of the study population *(Continued)*

Variables	Total		Mental health consultation				*P*-value*
			YES		NO		
	N	%	N	%	N	%	
Current	2462	18.6	379	15.4	2083	84.6	
Alcohol consumption							0.0023
Never or former	5289	39.9	908	17.2	4381	82.8	
Current (within a year)	7980	60.1	1212	15.2	6768	84.8	
Stress level							<.0001
Very	8441	63.6	1590	18.8	6851	81.2	
Little	4114	31.0	451	11.0	3663	89.0	
No	714	5.4	79	11.1	635	88.9	
Suicidal Thought							<.0001
Yes	7295	55.0	1472	20.2	5823	79.8	
No	5974	45.0	648	10.8	5326	89.2	
Sleeping duration							0.1173
Less than 7 h	7400	55.8	1193	16.1	6207	83.9	
7–8 h	5162	38.9	797	15.4	4365	84.6	
9 h or over	707	5.3	130	18.4	577	81.6	
Perceived health status							<.0001
Good	2488	18.8	262	10.5	2226	89.5	
Normal	4810	36.2	687	14.3	4123	85.7	
Bad	5971	45.0	1171	19.6	4800	80.4	

* *P*-values calculated by the chi-square test

1.62) than respondents who are married and cohabitate with their spouse.

Figure 1 presents the results for the subgroup analysis of the association between educational level and use of mental health consultation stratified by age. The analysis reveal that, compared to those 70 years or above in age, respondents in the 19 to 29 years old groups in the college or over educational level have a greater odds ratio for mental health consultation. Figure 2 presents the results for the subgroup analysis of the association between educational level and use of mental health consultation stratified according to suicidal thoughts. People who have suicidal thoughts have a stronger association between educational level and use of mental health consultation.

Discussion

The aim of this study is to identify factors associated with the use of mental health consultation in Korea. The findings reveal that educational level has a positive association with the use of mental health consultation services. Individuals aged 70 years or above tend to undergo mental health consultation less than those aged between 19 and 29 years. Females undergo more mental health consultations than males. Divorced people undergo the most mental health consultation, compared to respondents who are married and cohabitate with their spouse. There is no significant association between household income level and utilization of mental health consultation. Overall, younger people tend to show stronger correlation between educational level and the use of mental health consultation. People who have suicidal thoughts show a stronger association between educational level and use of mental health consultation.

In the present study, we note a significantly positive association between educational levels and the utilization of mental health services. This association may be explained by several reasons. First, highly educated people are more likely to have active attitudes toward mental health services. Individuals who achieve higher educational levels are better at managing their lives, compared to individuals with lower levels of education [31, 32]. The process of studying increases self-confidence and motivation [31]. These characteristics are essential for successful problem-solving, and highly-educated people tend to solve their difficulties using an active attitude approach [31–33]. Second, less educated people tend not to recognize their mental health problems [22]. Mental health services are a type of help-seeking process [21]. These help-seeking processes

Table 2 Factors associated with mental health consultation [a]

Variables	Mental health consultation	
	Adjusted OR	95%CI
Educational level - ISCED		
Low	1.00	–
Medium	1.32	(1.09–1.60)
High	1.35	(1.12–1.63)
College or over	1.49	(1.21–1.84)
Age		
19–29	1.00	–
30–39	0.89	(0.71–1.13)
40–49	0.88	(0.69–1.13)
50–59	0.80	(0.61–1.04)
60–69	0.86	(0.64–1.17)
70≤	0.46	(0.33–0.64)
Gender		
Male	1.00	–
Female	1.19	(1.02–1.38)
Household income level		
Quartile 1 (lowest)	1.00	–
Quartile 2	1.12	(0.96–1.31)
Quartile 3	1.16	(0.97–1.37)
Quartile 4 (highest)	1.17	(0.98–1.41)
Region		
Capital(Seoul, Gyeonggi)	1.00	–
Urban	0.98	(0.85–1.14)
Rural area	0.99	(0.88–1.12)
Marital status		
Married-cohabit	1.00	–
Married-no cohabit	1.29	(0.95–1.73)
Bereaved	1.23	(1.04–1.47)
Divorced	1.32	(1.08–1.62)
Unmarried	1.12	(0.91–1.38)
Occupation		
High-skilled white collar	1.00	–
Low-skilled white collar	1.08	(0.86–1.35)
High-skilled blue collar	0.92	(0.66–1.27)
Low-skilled blue collar	1.00	(0.78–1.27)
Others	1.54	(1.28–1.86)
Physical activity		
Inactive	1.00	–
Active	1.13	(0.99–1.28)
Smoking status		
Never or former	1.00	–
Current	0.98	(0.83–1.15)

Table 2 Factors associated with mental health consultation [a] *(Continued)*

Variables	Mental health consultation	
	Adjusted OR	95%CI
Alcohol consumption		
Never or former	1.00	–
Current (within a year)	0.81	(0.71–0.93)
Stress level		
Very	1.00	–
Little	0.65	(0.57–0.75)
No	0.78	(0.58–1.07)
Suicidal Thought		
Yes	2.15	(1.89–2.43)
No	1.00	–
Sleeping duration		
Less than 7 h	1.00	–
7–8 h	1.07	(0.95–1.20)
9 h or over	1.13	(0.91–1.41)
Perceived health status		
Good	1.00	–
Normal	1.31	(1.11–1.55)
Bad	1.89	(1.58–2.26)

[a] Logistic regression analysis was used to determine odds ratios (ORs) and 95% confidence intervals (CIs). A total of 13,269 participants were included in the analysis. An example of how to interpret this figure is as follows: 'respondents who received a college or over education are more likely to receive mental health consultation for depressive symptoms (OR = 1.49; 95% CI: 1.21–1.84), compared with respondents with low educational level'

consist of several steps, including recognizing the problem, realizing the necessary of help, and contacting health services [21]. Because educational level influences awareness of a health care problem, use of mental health services may differ according to the level of education. Third, highly educated people also have more knowledge about mental health services [34, 35]. They have more opportunities to obtain information about how to manage depression (e.g., receiving a mental health consultation) and access to mental health services [25, 26]. Finally, education may influence stigma about mental health services. Stigma of what others could think may be a common barrier for contacting mental health services [21]. The stigma associated with mental health consultation influences delays in seeking assistance [36]. Previous studies showed that highly educated people have less stigma about mental health services [37, 38]. Koreans with mental health problems may have more prejudice against mental health problem than normal people [39]. Also, they tend to avoid making their mental health problems known to other people [39]. Jang et al. identified that such stigma may be influenced by the cultural background in Korea [40].

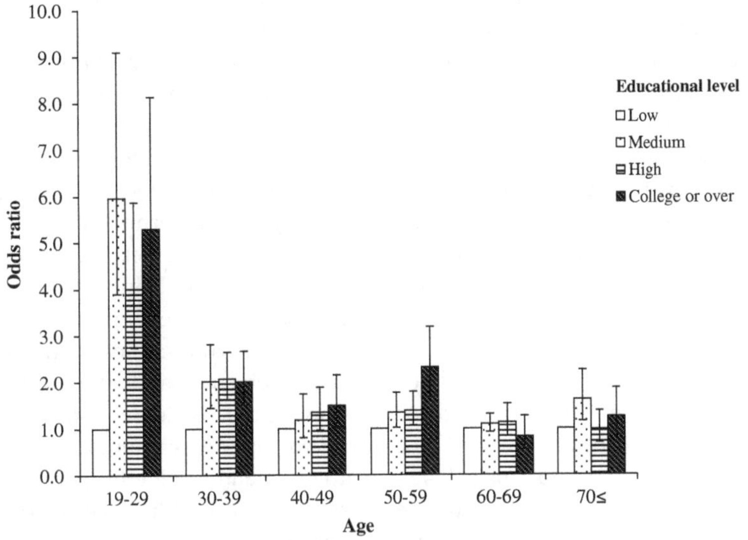

Fig. 1 Subgroup analysis of mental health consultation according to educational level stratified by age. An example of how to interpret this figure is as follows: 'compared with individuals 70 years or above in age, respondents in the 19 to 29 years old groups with college or over educational level have a greater odds ratio for mental health consultation.' Control variables include gender, region, house income level, marital status, occupation, physical activity, smoking status, alcohol consumption, stress level, suicidal thoughts, sleeping duration, and perceived health status

The present study shows that gender and marital status are associated with the utilization of mental health services, while income level has no significantly associations. The results of this study indicated that older adults were less likely to receive mental health consultation. This result was similar to the results of previous studies. Older adults may be less aware of a mental health problem, have a higher sense of self-sufficiency, and be more conscious of the disgrace associated with receipt of mental health services [41, 42]. Females are more likely to use mental health services than males. This correspond with previous studies [22, 43]. Females may be more likely to recognize their emotional problems than men who had similar symptoms [44]. Moreover, females tend to share their emotion with others and be more openness to acknowledging mental health problems [4, 22]. Divorced people are more likely to have mental health services than people who are married

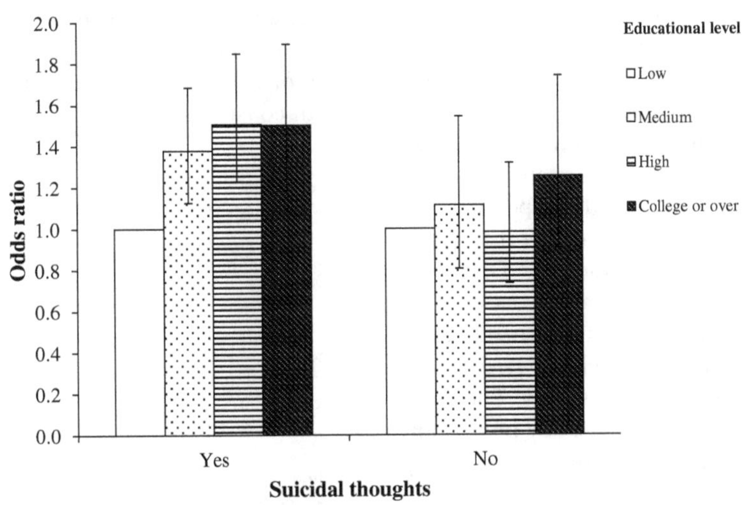

Fig. 2 Subgroup analysis of mental health consultation according to educational level stratified by suicidal thoughts. An example of how to interpret this figure is as follows: 'people who have suicidal thoughts have a stronger association between educational level and use of mental health consultation.' Control variables include age, gender, region, house income level, marital status, occupation, physical activity, smoking status, alcohol consumption, stress level, sleeping duration, and perceived health status

and cohabit in the study. In many cases, people seek consultation to receive advice for marital problems before divorce [45]. Also, pre-divorce counseling could influence access to mental health consultation. John. T. et al. also identified that separated or divorced people were the most likely to seek mental health services, and our study correspond with previous studies [22].

In the age group of individuals between 19 and 29 years, the association between educational level and use of mental health consultation is stronger than adults 70 years or older. Overall, younger people tend to show stronger correlation between educational level and the use of mental health consultation. This may be related to several factors. Older adults are more prejudiced about the use of mental health consultation and less aware of the severity of their depressive symptoms [41, 42]. Also, the fact that education level influences young people more could be implicated in developing mental health policies.

People who have suicidal thoughts show a stronger association between educational level and use of mental health consultation. People with suicidal thoughts have positive association between educational level and high rates of use of mental health consultation. Therefore, it is necessary to strengthen mental health policies in educational aspects, such as educating people how to manage the depressive symptoms and providing information on mental health services, especially those with suicidal thoughts.

This study has some limitations. First, the data were self-reported by the participants. It is possible that the responses did not correspond to actual consulting rates. Second, we could not examine the type of provider from which the respondents received the consultation, because questions about this factor were not included in the survey. There are also some differences between medical institutions, professional consulting institutions, and local health centres. Third, there was no use of psychometric instruments; the data were only based on participant's subjective view of their depression symptoms. However, the screenings question in the paper were included in the Korean version of the World Health Organization Composite International Diagnostic Interview-Short Form, and validated as a cost-effective screening instrument that could be easily integrated into health surveys [46]. Fourth, people with severe mental illnesses are less likely to respond to a survey. Therefore, it could introduce selection bias in the study population. Finally, the study was based on a cross-sectional survey. Causality could not be confirmed clearly and only association could be confirmed. Despite the above limitations, this study also has several strengths. We used nationally, multistage, stratified collected data that could be considered representative of the Korean population. Second, although most previous studies were conducted in Caucasians, we conducted research on an Asian society. Third, to the best of our knowledge, this study offers new insights into factors associated with the utilization of mental health services. In particular, Korea ranks highest in suicide rates among OECD countries, and the proportion of suicides due to depression is high. Additionally, the government has proposed policies to address depression rates and to recommend mental health consultation for depressive symptoms in Korea. Therefore, our results seem meaningful.

The most common cause of suicide in Korea is psychiatric problems, and the most typical mental illness people suffer is depression. It has been consistently reported that depression is a serious risk factor of suicide attempts and suicide in previous studies [41, 42]. Moreover, mental health services are considered a significant way of preventing suicide [47]. In this study, we examined factors affecting the use of mental health services to treat depressive symptoms and confirmed that educational level is correlated with the utilization of mental health services. The results could have implications for policies on the use of mental health services in Korea.

Conclusion

This study identified that only 16% of individuals with depressive symptoms obtain mental health consultation and that the rates of use of mental health consultation is lower for older adults men, and the divorced. In particular, educational level shows a significant positive association with mental health consultation in the Korea population. This study also presents information about the vulnerable classes of people receiving mental health consultation services. The government should pay more attention to providing public awareness about the symptoms of depression and increase accessibility of mental health consultation services.

Abbreviations

CHS: Community Health Survey; CI: Confidence interval; ISCED: International Standard Classification of Education; KSCO: Korean standard classification of occupations; OECD: Organisation for Economic Co-operation and Development; OR: Odds ratio; USA: United States of America; USD: United States dollar

Acknowledgements

We appreciate to the Korean Centers for Disease Control (KCDC) that provided meaningful data.

Funding

There is no funding.

Authors' contributions

JJ, SAL, ECP were involved in the study design. JJ, SAL prepared the manuscript. SAL, WK, YC, ECP critically revised the paper for important intellectual content. ECP had full access to the article and responsibility for the accuracy of analysis. All authors read and confirm the final version of article to be published. All authors read and approved the final manuscript.

Consent for publication
Not applicable.

Competing interests
The authors declare that they have no competing interests.

Author details
[1]Department of Public Health, Graduate School, Yonsei University, Seoul, Republic of Korea. [2]Institute of Health Services Research, Yonsei University, Seoul, Republic of Korea. [3]Department of Preventive Medicine & Institute of Health Services Research, Yonsei University College of Medicine, 50 Yonsei-ro, Seodaemun-gu, Seoul 120-752, Republic of Korea.

References

1. Wang PS, Aguilar-Gaxiola S, Alonso J, Angermeyer MC, Borges G, Bromet EJ, Bruffaerts R, De Girolamo G, De Graaf R, Gureje O. Use of mental health services for anxiety, mood, and substance disorders in 17 countries in the WHO world mental health surveys. Lancet. 2007;370(9590):841–50.
2. Thornicroft G. Most people with mental illness are not treated. Lancet. 2007; 370(9590):807–8.
3. World Health Organization. "Depression: let's talk" says WHO, as depression tops list of causes of ill health. Saudi Med J. 2017;38(5):565.
4. Mackenzie C, Gekoski W, Knox V. Age, gender, and the underutilization of mental health services: the influence of help-seeking attitudes. Aging Ment Health. 2006;10(6):574–82.
5. Segee PF, Maguire L, Ross J, Malik ML, Colket J, Davidson JR. Demographics, treatment seeking, and diagnoses of anxiety support group participants. J Anxiety Disord. 1999;13(3):315–34.
6. Rondet C, Parizot I, Cadwallader JS, Lebas J, Chauvin P. Why underserved patients do not consult their general practitioner for depression: results of a qualitative and a quantitative survey at a free outpatient clinic in Paris France. BMC Fam Pract. 2015;16(1):1.
7. Corrigan P. How stigma interferes with mental health care. Am Psychol. 2004;59(7):614.
8. Mathers CD, Loncar D. Projections of global mortality and burden of disease from 2002 to 2030. PLoS Med. 2006;3(11):e442.
9. Paykel ES. Depression: major problem for public health. Epidemiol Psychiatr Sci. 2006;15(1):4–10.
10. World Health Organization: The world health report 2001: mental health: new understanding, new hope; 2001.
11. Brent DA. Depression and suicide in children and adolescents. Pediatr Rev. 1993;14(10):380–8.
12. Lesage AD, Boyer R, Grunberg F, Vanier C, Morissette R, Loyer M. Suicide and mental disorders: a case-control study of young men. Am J Psychiatry. 1994;151(7):1063.
13. Cavanagh JT, Carson AJ, Sharpe M, Lawrie SM. Psychological autopsy studies of suicide: a systematic review. Psychol Med. 2003;33(3):395–405.
14. Henriksson MM, Aro HM, Marttunen MJ, Heikkinen ME, Isometsa E, Kuoppasalmi KE, Lonnqvist J. Mental disorders and comorbidity in suicide. Am J Psychiatry. 1993;150:935.
15. Kim C, Lesage A, Seguin M, Chawky N, Vanier C, Lipp O, Turecki G. Patterns of co-morbidity in male suicide completers. Psychol Med. 2003;33(7):1299–309.
16. Dumais A, Lesage A, Alda M, Rouleau G, Dumont M, Chawky N, Roy M, Mann JJ, Benkelfat C, Turecki G. Risk factors for suicide completion in major depression: a case-control study of impulsive and aggressive behaviors in men. Am J Psychiatry. 2005;162(11):2116–24.
17. OECD Publishing: OECD (2016), Society at a Glance 2016: OECD social indicators.
18. Uchida N, CHONG MY, Tan CH, Nagai H, Tanaka M, LEE MS, Fujii S, YANG SY, Si T, Sim K. International study on antidepressant prescription pattern at 20 teaching hospitals and major psychiatric institutions in East Asia: analysis of 1898 cases from China, Japan, Korea Singapore and Taiwan. Psychiatry Clin Neurosci. 2007;61(5):522–8.
19. World Health Organization. Investing in mental health evidence for action: World Health Organization; 2013.
20. Alvidrez J. Ethnic variations in mental health attitudes and service use among low-income African American, Latina, and European American young women. Community Ment Health J. 1999;35(6):515–30.
21. Howard KI, Cornille TA, Lyons JS, Vessey JT, Lueger RJ, Saunders SM. Patterns of mental health service utilization. Arch Gen Psychiatry. 1996;53(8):696–703.
22. Vessey JT, Howard KI. Who seeks psychotherapy? Psychother Theory Res Pract Train. 1993;30(4):546.
23. Trude S, Stoddard JJ. Referral gridlock. J Gen Intern Med. 2003;18(6):442–9.
24. Demyttenaere K, Bruffaerts R, Posada-Villa J, Gasquet I, Kovess V, Lepine J, Angermeyer M, Bernert SD, De Girolamo G, Morosini P. Prevalence, severity, and unmet need for treatment of mental disorders in the World Health Organization world mental health surveys. JAMA. 2004;291(21):2581–90.
25. Ross CE, Wu C-L. The links between education and health. Am Sociol Rev. 1995:719–45.
26. Chevalier A, Feinstein L. Sheepskin or Prozac: the causal effect of education on mental health. In: IZA discussion paper no 2231; 2006.
27. Gulliver A, Griffiths KM, Christensen H. Perceived barriers and facilitators to mental health help-seeking in young people: a systematic review. BMC Psychiatry. 2010;10(1):113.
28. Roh S, Lee S-U, Soh M, Ryu V, Kim H, Jang JW, Lim HY, Jeon M, Park J-I, Choi S. Mental health services and R&D in South Korea. Int J Ment Health Syst. 2016;10(1):45.
29. Ministry of Health and Welfare. 2017; Available from: http://www.mohw.go.kr/eng/sg/ssg0101mn.jsp?PAR_MENU_ID=1001&MENU_ID=100110. Accessed 22 Sept 2017.
30. Smith P, Nüsslin F. Benefits to medical physics from the recent inclusion of medical physicists in the international classification of standard occupation (ICSO-08). Med Phys Int J. 2013;1(1).
31. Mirowsky J, Ross CE. Education, personal control, lifestyle and health a human capital hypothesis. Res Aging. 1998;20(4):415–49.
32. Stansfeld SA, Head J, Marmot M. Explaining social class differences in depression and well-being. Soc Psychiatry Psychiatr Epidemiol. 1997;33(1):1–9.
33. Ross CE, Mirowsky J. Explaining the social patterns of depression: control and problem solving–or support and talking? J Health Soc Behav. 1989:206–19.
34. Ross CE, Wu C-L. Education, age, and the cumulative advantage in health. J Health Soc Behav. 1996;37:104–20.
35. Wood AL, Wahl OF. Evaluating the effectiveness of a consumer-provided mental health recovery education presentation. Psychiatr Rehabil J. 2006;30(1):46.
36. Corrigan PW. Mental health stigma as social attribution: implications for research methods and attitude change. Clin Psychol Sci Pract. 2000;7(1):48–67.
37. Holmes EP, Corrigan PW, Williams P, Canar J, Kubiak MA. Changing attitudes about schizophrenia. Schizophr Bull. 1999;25(3):447.
38. Corrigan PW, Watson AC. The stigma of psychiatric disorders and the gender, ethnicity, and education of the perceiver. Community Ment Health J. 2007;43(5):439–58.
39. Cho SJ, Lee JY, Hong JP, Lee HB, Cho MJ, Hahm BJ. Mental health service use in a nationwide sample of Korean adults. Soc Psychiatry Psychiatr Epidemiol. 2009;44(11):943.
40. Jang Y, Kim G, Hansen L, Chiriboga DA. Attitudes of older Korean Americans toward mental health services. J Am Geriatr Soc. 2007;55(4):616–20.
41. Byers AL, Arean PA, Yaffe K. Low use of mental health services among older Americans with mood and anxiety disorders. Psychiatr Serv. 2012;63(1):66–72.
42. Dalrymple KL, Zimmerman M. Treatment-seeking for social anxiety disorder in a general outpatient psychiatry setting. Psychiatry Res. 2011;187(3):375–81.
43. Regier DA, Narrow WE, Rae DS, Manderscheid RW, Locke BZ, Goodwin FK. The de facto US mental and addictive disorders service system: epidemiologic catchment area prospective 1-year prevalence rates of disorders and services. Arch Gen Psychiatry. 1993;50(2):85–94.

44. Wang PS, Lane M, Olfson M, Pincus HA, Wells KB, Kessler RC. Twelve-month use of mental health services in the United States: results from the National Comorbidity Survey Replication. Arch Gen Psychiatry. 2005;62(6):629–40.
45. Amato PR. The consequences of divorce for adults and children. J Marriage Fam. 2000;62(4):1269–87.
46. Gigantesco A, Morosini P. Development, reliability and factor analysis of a self-administered questionnaire which originates from the World Health Organization's composite international diagnostic interview–short form (CIDI-SF) for assessing mental disorders. Clin Pract Epidemiol Ment Health. 2008;4(1):8.
47. US Public Health Service. The surgeon General's call to action to prevent suicide. Washington, DC: author; 1999.

18

Building flexibility and managing complexity in community mental health: lessons learned in a large urban centre

Vicky Stergiopoulos[1,2,3*], Dima Saab[1], Kate Francombe Pridham[1], Anjana Aery[1] and Arash Nakhost[3,4]

Abstract

Background: Across many jurisdictions, adults with complex mental health and social needs face challenges accessing appropriate supports due to system fragmentation and strict eligibility criteria of existing services. To support this underserviced population, Toronto's local health authority launched two novel community mental health models in 2014, inspired by Flexible Assertive Community Team principles. This study explores service user and provider perspectives on the acceptability of these services, and lessons learned during early implementation.

Methods: We purposively sampled 49 stakeholders (staff, physicians, service users, health systems stakeholders) and conducted 17 semi-structured qualitative interviews and 5 focus groups between October 23, 2014 and March 2, 2015, exploring stakeholder perspectives on the newly launched team based models, as well as activities and strategies employed to support early implementation. Interviews and focus groups were audio recorded, transcribed verbatim and analyzed using thematic analysis.

Results: Findings revealed wide-ranging endorsement for the two team-based models' success in engaging the target population of adults with complex service needs. Implementation strengths included the broad recognition of existing service gaps, the use of interdisciplinary teams and experienced service providers, broad partnerships and collaboration among various service sectors, training and team building activities. Emerging challenges included lack of complementary support services such as suitable housing, organizational contexts reluctant to embrace change and risk associated with complexity, as well as limited service provider and organizational capacity to deliver evidence-based interventions.

Conclusions: Findings identified implementation drivers at the practitioner, program, and system levels, specific to the implementation of community mental health interventions for adults with complex health and social needs. These can inform future efforts to address the health and support needs of this vulnerable population.

Keywords: Mental health, Complex needs, Qualitative evaluation, Community mental health, Implementation, Flexible assertive community treatment

Background

Across jurisdictions, individuals with complex health, mental health and social needs face multiple barriers to accessing appropriate, integrated services and supports due to system fragmentation, strict eligibility criteria of existing services, stigma and discrimination.

* Correspondence: vicky.stergiopoulos@camh.ca
[1]Centre for Urban Health Solutions, Li Ka Shing Knowledge Institute, St. Michael's Hospital, 209 Victoria Street, Toronto, ON M5B 1W8, Canada
[2]Centre for Addiction and Mental Health, 100 Stokes Street, Toronto, ON M6J 1H4, Canada
Full list of author information is available at the end of the article

In western countries, individuals with serious mental illness (SMI) can access Assertive Community Treatment (ACT) or Intensive Case Management (ICM) services. Both ACT and ICM models have been studied in a wide range of contexts and for various subpopulations of adults with SMI [1–6]. ACT is a well-defined, team-based approach to care, with strong evidence in its favour [3, 5]. Its strict eligibility criteria, however, may exclude a subset of individuals with mental disorders and high support needs (e.g. individuals with primary substance use, or personality disorders) [7]. Furthermore, with few options for seamless participant transitions to lower levels of support during periods of stability, there are long waitlists for ACT services in several jurisdictions [8]. In contrast to ACT, with its well-developed fidelity criteria, ICM tends to be more variable in nature and implementation, yielding mixed findings in the evaluative literature [9, 10]. While ACT teams directly provide needed services to adults with SMI and high service utilization, ICM interventions deliver these same services in collaboration with other local service-providers [9], and generally provide a lower level of support to a broader group of adults with SMI.

To address some of these challenges, Flexible Assertive Community Treatment (FACT), a model that blends aspects of ACT and ICM services within a single team, emerged in the Netherlands in the past 10- years, and has been well described and adopted elsewhere [11–14]. Within a FACT team, service users retain the relationships with their care manager (nurse/social worker), their psychiatrist and other team members such as the peer expert, while stepping-up or down to higher (ACT-like) or lower (enriched ICM) levels of support as needed over time. As FACT eligibility criteria are more flexible than those of traditional ACT team criteria, ACT-ineligible individuals may access high levels of support services if needed. Early evaluations of the FACT model, relying primarily on observational studies and administrative data, have been promising, suggesting improvements in adherence rates, reduction in unmet needs and improved quality of life [12, 15–19].

This study describes the early implementation of two local community mental health teams, inspired by FACT principles, to address the needs of adults with complex health, mental health and social needs in Toronto, Canada's largest urban centre. The local service delivery context, and guidelines from the local health authority necessitated departures from full replication of FACT.

Service delivery context

Assertive Community Treatment (ACT) teams in the province of Ontario, Canada have been systematically implemented since 1998, with 79 ACT teams currently in operation [20]. Though Toronto has a high concentration of services, including ACT, individuals with complex health and social needs such as intellectual and developmental disabilities, traumatic brain injury, co-morbid substance use conditions, and co-morbid personality disorders, continue to face barriers in accessing community supports of high intensity. Similar to other jurisdictions, Ontario ACT standards prioritize adults with schizophrenia and bipolar affective disorder, creating access challenges for those not meeting diagnostic eligibility criteria or not having repeated and lengthy hospitalizations [21]. With ACT team wait lists averaging more than a year [22], local ICM services are often asked to step in while they are not resourced to serve individuals with complex health and social needs requiring more intensive interventions.

To address these challenges, Toronto's local health authority launched two "Integrated Service (IS) Teams", drawing from elements of FACT, in 2014. Although previous reviews have synthesized the factors that affect implementation of programs in general into a conceptual model [23, 24], and Fixsen et al. (2005) have developed the National Implementation Research Network (NIRN) framework for active implementation [25], these models are still evolving. Furthermore, research on how implementation unfolds in community based mental health services and systems at various stages of implementation is scant [26–28], including research on implementing ACT, or FACT [17, 18, 29, 30].

Study aims

This study aims to explore service user and provider perspectives on the acceptability of the IS team models, and to identify early implementation drivers. This information may be useful for future efforts to address the needs of adults with complex health, mental health and social needs in other jurisdictions facing similar challenges.

Methods

The integrated service teams: introducing team and organizational flexibility

Both Integrated Service (IS) teams, referred to throughout this paper as the "East" and "South" team, for their respective geographical areas in the city, were multidisciplinary, recovery oriented, and targeted individuals with complex needs (Table 1). Eligibility criteria focused on the social circumstances of service users, such as homelessness, criminal justice involvement, and service engagement, rather than strict diagnostic or past health service use criteria.

The East team, aiming to integrate hospital with community based expertise and resources, was implemented by adapting a pre-existing urban academic hospital ACT team serving a large homeless population [31]. Co-located with the hospital's primary care centre, the East team, enhanced by a clinical psychologist, as well as case managers and a personal support worker, focuses on hospital-primary care-community integration and the delivery of evidence-based interventions for a range of mental disorders. Service users, including those previously receiving ACT services as well as new referrals, can access a continuum of ACT and ICM services within the same team, with approximately 50-60% of service users requiring ACT level of support. The South team, implemented by a community mental health organization serving adults with a diversity of needs, was launched as a new team, triaging and assessing new referrals and coordinating their access to a range of pre-existing ICM, ACT, and crisis services in the host organization. Composed of nurses, addiction specialists, social workers, behavioural therapists, and

Table 1 East and South Team comparisons with ACT and FACT models

	ACT Standards in Ontario, Canada[a]	East Team	South Team	FACT in the Netherlands[b]
Target Population	Adults with serious mental illness (SMI) that seriously impairs their social functioning. Priority given to adults with schizophrenia, other psychotic disorders and bipolar disorder.	Adults meeting ACT admission criteria as well as adults experiencing complex mental, physical and social needs (including homelessness, criminal justice involvement, developmental and substance use disorders), with high utilization of acute care services and poor track record of system engagement.	Youth and adults (16-65 years) with complex mental, physical and emotional needs (including trauma, developmental and personality disorders), with high utilization of acute care services and poor track record of system engagement.	All patients with serious mental illness (SMI) in a particular district or region (including major axis I and severe limitations in social functioning).
Team size	60-100	190-208	90-100	220-250
Caseload	Urban - 1:10	1:13	1:13	1:20
Catchment area	1:200, 000	1:130,000-150,000	1:130,000-150,000	1: 40,000 -50,000
Clinical Human Resources	11 FTE clinical staff excluding team psychiatrist:	20.5 FTE clinical staff excluding team psychiatrists:	11 FTE clinical staff excluding consulting psychiatrist:	11 to 14 FTE clinical staff excluding team psychiatrist:
	1 FTE team coordinator; 3 FTE registered nurses; 1 FTE social worker; 1 FTE occupational therapist;1 FTE addiction specialist; 1 FTE vocational specialist;1 FTE peer support specialist; 2 FTE case managers; 0.8 FTE psychiatrist	1 FTE team coordinator;1 FTE psychologist; 5 FTE psychiatric nurses;2 FTE social workers; 2 FTE occupational therapists; 1.5 FTE peer support specialist; 1 FTE personal support worker; 1 FTE addiction specialist;1 FTE rehabilitation therapist;1 FTE vocational specialist;4.0 FTE case managers;1.3 FTE psychiatrists	2.0 FTE care coordinators; 1.0 FTE nurse practitioner, 2.0 FTE behavioral therapists; 0.5 FTE personal support worker; 2.0 FTE social workers; 2.0 FTE nurses; 1.0 FTE registered practical nurse; access to consulting psychiatrist	5 to 8 FTE psychiatric nurses;1 FTE psychologist;1 FTE employment specialist;1 FTE peer support worker; 1 FTE social worker; 2 FTE addiction specialists; 1.0 FTE psychiatrist
Team rounds	Daily meeting to discuss clients in crisis or update the team on ongoing issues.	Using the FACT board for daily morning meeting for 30–50 clients requiring daily attention.	Weekly meetings.	Using the FACT board for daily meetings for 20-30 clients requiring daily attention.
Team Vision	ACT services to clients who have not benefited from traditional out-patient programs.	Recovery focused ACT and ICM services within the same team. EBM interventions provided as core component of team function.	Recovery focused ICM level multidisciplinary support to clients, facilitating smooth care transitions within the organization as client support needs change. Select EBM interventions are provided.	Recovery focused ACT and ICM services within the same team. EBM interventions provided as core component of team function.
Step Down /Graduation	Transfer to less intensive service if demonstrated ability to function during gradual reduction in services over approximately 2 years.	Step down from board into the same team; able to move back onto the FACT board as needed. If stable for 2-3 years can be transferred to lower intensity of care in the local community.	Care coordinators facilitate transfer onto other teams within the same organization or other organizations as client support needs change over time.	Step down from board into the same team; able to move back onto board as needed. If stable for 2-3 years, step down to General Practitioner.
Continuity of care	Some teams may be hospital based. A small number may have psychiatrist with admission privileges. Most are community teams with varying types of relationships and arrangements with local hospitals.	Working in "transmural" integrated hospital /community services model. The team is not only a gatekeeper for the hospital, but also stays in touch with the client during his or her admission and retains the overall coordination of the client's treatment.	Team part of a community support services organization offering case management, ACT, justice prevention and diversion services, short term residential crisis services and group based services. No established relationships with local hospital inpatient units.	Working in "transmural" integrated hospital /community services model. The FACT team is not only a gatekeeper for the hospital, but also stays in touch with the client during his or her admission and retains the overall coordination of the client's treatment.

[a]Ministry of Health and Long Term Care, 2004
[b]van Veldhuizen J and Bahler M, 2013

care coordinators, the South team has access to a psychiatric consultant, and provides enhanced ICM support through multidisciplinary assessment and individual case management to service users with complex yet more moderate needs, while facilitating care transitions within the organization's various programs, including ACT, as support needs change over time.

Both IS teams accept referrals for adults aged 18-65 years (with the South Team additionally accepting youth older than 16 as appropriate) with a variety of health and social needs, including challenges in performing activities of daily living and functioning in the community, housing needs, criminal justice involvement, substance use, and acute or chronic medical illness, including developmental disabilities. The majority of early referrals to the East team were 25-54 years of age (74%), male (57%), had a history of violence/aggression (66%) and a substance use disorder (52%). Approximately 48% had no fixed address. Similarly, the majority of referrals to the South team were 25-54 years of age (73%), male (62%), with a history of self-harm/suicide attempts and psychotic disorders (56%). Approximately 17% had no fixed address.

Design and data collection

The evaluation included review of program documents (e.g. meeting minutes, program descriptions and policies), and qualitative data collection with a total of 49 stakeholders. We conducted two staff focus groups, three service user focus groups, and seventeen key informant interviews with program and system-level stakeholders. Data collection took place between October 23, 2014 and March 2, 2015.

All staff of the East and South IS teams were invited by the study coordinator to participate in a focus group, exploring staff ($n = 25$) perceptions of the new team based models and the early implementation process, including key program components and staff perspectives on what worked well and what were the challenges during early implementation [see Additional file 1]. Service user participants ($n = 17$) were recruited through convenience sampling. IS staff offered information on the study and directed potential participants to the study coordinator. One service user focus group was conducted with individuals who transitioned from the ACT team to the East team, while the other two focus groups engaged service users newly served by the two IS teams. Service user focus groups elicited information on the services and supports received by their respective teams and their experiences of these services [see Additional file 2]. Key informant interviews ($n = 17$) focused on key program ingredients and program and system-level factors influencing implementation [see Additional file 3]. Key informants were recruited through snowball sampling and included program managers, team leaders, psychiatrists, primary health care providers and relevant decision-makers.

Research staff, not involved in care provision, obtained written informed consent from all participants. Focus groups with staff and program participants lasted approximately 75 min; key informant interviews were approximately one hour in duration. All focus groups and interviews were audio recorded and transcribed verbatim; names and places were anonymized. The study was approved by the Research Ethics Board at St. Michael's Hospital.

Analysis

Interview and focus group transcripts were analyzed using thematic analysis, which involves the identification of common themes that span multiple interviews and focus groups [32, 33]. Two researchers independently examined a subset of the transcripts line-by-line, and grouped this qualitative data into codes or threads. They compared their approaches and resolved differences in coding strategies, arriving at a preliminary coding framework with the team's lead researcher. This coding framework was applied to an additional subset of transcripts and further expanded to accommodate new data. The final coding framework was used by research staff to code all transcripts and program documents. The research team met regularly to review coding categories and reduce them to a smaller number of higher level themes that were internally coherent, consistent and distinctive [32]. Research staff organized member-checking workshops with staff and management from both IS teams to establish the trustworthiness of the data. Analysis was facilitated by Nvivo 10.0 version software.

Results

Our findings of early implementation drivers are organized using Durlak and DuPre's conceptual framework [34], including the external context, provider characteristics, model characteristics, program delivery factors and support system factors. Findings support the two team-based models' success in engaging the target population. Implementation strengths included the broad recognition of existing service gaps, the use of interdisciplinary teams, experienced service providers, partnerships and collaboration across sectors and levels of care, training and team building activities. Emerging challenges included lack of complementary support services such as suitable housing, organizational contexts reluctant to embrace change and risk, and limited service provider and organizational capacity to deliver evidence-based interventions. Some challenges were shared, and others were unique to one or the other IS team as described below.

External context: system and community factors

Facilitator: an identified need for change to address the needs of underserviced populations

As noted earlier, the IS teams were funded by the local health authority, prioritizing adults in the urban core who were poorly served by available services. As one key informant said, "[Ontario] ACT teams have shied away from people that are homeless or have had criminal justice involvement, or developmental disabilities" (KI 16). This service user, in describing his situation, summarized the challenges facing many individuals prior to their referral to an IS team:

"My health was poor. I was sleeping on the street a lot. I was going through starvation periods, where I had no food...I was getting in trouble with the law, assaulting people... hearing voices and seeing things."

Recognition of the service gaps for this vulnerable population led to dedicated funding and incentives for provider organizations to work across services and sectors, helping launch new partnerships and collaborations: "I think we have to keep pushing our entire care system, to the point where we can really work together on [more] teams that cross organizations" (KI 15).

Challenge: Lack of complementary resources and supports

As several study participants identified, the complex challenges in service users' lives have deep, structural roots that community mental health services cannot address alone. Stakeholders recognized the limitations inherent in challenging the broader factors related to the social determinants of health: "Things like housing, things like a safe neighbourhood, access to quality food – there's a lot of food insecurity...We're dealing with issues of poverty... we're operating within a context of a macro system that doesn't promote recovery." Key informant participants further reflected on the implications of this context:

My anxieties were, you know, we are going to be only one team in a fairly hard-to-serve environment...I think there are a lot of systemic problems, that, you know, exist here ... it's good to have one flexible piece, but I think all pieces need to become flexible. (KI 1).

Team members identified the need for additional flexible resources in the community and systemic change, such as integrated primary care services, direct access to housing and rent supplements for those experiencing homelessness, or interim housing options for those referred upon exit from the criminal justice system.

Provider characteristics: a collaboration of the willing

Facilitator: commitment to learning and improvement

The organizations involved in IS team implementation had prior experience in serving adults with complex health and social needs, in service innovation and inter-sectoral partnerships, and were among few providers interested in exploring new approaches to service provision for this population. Stakeholders and managers at the organizational level were optimistic about the IS teams' potential for influencing systemic change, and were keen to evaluate their implementation and outcomes: "I do believe that we need more of this type of interventions ... than just more case management." (KI 4).

As implementation progressed, both teams encountered the need for process and practice improvements. Early on, the South team enlisted an external program consultant to engage staff in the development of team processes and protocols. Staff team members appreciated the opportunity to give feedback:

[The program consultant] would then be able to make those adjustments on whether – be it charts of how things would flow through, or whose role was going to be what, or what our care plan was going to look like, or our referral forms... he was able to kind of put that in place.

An East team key informant, similarly noted:

If we're successful or learn from the process and the system, we can influence the system ... we would have, then, a community partner and a hospital who have gained knowledge about how that [hospital community integration] works and could replicate. (KI 5).

Challenge: negotiating organizational shifts and change management

The East team transformed a pre-existing hospital based ACT team to develop a flexible approach to service delivery in partnership with a community agency, bringing together hospital and community expertise and resources. In doing so, they encountered challenges and tensions in integrating divergent operational and human resource policies between the partner organizations, including reporting structures, and staff compensation. A key informant reflected, "I think we needed to talk about it from the beginning, I think, and do more things in partnership" (KI 2). Stakeholders also discussed the need to offer adequate time and support for frontline staff during transitions of such scale. Summarizing the views of many frontline providers, one East team staff member said, "Things went so quickly and nobody slowed down ... it was so top-down and nobody came to talk to us."

Another key informant noted the benefits of having staff with a mix of clinical expertise and community knowledge in the hospital led East team:

We brought case managers [from a community mental health organization] who have a really good knowledge of the community, and they bring a different perspective to client care...I'm seeing a really nice blend, because [these case managers] are learning something about the medical model, which is important because our clients do have a lot of medical co-morbidities. (KI 14).

Introducing a flexible, recovery-focused model for individuals with complex mental health needs required large shifts in perspective and service delivery by frontline providers, who were hesitant to embrace new practice requirements. One key informant from the East team (KI 7) noted a gradual "culture shift happening, but I don't think we're all the way there." Some frontline staff members had difficulty adapting to the changes, and this contributed to high staff turnover in the East team during the early phases of implementation.

Model characteristics: compatibility with local contexts

Facilitator: non-diagnostic eligibility criteria and flexible level of support

The IS team's eligibility criteria enabled many service users to access care that has previously been denied to them. In the words of a service user: "I've been in the healthcare and mental healthcare system for many years... I just was continually falling through the cracks. [The IS team] was instant in getting me connected." Staff felt that the new teams allowed for the possibility of "fitting the model to the patient" rather than "fitting the patient to the model", thus reducing barriers to access and allowing for more timely and appropriate care. The teams aimed to work with adults who had, "not necessarily the diagnosis, but just [the] presentation" (KI 12). One provider stated:

I think as time passes we're looking less and less about you've got to meet A, B, C, D criteria... It's more, "Okay, you're very difficult to serve. Nobody else has been able to provide the services that you need. Maybe you 're appropriate for an IS team.

The ability to titrate the level of support over time was seen as necessary and valuable: "Not everyone needs that [ACT team] level of intensity, but at some point, most people do" (KI 4). A stakeholder with the East team described the potential for movement within the team, while noting this movement was still in its early stages:

We now have to start to see the flow and the movement on the other end... They are, you know, ACT clients we've seen every day, sometimes multiple times a day...and then, hopefully, they experience that period of stability. They move over to ICM case management. They are seen once a week ...and now, you know, we are actively looking at the discharge planning for people and we're moving them through that program and that system. (KI 3).

Challenge: balancing support needs with a recovery focus

Particularly in the initial stages of implementation, the exclusive focus on adults with complex needs resulted in a caseload with a large number of service users requiring high-intensity services. Staff suggested that "one client from the IS team would probably be equivalent to maybe three on an ACT team, in terms of management". Some staff felt this workload was not conducive to the recovery-focused service they wanted to provide:

We are supposed to be challenging discrimination in a recovery model but oftentimes what happens is that we just don't have the time to do that, so we just move on.

As another staff member described, "you are running around with your little garden hose trying to put out a forest fire." A key informant with the East team said, "I would have hoped to have a true FACT team, where... you have a mix of, you know, high needs, moderate needs, and low needs." Instead, this person felt the model, at least in its early stage, was more of a "super-ACT team... many too-complex clients, which makes it difficult for staff" (KI 16). Similarly, South team members explained the challenges with their case management approach: "Speaking on behalf of the nurses, we have other responsibilities for all the clients, not just our own caseload"; and, "I may have an entire caseload of people who require med observes, whereas somebody else doesn't have any" (KI 11). Despite having access to other ICM and ACT services within the organization, staff and stakeholders of this team recommended moving towards a "more ACT-like model", with more shared caseloads, similar to the East team, to distribute the work more equitably and facilitate recovery focused and evidence based care.

Program delivery system: organizational capacity

Facilitator: early and ongoing communication with key partner organizations

Both teams invested in relationship building and regular communication with key hospital and community organizations to ensure input, transparency and accountability. The hospital led East team described "a couple of meetings with all service organizations" in the geographical area, where the team would report on, "Here's where we are, here's the draft [eligibility] criteria at this point" (KI 7). This ensured that the program adaptations would address local service gaps, as well as "build positive relationships for the referral process" (KI 14). Likewise, community organization led South team staff described "working really diligently at making these connections". As a result, "they see us as being a really clean sort of resource and referral point" (South team staff). Stakeholders also noted that with more community outreach, working collaboratively with other agencies, the easier it would be for the teams to coordinate care for those receiving services from multiple agencies. One key informant emphasized that creating collaborative service user care plans with other agencies "provides an opportunity to engage with a range of other healthcare providers ... which then helps to create a culture spread around coordinated care planning to primary care, to community mental health, etc." (KI7).

Challenge: coordination with acute care resources

Often, the complexity of service user needs exceeded the IS team's or host community organization's expertise and resources. Both teams quickly recognized that management of medical conditions was particularly important for this population, facilitated in the East team by colocation with primary care services. Furthermore, service users frequently required acute psychiatric and medical care. Accessing hospital care and creating appropriate discharge plans could be challenging, especially for the South team, where the local hospital was not a direct partner in service delivery. One South team staff member summarized, "It's hard as a community team who services this clientele with these complexities to not have any type of say or privileges for admitting in, in hospitals." As one key informant explained, "What you don't want happening, and what happens sometimes is, 'We're going to discharge Tom on Thursday.' On Friday you get a call – 'Oh, well, actually we discharged him on Wednesday'" (KI 15). The South team saw opportunities for better communication when service users required hospitalization:

It would be really interesting to have a community person in the hospital that would kind of filter and control the information within the hospital system. Somebody consistent we could actually go to, to provide the information and feedback to. Almost like a back door. (South team staff).

Program support system: training and technical assistance

Facilitator: staff training and team building

Training on evidence-based practices such as Motivational Interviewing was provided to team members prior to service launch. This was perceived as helpful not only for supporting service users, but for building team cohesion. Speaking of their experience with full-team, intensive training on Dialectical Behavioural Therapy (DBT), a South team staff member noted,

I think it might contribute to the functioning of the team, because every single week we're reminded to be thinking dialectically. We are reminded to be working in this kind of approach...and so, I can't help but think that is influencing how we don't just engage with our clients, but how engage with ourselves.

Challenge: supporting delivery of evidence-based approaches

Participants from both teams noted the need for ongoing training and supervision to ensure consistent delivery of evidence-based practices. As one key informant said,

I think we do need, as a team, to get much more training in terms of how do we support clients in their recovery. I mean, I think theoretically we all know it, but I'm not so sure that we know it that much – how does it really play out in real life? How do we actually do that? (KI 14).

Stakeholders identified that training for all staff may be difficult to provide when simultaneously caring for an active caseload, but stressed the importance of building in time and resources for individual and team training and supervision, facilitated in the East team by team based psychiatrists and a clinical psychologist.

Discussion

Our findings suggest that it is possible to increase diagnostic and service flexibility of community mental health teams in response to service access barriers for individuals with complex health and social needs. In Toronto, Canada's largest urban centre, the implementation of novel approaches to serving this population was facilitated by recognition of the need for program adaptations and improvements to address existing service gaps, of the need for effective change management, as well as commitment and capacity to deliver flexible, multidisciplinary approaches to care. Although participating organizations were early champions of the need for improvement, our findings exposed significant provider, team and organizational challenges that need to be overcome in transformational efforts of this magnitude.

Community and political contexts can have large impacts on the implementation of health services [34–36]: our findings suggest that recognition of service gaps by both local health authorities and provider organizations facilitated the introduction and acceptability of the new teams. In supporting change and innovation, participants echoed concerns raised in many jurisdictions regarding service user tenure within high intensity teams, leading to services that quickly reach capacity and may not facilitate the provision of appropriate levels of care [8, 37]. Service providers and key informants also stressed the limitations of these services within inadequately resourced mental health service delivery systems, or without broader systemic change addressing lack of housing and adequate income supports for adults experiencing severe disabilities. These findings emphasize the importance of stakeholder engagement and of local needs assessment to assess readiness for change and implementation of new service approaches for this population.

The design and philosophies of the teams, and the importance placed by staff and stakeholders on the flexibility and adaptability of the models, as well as the competencies of frontline providers to deliver evidence based interventions echo findings from research on successful implementation of health care practices, including Assertive Community Treatment [26, 29, 30, 34, 35]. However, research has also identified that belief in, and the design of an intervention is not enough for successful implementation: "practices must be implemented actively" [26]. Initial and ongoing commitment to the development of community partnerships and inclusion of staff in decision-making facilitated the implementation of responsive and appropriate services. A study on key domains of successful implementation in community mental health suggested that engaged leaders can identify and put forth specific strategies to lead active implementation, such as redesigning workplace policies and adapting staff's assigned duties [26]. Our findings indicate instances where this was occurring within the IS teams, such as bringing in an external consultant to engage staff in service design, and providing full team training in evidence-based practices. The study also identified places in need of further attention, including the balancing of case management caseloads, revisiting operational policies and reporting structures in multi-agency service teams, providing ongoing training opportunities in team-building formats, and, for services delivered by community organizations, developing stronger partnerships with acute care facilities. Our findings have parallels with those in other contexts, and highlight the importance of effective team function and clinical leadership [29, 30].

Dedicating time and resources to these aspects of implementation may also improve staff capacity and comfort with delivering care to adults with complex needs, potentially preventing turnover and encouraging a work climate more open to change and innovation, mitigating the risk of burn out and emotional exhaustion that might result from inadequate training or resources [29]. Organizational support and leadership may be particularly critical when a new team is developed by transforming a previous program, such as the East team's transition from ACT. Positive service user outcomes from a similar ACT-to-FACT process in the UK suggest that growing pains and higher staff to service user ratios have not had a negative effect on service provision [12, 17], and a recent study highlighted positive mental health professional experiences of the FACT model [38], though, as others have noted, further evaluation of these approaches is needed [39–41]. As staff from the South team noted, adopting more "ACT-like" approaches by ICM teams by broader adoption of team based approaches to care and assumption of clinical responsibility across hospital and community settings may well be key ingredients of successfully engaging and supporting the target population.

Despite the use of rigorous qualitative methods, this research is limited in its generalizability due to the local service context in Toronto, Canada. Additionally, this study was completed during the early phase of program implementation, suggesting that examination of later phases of implementation and sustainability may be warranted, including purposive sampling of service user participants to increase trustworthiness of the data. In these early phases of program implementation, service user participation was limited to a convenience sample, introducing selection bias for this stakeholder group, and participant check in was not pursued with service user participants, given the focus of the study at this stage. Despite the limitations above, and the limitations of qualitative research in general, including researcher subjectivity in analysis and interpretation of data, our findings are relevant to many jurisdictions facing similar challenges, and may be helpful in efforts to innovate within existing community mental health models.

Conclusions

Stakeholders with a range of expertise and experiences offer important perspectives on the acceptability and implementation drivers of flexible models of service delivery for adults with complex health and social needs. Lessons learned can guide continued improvement in community mental health services and call for rigorous research to establish the effectiveness of novel interventions.

Abbreviations

ACT: Assertive Community Treatment; FACT: Flexible Assertive Community Treatment; ICM: Intensive Case Management; IS: Integrated Service; SMI: Serious Mental Illness

Acknowledgements

The authors would like to acknowledge the support of the service users, providers, and managers of the two IS teams in conducting this research.

Funding

Funding for this study was provided by the Ontario Ministry of Health and Long Term Care through "Building Bridges to Integrate Care", University of Toronto, Toronto, Canada. The funder was not involved in the design, collection, analysis or interpretation of data, or in writing of this manuscript.

Authors' contributions

KFP analyzed study data and contributed to manuscript preparation. DS assisted in study design, lead data collection and analysis, and contributed to manuscript preparation. AA assisted in data collection and analysis. AN guided interpretation of data and contributed to manuscript preparation. VS led study design, analysis, and interpretation of results, and oversaw the direction of this manuscript. All authors read and approved the final manuscript.

Consent for publication

All participants quoted in this article consented to the publication of anonymized quotations from their interviews in writing.

Competing interests

The authors declare that they have no competing interests.

Author details

[1]Centre for Urban Health Solutions, Li Ka Shing Knowledge Institute, St. Michael's Hospital, 209 Victoria Street, Toronto, ON M5B 1W8, Canada.
[2]Centre for Addiction and Mental Health, 100 Stokes Street, Toronto, ON M6J 1H4, Canada. [3]Department of Psychiatry, University of Toronto, 250 College Street, 8th Floor, Toronto, ON M5T 1R8, Canada. [4]Mental Health Services, St. Michael's Hospital, 30 Bond Street, Toronto, ON M5B 1W8, Canada.

References

1. Coldwell CM, Bender WS. The effectiveness of assertive community treatment for homeless populations with severe mental illness: a meta-analysis. Am J Psychiatr. 2007;164(3):393–9.
2. Killaspy H, Bebbington P, Blizard R, Johnson S, Nolan F, Pilling S, et al. The REACT study: randomised evaluation of assertive community treatment in North London. BMJ. 2006;332(7545):815–20.
3. Marshall M, Locjwood A. Assertive community treatment for people with severe mental disorders. Cochrane Database Syst Rev. 2011,Issuea. art. No.: CD001089. https://doi.org/10.1002/14651858.CD001089.pub2.
4. Morrissey J, Meyer P, Cuddeback G. Extending assertive community treatment to criminal justice settings: origins, current evidence, and future directions. Community Ment Health J. 2007;43(5):527–44.

5. Bond GR, Drake RE, Muser KT, Latimer E. Assertive community treatment for people with severe mental illness. Dis Manage Health Outcomes. 2001;9(3):141–59.
6. Nelson G, Aubry T, Lafrance A. A review of the literature on the effectiveness of housing and support, assertive community treatment, and intensive case management interventions for persons with mental illness who have been homeless. Am J Orthopsychiatry. 2007;77(3):350–61. https://doi.org/10.1037/0002-9432.77.3.350.
7. Reynolds SK, Wolbert R, Abney-Cunningham G, Patterson K. Dialectical behavior therapy for assertive community treatment teams. In: Dimeff LA, Koerner K, editors. Dialectical Behavior Therapy in Clinical Practice: Applications Across Disorders and Settings. New York: Guilford Press; 2007. p. 298-325.
8. Rosenheck R, Neale M, Mohamed S. Transition to low intensity case management in a VA assertive community treatment model program. Psychiatr Rehabilitaion J. 2010;33(4):288–96.
9. Dieterich M, Irving CB, Park B, Marshall M. Intensive case management for severe mental illness. Cochrane Database Syst Rev. 2010;(ID):CD007906. https://doi.org/10.1002/14651858.CD007906.pub2.
10. Ziguras SJ, Stuart GW. A meta-analysis of the effectiveness of mental health management over 20 years. Psychiatr Serv. 2000;51(11):1410–21.
11. van Veldhuizen JR. FACT: a Dutch version of ACT. Community Ment Health J. 2007;43(4):421–33.
12. Firn M, Hindhaugh K, Hubbeling D, Davies G, Jones B, White SJ. A dismantling study of assertive outreach services: comparing activity and outcomes following replacement with the FACT model. Soc Psychiatry Psychiatr Epidemiol. 2013;48(6):997–1003. https://doi.org/10.1007/s00127-012-0602-x.
13. van Veldhuizen JR, Bähler M. Flexible Assertive Community Treatment. Vision , model, practice and organization. Groningen, the Netherlands. 2013. Available from: https://www.eaof.org/factmanual.pdf, https://doi.org/10.13140/RG.2.1.3925.1683.
14. The CCAF: Certification Centre for ACT and Flexible ACT. Available from: https://ccaf.nl/international. Accessed 14 Jan 2018.
15. Nugter MA, Engelsbel F, Bähler M, Keet R, van Veldhuizen R. Outcomes of FLEXIBLE assertive community treatment (FACT) implementation: a prospective real life study. Community Ment Health J. 2016;52(8):898–907. https://doi.org/10.1007/s10597-015-9831-2.
16. Drukker M, Visser E, Sytema S, van Os J. Flexible assertive community treatment, severity of symptoms and psychiatric health service use, a real life observational study. Clin Pract Epidemiol Ment Health. 2013;9:202–9. https://doi.org/10.2174/1745017901309010202.
17. Firn M, White S, Hubbeling D, Jones B. The replacement of assertive outreach services by reinforcing local community teams: a four year observational study. J Ment Health. 2016;5:1–6.
18. Svensson B, Hansson L, Markstrom U, Lexen A. What matters when impementing flexible assertive community treatment in a Swedish healthcare context: a two-year implementation study. Int J Ment Health 2017. https://doi.org/10.1080/00207411.2017.1345041.
19. Bak M, van Os J, Delespaul P, de Bie A, á Campo J, Poddighe G, et al. An observational, "real life" trial of the introduction of assertive community treatment in a geographically defined area using clinical rather than service use outcome criteria. Soc Psychiatry Psychiatr Epidemiol. 2007;42(2):125–30. https://doi.org/10.1007/s00127-006-0147-y.
20. George L, Kidd S, Wong M, Harvey R, Browne G. ACT fidelity in Ontario: measuring adherence to the model. Can J Community Ment Health. 2010; 29(S5):87–96. https://doi.org/10.7870/cjcmh-2010-0036.
21. Ontario ACT Association. Ontario program standards for ACT teams. Ontario, Canada: Ontario Ministry of Health and Long Term Care; 2004.
22. Access Point. Frequently asked questions. 2015. http://theaccesspoint.ca/frequently-asked-questions/. Accessed 14 Jan 2018.
23. Damschroder LJ, Aron DC, Keith RE, Kirsh SR, Alexander JA, Lowery JC. Fostering implementation of health services research findings into practice: a consolidated framework for advancing implementation science. Implement Sci. 2009;4(1):50. https://doi.org/10.1186/1748-5908-4-50.
24. Greenhalgh T, Robert G, Macfarlane F, Bate P, Kyriakidou O. Diffusion of innovations in service organizations: systematic review and recommendations. Milbank Q. 2004;82(4):581–629. https://doi.org/10.1111/j.0887-378X.2004.00325.x.
25. Fixsen DL, Naoom SF, Blase KA, Friedman RM, Wallace F. Implementation research: a synthesis of the literature. Tampa: National Implementation Research Network, Louis de la Parte Florida Mental Health Institute, University of South Florida; 2005.
26. Torrey WC, Bond GR, McHugo GJ, Swain K. Evidence-based practice implementation in community mental health settings: the relative importance of key domains of implementation activity. Admin Pol Ment Health. 2012;39(5):353–64. https://doi.org/10.1007/s10488-011-0357-9.
27. Kimberly J, Cook JM. Organizational measurement and the implementation of innovations in mental health services. Adm Policy Ment Health Ment Health Serv Res. 2008;35(1):11–20. https://doi.org/10.1007/s10488-007-0143-x.
28. Aarons GA, Hurlburt M, Horwitz SM. Advancing a conceptual model of evidence-based practice implementation in public service sectors. Adm Policy Ment Health Ment Health Serv Res. 2011;38(1):4–23. https://doi.org/10.1007/s10488-010-0327-7.
29. Billings J, Johnson S, Bebbington P, Greaves A, Priebe S, Muijen M, Ryrie I, Watts J, White I, Wright C. Assertive outreach teams in London: staff experiences and perceptions. Br J Psychiatry. 2003;183:139–47.
30. Harvey C, Killaspy H, Martino S, Johnson S. Implementation of assertive community treatment in Australia: model fidelity, patient characteristics and staff experiences. Community Ment Health J. 2012;48(5):652–61.
31. Nakhost A, Law SF, KMF P, Stergiopoulos V. Addressing complexity and improving access in community mental health services: an inner city adaptation of flexible ACT. Psychiatr Serv. 2017;68:867–9. https://doi.org/10.1176/appi.ps.201700195.
32. Braun V, Clarke V. Using thematic analysis in psychology. Qual Res Psychol. 2006;3(2):77–101.
33. Morse J, Field P. Qualitative research methods for health professions. 2 ed. 1995.
34. Durlack JA, DuPre EP. Implementation matters: a review of research on the influence of implementation on program outcomes and the factors affecting implementation. Am J Community Psychol. 2008;41(3-4):327–50.
35. Mancini AD, Moser LL, Whitley R, McHugo GJ, Bond GR, Finnerty MT, et al. Assertive community treatment: facilitators and barriers to implementation in routine mental health settings. Psychiatr Serv. 2009;60(2):189–95. https://doi.org/10.1176/appi.ps.60.2.189.
36. Rosenheck RA. Organizational process: a missing link between research and practice. Psychiatr Serv. 2001;52(12):1607-1612.
37. Donahue S, Manuel J, Herman D, Fraser L, Chen H, Essock S. Development and use of a transition readiness scale to help manage ACT team capacity. Psychiatr Serv. 2012;63(3):223–9. https://doi.org/10.1176/appi.ps.201100041.
38. Lexen A, Svensson B. Mental health professional experiences of the flexible assertive community treatment model: a grounded theory study. J Ment Health. 2016;25(4):379–84. https://doi.org/10.1080/09638237.2016.1207236.
39. Bond G, Drake R. Should we adopt the Dutch version of ACT? Commentary on "FACT: a Dutch version of ACT". Community Ment Health J. 2007;43(4):435–7.
40. Norden T, Norlander T. Absence of positive results for flexible assertive community treatment. What is the next approach? Clin Pract Epidemiol Ment Health. 2014;10(September):87–91.
41. van Veldhuizen JR, Delespaul P, Kroon H, Mulder N. Flexible ACT & resource-group ACT: different working procedures which can supplement and strengthen each other. A response. Clinical Practice & Epidemiology in Mental Health. 2015;11:12–5.

19

Gender differences in mental health problems among adolescents and the role of social support: results from the Belgian health interview surveys 2008 and 2013

Filip Van Droogenbroeck*, Bram Spruyt and Gil Keppens

Abstract

Background: To investigate how social support relates to mental health problems for Belgian late adolescents and young adults 15–25 years of age. Additionally, we examine changes in mental health problems between 2008 and 2013 and investigate gender differences.

Methods: Multivariate analysis of variance was used to investigate (1) psychological distress, (2) anxiety and (3) depression among 713 boys and 720 girls taken from two successive waves (2008 and 2013) of a representative sample of the Belgian population (Belgian Health Interview survey). Psychological distress was measured by the General Health Questionnaire, anxiety and depression by the Symptom Check-List-90-Revised.

Results: Gender differences were found for psychological distress, anxiety and depression with girls reporting significantly higher scores than boys. Multivariate analysis of variance (MANOVA) revealed that adolescents who are dissatisfied with their social contacts and experience poor social support reported more psychological distress, anxiety and depression. In addition, young adult boys (20–25 years of age) were more likely to experience psychological distress when compared to late adolescent boys (15–19 years of age). Finally, the prevalence of anxiety and depression increased substantially between 2008 and 2013 for girls and to a lesser extent for boys.

Conclusions: Especially girls and young people with poor social support experience mental health problems more frequently than boys and those with strong social support. Improving social support among young people may serve as a protective buffer to mental health problems.

Keywords: Psychological distress, Anxiety, Depression, Gender, trends, social support, adolescent mental health

Background

Mental health has become a priority in public health policy. In 2013 a World Health Assembly resolution was passed by the World Health Organization (WHO) that called for a comprehensive mental health action plan at the national level [1]. In this regard, late adolescents and young adults deserve special attention. Half of all mental health disorders in adulthood start by the age of 14 and three-quarter by the age of 25 [2]. According to the most recent statistics, in any given year 20% of adolescents worldwide experience mental disorders, most commonly anxiety or depression (WHO, 2012). Mental health problems are considered to be some of the most common and yet most stigmatising of conditions [3].

Defining mental health is challenging as it is conceptually ambiguous. In this article we adopt the holistic definition from the World Health Organization [4] which describes mental health as "a state of well-being in which every individual realizes his or her own potential, can cope with the normal stresses of life, can work productively and fruitfully, and is able to make a contribution to her or his community." Mental health problems in adolescents result from the complex and dynamic

* Correspondence: Filip.Van.Droogenbroeck@vub.be
Sociology Department, Vrije Universiteit Brussel, Pleinlaan 2, 1050 Brussel, Belgium

interplay between individual attributes and behaviours (e.g., genetic factors, emotional and social intelligence), social and economic circumstances (e.g., experienced social support, poverty, education opportunities), and wider sociocultural environmental factors (e.g., social and economic policies at the national level, discrimination) [5]. These aspects interact with each other in a dynamic way that can either protect, or pose a risk to, mental health. In this article we will investigate how social support and socioeconomic status (SES) are related to three common mental health problems (i.e., psychological distress, anxiety and depression) across gender amongst a representative sample of Belgian young people between 15 and 25 years of age. This age group allows us to compare late adolescents (15–19) with young adults (20–25). Earlier research suggests that the transitional period from adolescence to young adulthood is characterised by changes in people's psychological attachment styles [6].

Social support can be considered as a form of social capital and is usually defined by structural aspects of people's relationships (e.g., number of ties, group memberships, etc.) and explicit functions (e.g., emotional, informational, instrumental assistance) they may serve. Social support has been identified as a key protective factor for mental well-being [7–11]. Positive relationships with family and friends are thought to serve as buffers to the negative influences within one's immediate environment. Although there is no consensus on the mechanisms of how social support positively influences mental health, generally, two broad categories of supportive behaviors are distinguished: emotional sustenance and active coping assistance. Emotional sustenance are demonstrations of caring, valuing, and understanding by (significant) others while active coping assistance relates to supporters giving advice or implementing problem-focused and emotion-focused coping strategies that they would use themselves [7, 12]. Both influence mental health differently, emotional sustenance has primarily an indirect influence through social psychological mechanisms (e.g., social influence/comparison, social control, role-based purpose and meaning, self-esteem, sense of control, belonging) while active coping assistance primarily has a direct influence on mental health (see [12] for an overview of the mechanisms of social support to mental health). Some studies found gender differences for the relationship between social support and mental health problems. Schraedley and colleagues found that the mental health problems of girls were more related to the level of social support than for boys [13]. Furthermore, well-established gender differences exist for mental health problems in general. Depression, anxiety, and psychological distress affect girls to a greater extent than boys across different countries and varying contexts [14, 15]. For these reasons we will pay specific attention to gender differences in the empirical analyses.

We contribute to the existing literature in three ways. First, poor mental health has important consequences for the broader health and long-term development of adolescents and is associated with several health and social outcomes such as unemployment, higher alcohol, tobacco and illicit substances use, adolescent pregnancy, school dropout and delinquent behaviours [16, 17]. In health terms, mental health problems are related to premature mortality (up to 20 years due to suicide or from other diseases that are often left unattended such as HIV, cancers, cardiovascular disease, and diabetes [5, 18]. Suicide is in the top three causes of death for young people between 10 and 25 years of age [19]. The long-term consequences of poor mental health make it important to investigate the determinants of mental health problems at the age when they are known to most likely develop. We adopt a broad focus by studying not only depression but also distress and anxiety for boys and girls separately. Second, to the best of our knowledge this is the first Belgian population-based study on adolescent mental health problems and adds to the scarce population-based research on the relation between social support and mental health problems among adolescents. Third, by using two successive waves of the Belgian Health Survey, we are able to study the evolution in the prevalence of three mental health problems across gender and in this way contribute to the literature that documents evolutions in mental problems [20]. In this regard, several studies indicated an increase in mental health problems over time for girls but not necessarily for boys [20–23]. A recent study by Fink et al. in England indicated that girls but not boys reported more emotional problems in 2014 than in 2009 [20]. More research is needed to assess if these gender-specific trends are also observable in other countries. The period covered by our data (2008–2013) is particularly interesting because it concerns one of the most severe financial and economic crises since WWII with high unemployment rates especially among young people.

Methods

Data

The data are based on two successive cross-sectional waves (2008 and 2013) of the Belgian Health Interview Survey (B-HIS) (https://his.wiv-isp.be/). The research protocol was approved by the High Council of Statistics, the ethical committee of the Scientific Institute of Public Health and the Commission for the Protection of Private Life. This ensured that the privacy of the respondents was protected (for more information see https://his.wiv-isp.be/Shared%20Documents/protocol2004.pdf). The B-HIS is held among a representative sample of the Belgian population (15 to 105 years of age) and aims to give an overview of the health status of the Belgian population. It is repeated every 3–5 years and each wave has to result in a net sample of at least 10,000 participants. A multistage sampling design is used, which involves geographical stratification (regions, municipalities), a selection of households within each cluster, and a selection of respondents within each household. The methodology has been described in detail by Demarest and colleagues [24]. Face-to-face interviews with PAPI (paper and pencil interviewing) are used. In addition, self-administered questionnaires were given to the participants older than 15 years, which dealt with more sensitive topics such as mental health problems and alcohol consumption. Instruments were constructed following strict procedures, including mainly standardised instruments from the WHO Consensus on Harmonising Methods and Instruments for Health Surveys, the Dutch Central Bureau of Statistics, the Belgian Centre for Social Policy, and the French National Institute for Health and Medical Research.

Measures

We focus on three mental health problems: psychological distress, depression and anxiety. These were measured by widely validated scales such as the Symptom Check-List-90-Revised (SCL-90-R) and the General Health Questionnaire (GHQ12). Research has demonstrated that both the SCL-90-R and GHQ12 can be successfully used as a screening instrument to identify mental disorders among young people [25–27].

Depression and anxiety were measured by the SCL-90-R, a 90-item instrument which assesses the presence and severity of a wide range of symptoms in an individual in the week prior to the interview [28]. Although the original SCL-90-R instrument comprises nine subscales, several studies failed to identify the nine-factor structure [29–31]. Instead the SCL-90-R shows a better fit as one global index. Still there are good reasons to use the anxiety and depression subscales as separate constructs. First, several studies indicate that the anxiety and depression subscales have been used separately and successfully to screen clients for depression and anxiety [32–35]. Second, previous research has also revealed a frequent temporal sequence where anxiety comes first and subsequently depression [36, 37]. Therefore, using anxiety as a separate construct might facilitate insight into the early identification of depression. In general, anxiety and depression are commonly considered to be comorbid conditions and are correlated [38–40]. Third, we performed confirmatory factor analysis to test a one-factor and two-factor solution. Although both scales have a strong correlation as expected ($r = .79$; $p < .000$) the two-factor model ($\chi^2(226) = 1583.3$; RMSEA = 0.065 (upper limit 90% 0.068); CFI = 0.910; TLI = 0.900; SRMR = 0.042 – three error-covariances) reveals a better fit than the one factor solution ($\chi^2(227) = 1909.2$; RMSEA = 0.069 (upper limit 90% 0.075); CFI = 0.889; TLI = 0.876; SRMR = 0.045 – three error-covariances). Based on these three considerations, we report the results for the depression and anxiety subscales separately in this article.[1]

Depression was measured by 13 items (e.g., "Repeated unpleasant thoughts that won't leave your mind," $\alpha = .89$[2]). Anxiety was measured by 10 items (e.g., "Spells of terror or panic," $\alpha = .88$[3]). Respondents were asked to rate the intensity of distress by the symptom on a 5-point Likert scale, ranging from 1 "not at all" to 5 "extremely," with higher scores indicating more complaints. For each indicator, the relevant items were summed and divided by the number of items resulting in sum scales ranging from 1 to 5.

Psychological Distress was assessed by the GHQ12 which is designed to detect non-psychotic psychiatric problems [41, 42]. It is a composed index of 12 items (e.g., "Felt constantly under strain?"; $\alpha = .83$), which are rated by respondents on a 5-point Likert scale ranging from 0 "not at all" to 4 "much more than usual". The recommended traditional scoring method was used to recode the initial Likert scores in a summed score ranging between 0 and 12 [41].

We included six independent variables. *Age* (0 "15–19 years of age", 1 "20–25 years of age") was used as a control variable. We also included *year of the survey* (0 "2008", 1 "2013") to assess trends between survey years.

The *highest educational level within the household* (0 "Higher secondary education or lower", 1 "At least higher education") and *household income* were considered as a proxy for different levels of SES of the family. The household income variable was divided in quintiles which are based on the income distribution at the Belgian level. Higher scores reflect higher household incomes relative to the Belgian income distribution.

To measure social capital two variables where constructed. The *appreciation of social contacts* (0 "Rather unsatisfied", 1 "Rather satisfied") and the *perceived quality of social support* (0 "Poor support", 1 "Intermediate or strong support"). The correlation between both indicators was .242 ($p < .001$).

Participants

Currently, five waves of the Belgian Health Interview Survey (B-HIS) are available. For the purpose of our study, only waves which had indicators on social support were used. The response rates for the consecutive waves are: 55% (2008; $N = 11,254$) and 57% (2013; $N = 10,829$). In addition, young people between 15 and 25 years of age ($N_{total} = 1433$) were selected. Baseline participation for our age range was ($N = 1976$) which implies an item non-response of ($N = 543$). Item non-response analysis indicated that respondents from households with a lower education level were more likely to have missing values for the items concerning health and the other independent variables. This item non-response is closely related to the unit non-response (i.e. failure to participate) as observed in the B-HIS and other national health surveys [24]. In general, the relationship between socially and economically deprived respondents and non-response bias has been well established [43]. Given the positive relationship between being socially and economically deprived and mental health problems the item non-response in the B-HIS might underestimate the prevalence of and social differences in mental health problems and influence our general estimations.

Analysis

Our analysis is borne out of two parts: first, descriptive statistics are given for all dependent variables. Second, multivariate analysis of variance (MANOVA) was used to assess differences in mental health problems for age, household income, highest educational level in the household, and social support for boys and girls separately. In addition, a dummy variable was constructed to control for the year of the survey and to assess trends. Coefficients with 95% confidence intervals (CIs) were calculated for each predictor. All analyses were carried out in Stata-MP (version 13) [44].

Results

Descriptive statistics

Table 1 presents the descriptive statistics for young people in the age group of 15–25 years. Approximately 60% of the investigated young people were between 20 and 25 years, half the sample consisted of girls and about 60% came from a household where the parents' educational level was not higher than secondary education. The majority of the investigated young people were rather satisfied with the appreciation of their social contacts (94.2%) and perceived an intermediate or strong

Table 1 Descriptive statistics (column percentages)

	Male %	Female %	Total %
Year			
2008	60.6	56.1	58.3
2013	39.4	43.9	41.7
Gender			
Male	/	/	49.8
Female	/	/	50.2
Age			
15–19	42.4	38.6	40.5
20–25	57.6	61.4	59.5
Highest educational level within the household			
Secondary education or lower	58.8	58.6	58.7
At least higher education	41.2	41.4	41.3
Appreciation social contact			
Rather unsatisfied	6.2	5.4	5.8
Rather satisfied	93.8	94.6	94.2
Quality of social support			
Poor support	12.3	13.6	13.0
Intermediate/strong support	87.7	86.4	87.0
Reported equivalent household income (Belgian Weighted quintiles – m(S.D.))	2.86 (1.44)	2.81 (1.44)	2.84 (1.44)
Psychological distress[a] (1–12) M(S.D.)	1.13 (2.11)	1.71 (2.48)	1.42 (2.32)
Depression[a] (1-5) M(S.D.)	1.27 (0.40)	1.45 (0.57)	1.36 (0.50)
Anxiety[a] (1-5) M(S.D.)	1.21 (0.37)	1.35 (0.55)	1.28 (0.47)
Total N	713	720	1433

[a]Means between girls and boys on these scales differ significantly, that is, $p < 0.000$ (ANOVA with *post hoc* Bonferroni test)

quality of social support (87%). Anova with post hoc Bonferonni corrections indicated that girls score significantly higher on psychological distress, depression and anxiety than boys. Gender differences for the social economic background and social capital indicators were very small.

Multivariate results

Table 2 shows the results for the selected variables using a multivariate analysis of variance for boys and girls separately. We found similar results for boys and girls. Psychological distress, depression and anxiety was strongly related with our indicators for social capital. In addition, young people who are dissatisfied with their social contacts and experience poor social support were more likely to report psychological distress, anxiety and depression. Although the point estimates of the effect parameters vary, the overlapping confidence intervals indicate that in general the strength of these relations is comparable across the different outcomes. There was no significant relationship for boys or girls between our indicators of social position and the three mental health problems. For other indicators, however, we did find interesting gender differences. Psychological distress was more common among young adult boys (20–25 years old) when compared to late adolescent boys (15–19 years old). No such age differences were found among girls. In addition, the results showed significant and substantial differences in depression and anxiety scores across the two waves between girls and to a lesser extent for boys. The relationship between depression, anxiety and survey year was twice as large for girls when compared to boys. In order to test whether the effect-size for the waves differed between boys and girls, we used the formula proposed by Paternoster et al. to test for the equality of regression coefficients [45]. We found that in a multivariate model the strength of the effect of the year of the survey differed significantly at the $p < 0.100$ level between girls and boys for depression ($z = -1.71$; $p = 0.087$) and anxiety ($z = -1.79$; $p = 0.073$). In addition, girls reported more psychological distress, anxiety and depression than boys in a combined multivariate model which controlled for the independent variables (not shown in table).

Conclusion

Late adolescence and young adulthood are phases in life characterised by profound transitions and changes. The quest for one's own identity and the search for a way to stand on one's own feet goes along with feelings of uncertainty and anxiety. While most adolescents are able to successfully cope with these feelings, a considerable group suffers from more serious mental health problems. In this study, we used high-quality representative data from 1433 Belgian late adolescents and young adults gathered in 2008 and 2013. The GHQ12 and SCL-90-R measures showed gender differences in the prevalence of mental health problems which is consistent with previous studies [5, 13, 15, 20, 46]. Boys reported less psychological distress, anxiety and depression than girls. These results are important especially if one takes into account the fact that mental health problems that manifest themselves during late adolescence and young adulthood prove to be good predictors for mental health disorders in adulthood [2]. For this reason health policies should closely monitor the evolutions in the mental health of youth and develop effective prevention strategies. This seems particularly applicable for depression and anxiety among girls for which we found that anxiety and depression increased substantively in comparison to boys in the span of only 5 years' time. The observed increase in depression and anxiety for girls and to a lesser extent for boys is consistent with previous research in England [20]. On the other hand, boys reported less psychological distress in 2013 when compared to 2008 while for girls we did not find this for psychological distress. These opposite results illustrate the importance of investigating different aspects of mental health and how these are differentially related to gender. The causes of gender differences in mental health problems among adolescents are not fully understood but previous research has indicated that boys may have more difficulties in acknowledging their mental health problems and tend to mask their mental health problems by acting out their difficulties resulting in more externalising disorders that are problematic for others such as antisocial personality disorders and substance abuse or dependence [17]. Girls, on the other hand, report more internalising disorders such as depression and anxiety. These differences between boys and girls may be related to gender conceptions and the socially defined role of women and men which in many societies exposes them to gender-specific stressors. Girls are expected to be more emotionally sensitive [47], suffer more from stressors which involve significant others such as the death of friends or relatives [48], experience more restricted gender roles and body dissatisfaction [49, 50], ruminate more as a coping strategy [51], experience more family violence, abuse and school performance pressure [15, 52], which all have been associated with a greater likelihood of mental health problems. Given that the trend patterns which we found for girls are similar to a recent study in England covering the same time period this might point to the influence of the economic and financial crisis which has been associated with higher levels of mental health problems among adolescents due to increasing youth unemployment and cuts to mental health services [20, 53, 54]. If these

Table 2 MANOVA on psychological distress, depression and anxiety – Unstandardized coefficients and 95% confidence intervals (CI)

	Psychological distress (GHQ 1–12)				Depression subscale (1–5)				Anxiety subscale (1–5)			
	Male		Female		Male		Female		Male		Female	
	b	95% CI	b	95% CI	b	95% CI	b	95% CI	b	95% CI	b	95% CI
Survey year (2013 vs. 2008)	−0.40*	[−0.71;−0.09]	-0.09	[−0.44;0.27]	0.08**	[0.03;0.14]	0.17***	[0.09;0.24]	0.06*	[0.01;0.12]	0.15***	[0.07;0.23]
Highest educational level within the household (At least higher education vs. Higher secondary education or lower)	0.09	[−0.25;0.42]	0.31	[−0.09;0.71]	0.01	[−0.05;0.07]	−0.02	[−0.11;0.07]	−0.02	[−0.07;0.04]	0.01	[−0.08;0.1]
Age (20–25 vs. 15–19)	0.46**	[0.15;0.76]	0.10	[−0.26;0.46]	0.02	[−0.04;0.07]	0.02	[−0.06;0.1]	0.03	[−0.03;0.08]	0.07	[−0.01;0.15]
Reported equivalent household income (Belgian weighted quintiles)	−0.05	[−0.16;0.07]	0.03	[−0.11;0.16]	0.00	[−0.02;0.02]	0.00	[−0.03;0.03]	0.01	[−0.01;0.03]	−0.01	[−0.04;0.02]
Appreciation social contacts (Rather satisfied vs. Rather unsatisfied)	−1.85***	[−2.5;-1.21]	−1.94***	[−2.73;-1.15]	−0.52***	[−0.64;-0.4]	−0.49***	[−0.67;-0.32]	−0.41***	[−0.52;-0.3]	−0.20*	[−0.38;-0.03]
Quality of social support (Poor support vs. Intermediate/strong support)	−0.48	[−0.97;0]	−1.39***	[−1.91;-0.86]	−0.24***	[−0.33;-0.15]	−0.44***	[−0.55;-0.32]	−0.15**	[−0.23;-0.07]	−0.28***	[−0.4;-0.16]
Constant	3.29***	[2.56;4.02]	4.52***	[3.61;5.43]	1.92***	[1.79;2.05]	2.22***	[2.02;2.43]	1.67***	[1.55;1.8]	1.71***	[1.51;1.92]
N	713		720		713		720		713		720	
R^2 (%)	8.3%		8.4%		18.1%		15.0%		11.9%		6.7%	

* $p < 0.05$, ** $p < 0.01$, *** $p < 0.001$

societal and economic changes are influencing the mental health of adolescents, the key question raised by our results concerns whether and why these would have a differential impact on boys and girls. Our data does not allow us to answer this question but at least suggest that the impact of societal changes associated with the economic and financial crisis may be much more far-reaching than what is often assumed in the public debates. Biological gender differences and the different societal expectations towards boys and girls which are related to mental health problems call for effective mental health promotion strategies that are adapted to the needs of boys and girls (e.g., see [5, 14] for effective promotion strategies of women's mental health).

Schraedley and colleagues found that among adolescents the prevalence of mental health problems increase with increasing age [13]. We found that young adult boys (20–25 years old) suffered from more psychological distress when compared to late adolescent boys (15–19 years old). No significant differences were found for girls or for the other mental health problems for boys, but the parameter estimates point towards the same direction. A plausible explanation for these findings is that the border between late adolescence and young adult almost coincides with the end of compulsory education in Belgium (18 years of age). People who leave compulsory education either go to higher tertiary education or enter the labour market. In both cases young people are confronted with many new experiences, expectations, potential unemployment, and responsibilities which may result in increased stress and along this way affect mental health. Although our data does not allow a strict empirical test of this idea, several other studies provide empirical support for the latter reasoning [53, 55]. These findings illustrate the importance to investigate these mental health problems separately and not combine them into a general construct.

In stressful situations it is good to have people to rely on. Indeed, one of the main contributions of this study is that it shows the crucial importance of a rewarding social network regarding young people's mental health problems. Late adolescents and young adults who are satisfied with their social contacts and/or feel strongly supported by others, report a less anxiety, depression, and psychological distress. In this context it is important to stress that social relationships do not only provide support in case of problems (curative function) but also opportunities for (different kinds of) voluntary action. Doing something meaningful for others and/or society is an effective means to search for one's own identity and is associated with greater (mental) health (prevention function) [56]. This is important because mental health problems often prove to be difficult to cure.

Limitations and further research

Our results raise three questions which cannot be answered with the data we have at our disposal but provide an excellent starting point for further research. *First,* as our results are based on correlational data caution is warranted when interpreting our results. This implies that there could be reversed causality. Social support can influence mental health but existing mental health problems are also likely to affect the number of social ties and type of support an individual receives. Developing effective prevention strategies require that we get a better grip on the causal mechanism behind the observed differences and evolutions. Our results suggest that especially the transition from compulsory education to tertiary education/entering the labour market seems to be a particularly relevant life change to study with a longitudinal design that allows the assessment of differences within individuals over time.

Second, the importance of having a rewarding social network for young people's mental health raises questions concerning which social relationships are more important than others, how different social relationships interact, and what aspects of social relationships are beneficial for mental health. Indeed, late adolescents and young adults have relationships with many other people. Especially the relative importance between adults (i.e. parents, family, teachers...) and peers seems worthy to investigate [10]. To answer these questions network data provide much more opportunities when compared to the common samples of individuals as used in classical health surveys. In addition, the relationship between the different components of social support and mental health problems can be disentangled. Research from Van Voorhees suggests that for young people's mental health the feeling to be accepted among peers rather than warmth or support is a critical protective factor in the peer context. For the relationship with the parents on the other hand, a sense of closeness and warm relations play an important protective role [46].

Third, quite surprisingly no important net differences were found according to indicators that reflect the social position (i.e., highest educational level in the household and household income). One possible explanation for this is the selection bias and higher non-response among socially and economically deprived respondents. This potentially flattens differences between social strata and underestimates the general prevalence of mental health problems because research has indicated that people from socially disadvantaged backgrounds are more likely to report worse (mental) health. This is a problem most (national health) surveys are confronted with. The B-HIS takes measures both in the design and management of the survey to reduce the impact of unit non-response on the representativeness of the survey results but still this selection bias potentially affects our results and should be taken into account when interpreting our findings. A second explanation could be that the measures we relied on mainly refer to the social *context* in which late adolescents and young adults live. While young people who live in socially and economically deprived families can be expected to have to cope with more (severe) problems, the extent to which they successfully manage to do so may be stronger related to their *own* social position. Indeed, one of the distinguishing features of late adolescence and young adulthood is that people find themselves at the crossroad of the ascribed (family) status and the achieved personal status. Although sociological research continues to show persistent social reproduction, the intergenerational transmission of social position is far from perfect [57]. Further research should deepen our understanding of the impact of social mobility on young people's mental health [58]. Another reason why social differences in mental health problems may be rather modest among young people is that mental health is the outcome of the balance between personal experiences *and* expectations. It is known that parents in middle and higher class families often have very high expectations regarding their children' educational and labour market success [59]. This renders it plausible that the absence of a uniform relationship between indicators for social position and mental health problems may conceal that in different social environments poor mental health is caused by different factors (e.g., material deprivation in lower classes; unrealistically high expectations among the middle and higher classes). At this point only research that includes more fine measures of expectations are able to enhance our understanding of the relationship between social position and mental health problems.

Endnotes

[1]Results for a composed depression/anxiety indicator will be made available upon simple request.

[2]Fit indices from confirmatory factor analysis: (χ^2 (65) = 535.664, RMSEA = 0.071 CFI = 0.935, TLI = 0.922, SRMR = 0.036).

[3]Fit indices from confirmatory factor analysis: (χ^2 (62) = 328.207, RMSEA = 0.055, CFI = 0.963, TLI = 0.954, SRMR = 0.028).

Acknowledgements
Not applicable.

Funding
The authors declare that there was no external funding.

Authors' contributions
FVD undertook data management, statistical analysis and drafted the manuscript. FVD, BS, GK interpreted the data, critically revised the manuscript, contributed to the review process and the final draft of the manuscript. All authors gave their final approval for submission.

Consent for publication
Not applicable.

Competing interests
The authors declare that they have no current or potential conflicts interests.

References

1. WHO, editor. Mental health action plan 2013–2020. Geneva, Switzerland: World Health Organization; 2014.
2. OECD. Making mental health count: the social and economic costs of neglecting mental health care. Paris: OECD; 2014.
3. Williams B, Pow J. Gender differences and mental health: an exploratory study of knowledge and attitudes to mental health among Scottish teenagers. Child Adolesc Mental Health. 2007;12:8–12.
4. WHO. Promoting mental health: concepts, emerging evidence, practice : summary report. Geneva: World Health Organization; 2004.
5. Women's Mental Health. An evidence based review. Geneva, Switzerland: World Health Organization; 2000.
6. Cook SH, Heinze JE, Miller AL, Zimmerman MA. Transitions in friendship attachment during adolescence are associated with developmental trajectories of depression through adulthood. J Adolesc Health. 2016;58: 260–6.
7. Almedom AM. Social capital and mental health: an interdisciplinary review of primary evidence. Soc Sci Med. 2005;61:943–64.
8. Åslund C, Starrin B, Nilsson KW. Social capital in relation to depression, musculoskeletal pain, and psychosomatic symptoms: a cross-sectional study of a large population-based cohort of Swedish adolescents. BMC Public Health. 2010;10:715.
9. Beeri A, Lev-Wiesel R. Social rejection by peers: a risk factor for psychological distress. Child Adolesc Mental Health. 2012;17:216–21.
10. Cheng Y, Li X, Lou C, Sonenstein FL, Kalamar A, Jejeebhoy S, et al. The association between social support and mental health among vulnerable adolescents in five cities: findings from the study of the well-being of adolescents in vulnerable environments. J Adolesc Health. 2014;55(6 Suppl): S31–8.
11. Oldfield J, Humphrey N, Hebron J. The role of parental and peer attachment relationships and school connectedness in predicting adolescent mental health outcomes. Child Adolesc Ment Health. 2016;21:21–9.
12. Thoits PA. Mechanisms linking social ties and support to physical and mental health. J Health Soc Behav. 2011;52:145–61.
13. Schraedley PK, Gotlib IH, Hayward C. Gender differences in correlates of depressive symptoms in adolescents. J Adolesc Health. 1999;25:98–108.
14. WHO. Gender disparities in mental health. In: Mental health. Ministerial Round Tables 2001, 54th World Health Assemble, 200. Geneva: World Health Organization; 2001.
15. Wiklund M, Malmgren-Olsson E-B, Öhman A, Bergström E, Fjellman-Wiklund A. Subjective health complaints in older adolescents are related to perceived stress, anxiety and gender – a cross-sectional school study in northern Sweden. BMC Public Health. 2012;12:993.
16. Kashdan TB, Herbert JD. Social anxiety disorder in childhood and adolescence: current status and future directions. Clin Child Fam Psychol Rev. 2001;4:37–61.
17. Patel V, Flisher AJ, Hetrick S, McGorry P. Mental health of young people: a global public-health challenge. Lancet. 2007;369:1302–13.
18. Wahlbeck K, Westman J, Nordentoft M, Gissler M, Laursen TM. Outcomes of Nordic mental health systems: life expectancy of patients with mental disorders. Br J Psychiatry. 2011;199:453–8.
19. Kõlves K, Leo DD. Adolescent suicide rates between 1990 and 2009: analysis of age group 15–19 years worldwide. J Adolesc Health. 2016; 58:69–77.
20. Fink E, Patalay P, Sharpe H, Holley S, Deighton J, Wolpert M. Mental health difficulties in early adolescence: a comparison of two cross-sectional studies in England from 2009 to 2014. J Adolesc Health. 2015;56:502–7.
21. Tick NT, van der Ende J, Verhulst FC. Ten-year trends in self-reported emotional and behavioral problems of Dutch adolescents. Soc Psychiatry Psychiatr Epidemiol. 2008;43:349–55.

22. Torikka A, Kaltiala-Heino R, Rimpelä A, Marttunen M, Luukkaala T, Rimpelä M. Self-reported depression is increasing among socio-economically disadvantaged adolescents – repeated cross-sectional surveys from Finland from 2000 to 2011. BMC Public Health. 2014;14:408.
23. West P, Sweeting H. Fifteen, female and stressed: changing patterns of psychological distress over time. J Child Psychol Psychiatry. 2003;44: 399–411.
24. Demarest S, der Heyden JV, Charafeddine R, Drieskens S, Gisle L, Tafforeau J. Methodological basics and evolution of the Belgian health interview survey 1997–2008. Archives of. Public Health. 2013;71:24.
25. Holi MM, Marttunen M, Aalberg V. Comparison of the GHQ-36, the GHQ-12 and the SCL-90 as psychiatric screening instruments in the Finnish population. Nord J Psychiatry. 2003;57:233–8.
26. Navarro P, Ascaso C, Garcia-Esteve L, Aguado J, Torres A, Martín-Santos R. Postnatal psychiatric morbidity: a validation study of the GHQ-12 and the EPDS as screening tools. Gen Hosp Psychiatry. 2007;29:1–7.
27. Starcevic V, Bogojevic G, Marinkovic J. The SCL-90-R as a screening instrument for severe personality disturbance among outpatients with mood and anxiety disorders. J Personal Disord. 2000;14:199–207.
28. Derogatis L. SCL-90-R: administration, scoring and procedures manual for the R(evised) version. Baltimore, MD: John Hopkins University, School of Medicine; 1977.
29. Rauter UK, Leonard CE, Swett CP. SCL-90-R factor structure in an acute, involuntary, adult psychiatric inpatient sample. J Clin Psychol. 1996;52:625–9.
30. Schmitz N, Hartkamp N, Kiuse J, Franke GH, Reister G, Tress W. The symptom check-List-90-R (SCL-90-R): a German validation study. Qual Life Res. 2000;9:185–93.
31. Hardt J, Gerbershagen HU, Franke P. The symptom check-list, SCL-90-R: its use and characteristics in chronic pain patients. Eur J Pain. 2000;4:137–48.
32. Morgan CD, Wiederman MW, Magnus RD. Discriminant validity of the SCL-90 dimensions of anxiety and depression. Assessment. 1998;5:197–201.
33. Aben I, Verhey F, Lousberg R, Lodder J, Honig A. Validity of the Beck depression inventory, hospital anxiety and depression scale, SCL-90, and Hamilton depression rating scale as screening instruments for depression in stroke patients. Psychosomatics. 2002;43:386–93.
34. Schmitz N, Kruse J, Heckrath C, Alberti L, Tress W. Diagnosing mental disorders in primary care: the general health questionnaire (GHQ) and the symptom check list (SCL-90-R) as screening instruments. Soc Psychiatry Psychiatr Epidemiol. 1999;34:360–6.
35. Kennedy BL, Morris RL, Pedley LL, Schwab JJ. The ability of the symptom checklist SCL-90 to differentiate various anxiety and depressive disorders. Psychiatr Q. 2001;72:277–88.
36. Preisig M, Merikangas KR, Angst J. Clinical significance and comorbidity of subthreshold depression and anxiety in the community. Acta Psychiatr Scand. 2001;104:96–103.
37. Wittchen HU, Kessler RC, Pfister H, Lieb M. Why do people with anxiety disorders become depressed? A prospective-longitudinal community study. Acta Psychiatr Scand Suppl. 2000;102:14–23.
38. Endler NS, Cox BJ, Parker JD, Bagby RM. Self-reports of depression and state-trait anxiety: evidence for differential assessment. J Pers Soc Psychol. 1992; 63:832–8.
39. McWilliams LA, Cox BJ, Enns MW. Self-report differentiation of anxiety and depression in a mood disorders sample. J Psychopathol Behav Assess. 2001;23:125–31.
40. VanDyke MM, Parker JC, Smarr KL, Hewett JE, Johnson GE, Slaughter JR, et al. Anxiety in rheumatoid arthritis. Arthritis & Rheumatism. 2004;51: 408–12.
41. Goldberg DP, Williams P. The general health questionnaire. Windsor, England: NFER Publishing; 1988.
42. Jackson C. The general health questionnaire. Occup Med (Lond). 2007;57:79.
43. Van Der Heyden J, Demarest S, Herck KV, Bacquer DD, Tafforeau J, Oyen HV. Association between variables used in the field substitution and post-stratification adjustment in the Belgian health interview survey and non-response. Int J Public Health. 2014;59:197–206.
44. Statacorp. Stata statistical software: release 13. College Station, TX: StataCorp LP; 2013.
45. Paternoster R, Brame R, Mazerolle P, Piquero A. Using the correct statistical test for the equality of regression coefficients. Criminology. 1998;36:859–66.
46. Van Voorhees BW, Paunesku D, Kuwabara SA, Basu A, Gollan J, Hankin BL, et al. Protective and vulnerability factors predicting new-onset depressive episode in a representative of U.S. adolescents. J Adolesc Health. 2008;42: 605–16.
47. Rosenfield S, Mouzon D. Gender and mental health. In: Aneshensel CS, Phelan JC, Bierman A, editors. Handbook of the sociology of mental health: Springer Netherlands; 2013. p. 277–96. https://doi.org/10.1007/978-94-007-4276-5_14.
48. Matud MP. Gender differences in stress and coping styles. Personal Individ Differ. 2004;37:1401–15.
49. Haugen T, Johansen BT, Ommundsen Y. The role of gender in the relationship between physical activity, appearance evaluation and psychological distress. Child Adolesc Ment Health. 2014;19:24–30.
50. Rodríguez-Cano T, Beato-Fernández L, Llario AB. Body dissatisfaction as a predictor of self-reported suicide attempts in adolescents: a Spanish community prospective study. J Adolesc Health. 2006;38:684–8.
51. Nolen-Hoeksema S, Larson J, Grayson C. Explaining the gender difference in depressive symptoms. J Pers Soc Psychol. 1999;77:1061–72.
52. Elliott M. Gender differences in causes of depression. Women Health. 2001; 33:163–77.
53. Hammarström A. Health consequences of youth unemployment—review from a gender perspective. Soc Sci Med. 1994;38:699–709.
54. OECD. Rising youth unemployment during the crisis. OECD social, employment and migration working papers. Paris: Organisation for Economic Co-operation and Development; 2010.
55. McKee-Ryan F, Song Z, Wanberg CR, Kinicki AJ. Psychological and physical well-being during unemployment: a meta-analytic study. J Appl Psychol. 2005;90:53–76.
56. Post SG. Altruism, happiness, and health: it's good to be good. Int J Behav Med. 2005;12:66–77.
57. Bernardi F, Ballarino G, editors. Education, occupation and social origin: a comparative analysis of the transmission of socio-economic inequalities. Northampton, MA: Edward Elgar Pub; 2016.
58. Tiffin P, Pearce M, Parker L. Social mobility over the lifecourse and self reported mental health at age 50: prospective cohort study. J Epidemiol Community Health. 2005;59:870–2.
59. Bradley RH, Corwyn RF. Socioeconomic status and child development. Annu Rev Psychol. 2002;53:371–99.

Permissions

All chapters in this book were first published in PSYCHIATRY, by BioMed Central; hereby published with permission under the Creative Commons Attribution License or equivalent. Every chapter published in this book has been scrutinized by our experts. Their significance has been extensively debated. The topics covered herein carry significant findings which will fuel the growth of the discipline. They may even be implemented as practical applications or may be referred to as a beginning point for another development.

The contributors of this book come from diverse backgrounds, making this book a truly international effort. This book will bring forth new frontiers with its revolutionizing research information and detailed analysis of the nascent developments around the world.

We would like to thank all the contributing authors for lending their expertise to make the book truly unique. They have played a crucial role in the development of this book. Without their invaluable contributions this book wouldn't have been possible. They have made vital efforts to compile up to date information on the varied aspects of this subject to make this book a valuable addition to the collection of many professionals and students.

This book was conceptualized with the vision of imparting up-to-date information and advanced data in this field. To ensure the same, a matchless editorial board was set up. Every individual on the board went through rigorous rounds of assessment to prove their worth. After which they invested a large part of their time researching and compiling the most relevant data for our readers.

The editorial board has been involved in producing this book since its inception. They have spent rigorous hours researching and exploring the diverse topics which have resulted in the successful publishing of this book. They have passed on their knowledge of decades through this book. To expedite this challenging task, the publisher supported the team at every step. A small team of assistant editors was also appointed to further simplify the editing procedure and attain best results for the readers.

Apart from the editorial board, the designing team has also invested a significant amount of their time in understanding the subject and creating the most relevant covers. They scrutinized every image to scout for the most suitable representation of the subject and create an appropriate cover for the book.

The publishing team has been an ardent support to the editorial, designing and production team. Their endless efforts to recruit the best for this project, has resulted in the accomplishment of this book. They are a veteran in the field of academics and their pool of knowledge is as vast as their experience in printing. Their expertise and guidance has proved useful at every step. Their uncompromising quality standards have made this book an exceptional effort. Their encouragement from time to time has been an inspiration for everyone.

The publisher and the editorial board hope that this book will prove to be a valuable piece of knowledge for researchers, students, practitioners and scholars across the globe.

List of Contributors

Lizhang Chen
Department of Epidemiology and Health Statistics, School of Public Health, Central South University, Changsha, China

Wei Zhou
Department of Epidemiology and Health Statistics, School of Public Health, Central South University, Changsha, China
Hospital Administration Institute, Xinagya Hospital, Central South University, Changsha, China

Yu Yu
Evaluation Department, Xiangya Hospital, Central South University, Changsha, China

Mei Yang
Department of Addiction Medicine, Shenzhen Kangning Hospital, Shenzhen Mental Health Center, Shenzhen, China

Shuiyuan Xiao
Department of Social Medicine and Health Management, School of Public Health, Central South University, Changsha, China

Sarah M. Murray
Department of Mental Health, Johns Hopkins Bloomberg School of Public Health, 624 N Broadway, Baltimore, MD 21205, USA

Amanda J. Nguyen
University of Virginia Curry School of Education, 405 Emmet St S, Charlottesville, VA 22904, USA

Brandon A. Kohrt
Department of Psychiatry and Behavioral Sciences, George Washington University, 2120 L St NW Suite 600, Washington, DC 20037, USA

Sheila Ndyanabangi
Ministry of Health, Republic of Uganda, Plot 6, Lourdel Road, Nakasero, Kampala, Uganda

Stephen Alderman
Peter C. Alderman Foundation, New York, NY, USA

Susanne Montgomery, Gagandeep Sandhu, Jessica Requejo and Qais Alemi
Department of Social Work & Social Ecology, School of Behavioral Health, Loma Linda University, 1898 Business Center Drive, San Bernardino, CA 92408, USA

Carl Stempel
Department of Sociology and Social Services, California State University, East Bay, 25800 Carlos Bee Blvd, Hayward, CA 94542, USA

Patrick Marius Koga
Department of Public Health Sciences, UCD School of Medicine, University of California, One Shields Avenue, Med Sci 1-C, Davis, CA 95616, USA

Valerie Smith
Department of Health Sciences, California State University, East Bay, 25800 Carlos Bee Blvd, Hayward, CA 94542, USA

Bianca Villegas
Department of Epidemiology, School of Public Health, Loma Linda University, 24951 North Circle Drive, Loma Linda, CA 92350, USA

Gearoid Moynihan and Jane O'Connor
National Forensic Mental Health Service, Central Mental Hospital, Dundrum, Dublin 14, Ireland

Ken O'Reilly and Harry G. Kennedy
National Forensic Mental Health Service, Central Mental Hospital, Dundrum, Dublin 14, Ireland
Department of Psychiatry, Trinity College Dublin, Dublin 2, Ireland

Debbie C. Hocking
Cabrini Institute, 154 Wattletree Road, Malvern, VIC 3144, Australia
Florey Institute of Neuroscience and Mental Health, 30 Royal Parade (Cnr Genetics Lane), Parkville, VIC 3052, Australia
Department of Psychiatry, School of Clinical Sciences, Monash University, Clayton, VIC 3168, Australia

Suresh Sundram
Florey Institute of Neuroscience and Mental Health, 30 Royal Parade (Cnr Genetics Lane), Parkville, VIC 3052, Australia
Department of Psychiatry, Faculty of Medicine, Dentistry and Health Sciences, University of Melbourne, Parkville, VIC 3010, Australia
Department of Psychiatry, School of Clinical Sciences, Monash University, Clayton, VIC 3168, Australia
Adult Psychiatry, Monash Medical Centre, Clayton, VIC 3168, Australia

Serafino G. Mancuso
Department of Psychiatry, Faculty of Medicine, Dentistry and Health Sciences, University of Melbourne, Parkville, VIC 3010, Australia

Nicola Hancock, Jennifer Smith-Merry and Glenda Jessup
The University of Sydney, Sydney, Australia

Sarah Wayland
University of Technology, Sydney, Sydney, Australia

Allison Kokany
WentWest, Blacktown, Australia

BreeOna Ebrecht and Rebecca Aiyo
Peter C. Alderman Foundation, plot 855, Mawanda Road, Nakawa, Kampala, Uganda

Wietse A. Tol
Peter C. Alderman Foundation, plot 855, Mawanda Road, Nakawa, Kampala, Uganda
Department of Mental Health, Johns Hopkins Bloomberg School of Public Health, 624 N Broadway, Baltimore, MD 21205, USA

Seggane Musisi
Peter C. Alderman Foundation, plot 855, Mawanda Road, Nakawa, Kampala, Uganda
Department of Psychiatry, Makerere University College of Health Sciences, Kampala, Uganda

Juliet Nakku
Peter C. Alderman Foundation, plot 855, Mawanda Road, Nakawa, Kampala, Uganda
Butabika National Psychiatric Referral Hospital, Butabika Rd, Kampala, Uganda

Peter McPherson, Joanna Krotofil and Helen Killaspy
Division of Psychiatry, Faculty of Brain Sciences, UCL, 6th Floor, Maple House, 149 Tottenham Court Road, London W1T 7NF, UK

Jingyi Wang, Farhana Mann, Brynmor Lloyd-Evans and Ruimin Ma
Division of Psychiatry - University College London, 6th Floor, Maple House, 149 Tottenham Court Road, London W1T 7NF, England

Sonia Johnson
Division of Psychiatry - University College London, 6th Floor, Maple House, 149 Tottenham Court Road, London W1T 7NF, England
Camden and Islington NHS Foundation Trust, St Pancras Hospital, 4 St Pancras Way, London NW1 0PE, England

Helen Jennings
Department of Occupational Therapy, School of Health Sciences, York St. John University, York, UK

Mike Slade and Rebecca Toney
School of Health Sciences, Institute of Mental Health, University of Nottingham, Triumph Road, Nottingham NG7 2TU, UK

Peter Bates
Peter Bates Associates Ltd, Nottingham, UK

Emma Munday
RECOLLECT Lived Experience Advisory Panel, Nottingham, UK

Marijke Schotanus-Dijkstra, Constance H. C. Drossaert, Marcel E. Pieterse, Jan A. Walburg and Ernst T. Bohlmeijer
Centre for eHealth and Well-being Research, Department of Psychology, Health and Technology, University of Twente, 7500 AE Enschede, The Netherlands

Filip Smit
Department of Public Mental Health, Trimbos Institute, Utrecht, The Netherlands
Department of Epidemiology and Biostatistics, EMGO Institute for Health and Care Research, VU University Medical Centre, Amsterdam, The Netherlands
Department of Clinical, Neuro and Developmental Psychology, EMGO Institute for Health and Care Research, VU University, Amsterdam, The Netherlands

Mary Gemma Cherry
Division of Clinical Psychology, University of Liverpool, Whelan Building, Quadrangle, Brownlow Hill, Liverpool L69 3GB, UK

Peter James Taylor
Division of Clinical Psychology, University of Liverpool, Whelan Building, Quadrangle, Brownlow Hill, Liverpool L69 3GB, UK
Division of Psychology & Mental Health, University of Manchester, Zochonis building, Manchester M13 9PL, UK

Stephen Lloyd Brown
Department of Psychological Sciences, University of Liverpool, Whelan Building, Quadrangle, Brownlow Hill, Liverpool L69 3GB, UK

William Sellwood
Division of Health Research, University of Lancaster, Furness Building, Bailrigg, Lancaster LA1 4YW, UK

Chika Tanaka and Hiroya Matsuo
Graduate School of Health Sciences, Kobe University, 701, 2-6-2, Yamamoto-dori, Chuo-ku, Kobe, Hyogo 650-0003, Japan

Maria Teresa Reyes Tuliao
City Health Office, City Government of Muntinlupa, Muntinlupa, Philippines

Eizaburo Tanaka
Hyogo Institute for Traumatic Stress, Kobe, Japan

Tadashi Yamashita
Kobe City College of Nursing, Kobe, Japan

Judith Osok and Anastasia Polkonikova-Wamoto
Department of Psychiatry, University of Nairobi, Nairobi, Kenya

Manasi Kumar
Department of Psychiatry, University of Nairobi, Nairobi, Kenya
Research Department of Clinical Health and Educational Psychology, University College London, London, UK

Beatrice Amugune
Department of Pharmacy, University of Nairobi, Nairobi, Kenya

Beatrice Madeghe
Department of Food and Nutrition Sciences, University of Nairobi, Nairobi, Kenya

Grace Nduku Wambua
Department of Clinical, Neuro- & Developmental Psychology, Vrije University of Amsterdam, Amsterdam, Netherlands

David Bukusi
Head VCT and HIV Care, Kenyatta National Hospital, Nairobi, Kenya

Fred Were
College of Health Sciences, University of Nairobi, Nairobi, Kenya

Keng-Yen Huang
Department of Population Health, New York University School of Medicine, New York, USA

M. von Werthern, K. Robjant, Z. Chui, R. Schon and C. Mason
Helen Bamber Foundation, Bruges Place, 15-20 Baynes Street, London NW1 0TF, UK

C. Katona
Helen Bamber Foundation, Bruges Place, 15-20 Baynes Street, London NW1 0TF, UK
Division of Psychiatry, University College London, London, UK

L. Ottisova
Health Services and Population Research Department, Kings College London, London, UK

M. de Courten
Centre for Chronic Disease, College of Health and Biomedicine, Victoria University, Melbourne, Australia

K. T. Hallam
Centre for Chronic Disease, College of Health and Biomedicine, Victoria University, Melbourne, Australia
Outlook Matters, Pty Ltd, Melbourne, Australia

S. Bilsborough
Stepathlon Private Limited, No. 2B 25E, Lorette Ville, Ground Floor, Village Bandra, Santacruz West, Main Avenue, Mumbai, India

Dima Saab, Kate Francombe Pridham and Anjana Aery
Centre for Urban Health Solutions, Li Ka Shing Knowledge Institute, St. Michael's Hospital, 209 Victoria Street, Toronto, ON M5B 1W8, Canada

Vicky Stergiopoulos
Centre for Urban Health Solutions, Li Ka Shing Knowledge Institute, St. Michael's Hospital, 209 Victoria Street, Toronto, ON M5B 1W8, Canada
Centre for Addiction and Mental Health, 100 Stokes Street, Toronto, ON M6J 1H4, Canada
Department of Psychiatry, University of Toronto, 250 College Street, 8th Floor, Toronto, ON M5T 1R8, Canada

Arash Nakhost
Department of Psychiatry, University of Toronto, 250 College Street, 8th Floor, Toronto, ON M5T 1R8, Canada
Mental Health Services, St. Michael's Hospital, 30 Bond Street, Toronto, ON M5B 1W8, Canada

Ken O' Reilly and Harry G Kennedy
National Forensic Mental Health Service, Central Mental Hospital, Dundrum, Dublin, Ireland
Department of Psychiatry, Trinity College, Dublin, Ireland

Padraic O' Flynn and Roisin O' Regan
National Forensic Mental Health Service, Central Mental Hospital, Dundrum, Dublin, Ireland

Jieun Jang, Sang Ah Lee, Woorim Kim and Young Choi
Department of Public Health, Graduate School, Yonsei University, Seoul, Republic of Korea
Institute of Health Services Research, Yonsei University, Seoul, Republic of Korea

Eun-Cheol Park
Institute of Health Services Research, Yonsei University, Seoul, Republic of Korea
Department of Preventive Medicine & Institute of Health Services Research, Yonsei University College of Medicine, 50 Yonsei-ro, Seodaemun-gu, Seoul 120-752, Republic of Korea

Filip Van Droogenbroeck, Bram Spruyt and Gil Keppens
Sociology Department, Vrije Universiteit Brussel, Pleinlaan 2, 1050 Brussel, Belgium

Index

www.ingramcontent.com/pod-product-compliance
Lightning Source LLC
LaVergne TN
LVHW080703210926
848485LV00003B/411